Current Trends in Oncology Nursing

Edited by
Judith K. Payne, PhD, RN, AOCN®

D1608985

Oncology Nursing Society
Pittsburgh, Pennsylvania

ONS Publications Department
Executive Director, Professional Practice and Programs: Elizabeth M. Wertz Evans, RN, MPM,
CPHQ, CPHIMS, FACMPE
Publisher and Director of Publications: Barbara Sigler, RN, MNEd
Managing Editor: Lisa M. George, BA
Technical Content Editor: Angela D. Klimaszewski, RN, MSN
Staff Editor II: Amy Nicoletti, BA
Copy Editor: Laura Pinchot, BA
Graphic Designer: Dany Sjoen

Library of Congress Cataloging-in-Publication Data

Current trends in oncology nursing / edited by Judith K. Payne.
   p. ; cm.
Includes bibliographical references.
ISBN 978-1-935864-25-7 (alk. paper)
I. Payne, Judith K. (Judith Kay) II. Oncology Nursing Society.
[DNLM: 1. Oncologic Nursing--methods. 2. Neoplasms--nursing. 3. Oncologic Nursing--trends. WY 156]
616.99′40231--dc23

2012020352

Publisher's Note

This book is published by the Oncology Nursing Society (ONS). ONS neither represents nor guarantees that the practices described herein will, if followed, ensure safe and effective patient care. The recommendations contained in this book reflect ONS's judgment regarding the state of general knowledge and practice in the field as of the date of publication. The recommendations may not be appropriate for use in all circumstances. Those who use this book should make their own determinations regarding specific safe and appropriate patient-care practices, taking into account the personnel, equipment, and practices available at the hospital or other facility at which they are located. The editor and publisher cannot be held responsible for any liability incurred as a consequence from the use or application of any of the contents of this book. Figures and tables are used as examples only. They are not meant to be all-inclusive, nor do they represent endorsement of any particular institution by ONS. Mention of specific products and opinions related to those products do not indicate or imply endorsement by ONS. Web sites mentioned are provided for information only; the hosts are responsible for their own content and availability. Unless otherwise indicated, dollar amounts reflect U.S. dollars.

ONS publications are originally published in English. Publishers wishing to translate ONS publications must contact ONS about licensing arrangements. ONS publications cannot be translated without obtaining written permission from ONS. (Individual tables and figures that are reprinted or adapted require additional permission from the original source.) Because translations from English may not always be accurate or precise, ONS disclaims any responsibility for inaccuracies in words or meaning that may occur as a result of the translation. Readers relying on precise information should check the original English version.

Printed in the United States of America

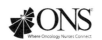

Oncology Nursing Society
Integrity • Innovation • Stewardship • Advocacy • Excellence • Inclusiveness

Contributors

Editor

Judith K. Payne, PhD, RN, AOCN®
Program Director, Nursing Research
University of Wisconsin Hospital and Clinics
Madison, Wisconsin
Chapter 1. Introduction; Chapter 6. Basic Science of Genetics; Chapter 16. Contemporary Issues in Oncology Nursing

Authors

Carlton G. Brown, PhD, RN, AOCN®
Director of Nursing
Evidence-Based Practice
Memorial Sloan-Kettering Cancer Center
New York, New York
Chapter 5. Oncology Nursing Leadership and Healthcare Policy

Wendy C. Budin, PhD, RN-BC, FAAN
Director of Nursing Research
NYU Langone Medical Center
Adjunct Professor, New York University College of Nursing
New York, New York
Chapter 4. Theoretical Frameworks and Philosophies of Care

Carlin A.M. Callaway, MSN, MS, RN, ACNP-BC, ACNS-BC, OCN®
Advanced Practice Nurse
Naval Medical Center San Diego
San Diego, California
Chapter 9. Ethics

Frances Cartwright-Alcarese, PhD, RN, AOCN®
Senior Director of Nursing, Oncology Services and Medicine
NYU Langone Medical Center
New York, New York
Chapter 4. Theoretical Frameworks and Philosophies of Care

Regina S. Cunningham, PhD, RN, AOCN®
Associate Chief Nursing Officer, Cancer Services
Abramson Cancer Center
Adjunct Associate Professor
School of Nursing
University of Pennsylvania
Philadelphia, Pennsylvania
Chapter 8. Systems and Safety in the Oncology Practice Environment

Jeanne M. Erickson, PhD, RN, AOCN®
Assistant Professor
University of Virginia School of Nursing
Charlottesville, Virginia
Chapter 9. Ethics

Marilyn J. Hammer, PhD, DC, RN
Assistant Professor
New York University College of Nursing
New York, New York
*Chapter 4. Theoretical Frameworks and
Philosophies of Care*

Sookyung Hyun, DNSc, RN
Assistant Professor
College of Nursing and Department of
Biomedical Informatics
The Ohio State University
Columbus, Ohio
Chapter 15. Cancer Care and Informatics

Mary Pat Johnston, RN, MS, AOCN®
Oncology Clinical Nurse Specialist
Pro Health Care Regional Cancer Center
Waukesha Memorial Hospital
Waukesha, Wisconsin
Chapter 11. Oncology Community Health

Sarah H. Kagan, PhD, RN, AOCN®
Lucy Walker Honorary Term Professor
of Gerontological Nursing, School of
Nursing
Secondary Faculty
Division of Hematology-Oncology
School of Medicine
University of Pennsylvania
Philadelphia, Pennsylvania
*Chapter 10. The Reality of Gero-Oncology
for Nursing in an Aging Society*

Sandra Kurtin, RN, MS, AOCN®, ANP-C
Nurse Practitioner
Assistant Professor of Clinical Medicine
The University of Arizona Cancer Center
Tucson, Arizona
*Chapter 13. Primary Care of the Cancer
Survivor: A Collaborative Continuum-
Based Model for Care*

Kathleen Murphy Ende, RN, PsyD, PhD,
AOCNP®
Clinical Psychologist and Nurse
Practitioner, Palliative Care Service
Meriter Hospital
Madison, Wisconsin
Chapter 12. Mental Health Issues in Cancer

Margaret Quinn Rosenzweig, PhD, FNP-
BC, AOCNP®
Associate Professor
University of Pittsburgh
Pittsburgh, Pennsylvania
*Chapter 2. Advanced Practice Nursing in
Cancer Care*

Leah L. Shever, PhD, RN
Director of Nursing Research, Quality, and
Innovation
University of Michigan Health System
Ann Arbor, Michigan
Chapter 3. Modeling Research for Practice

Sandra Millon Underwood, RN, PhD,
FAAN
Professor
College of Nursing
University of Wisconsin, Milwaukee
Milwaukee, Wisconsin
*Chapter 14. Reducing Cancer-Related Health
Disparities: What Nurses Can Do to Effect
Change*

Kristi L. Wiggins, MSN, RN, ANP-BC,
AOCNP®, CCRC
Adult Nurse Practitioner—Adult Bone
Marrow Transplant/Cellular Therapy
Duke University Medical Center
Durham, North Carolina
*Chapter 6. Basic Science of Genetics;
Chapter 7. Nursing in Genetics*

Disclosure

Editors and authors of books and guidelines provided by the Oncology Nursing Society are expected to disclose to the readers any significant financial interest or other relationships with the manufacturer(s) of any commercial products.

A vested interest may be considered to exist if a contributor is affiliated with or has a financial interest in commercial organizations that may have a direct or indirect interest in the subject matter. A "financial interest" may include, but is not limited to, being a shareholder in the organization; being an employee of the commercial organization; serving on an organization's speakers bureau; or receiving research from the organization. An "affiliation" may be holding a position on an advisory board or some other role of benefit to the commercial organization. Vested interest statements appear in the front matter for each publication.

Contributors are expected to disclose any unlabeled or investigational use of products discussed in their content. This information is acknowledged solely for the information of the readers.

The contributors provided the following disclosure and vested interest information:

Regina S. Cunningham, PhD, RN, AOCN®: Amgen, Merck, honoraria

Mary Pat Johnston, RN, MS, AOCN®: ONS Board of Directors, Director at Large, Liaison to ONCC; Amgen, Novartis, ONS, honoraria

Sandra E. Kurtin, RN, MS, AOCN®, ANP-C: Bristol-Myers Squibb, Celgene, Novartis, Millennium, consultant; Celgene, Novartis, Millennium, honoraria

Contents

Preface..xi

Chapter 1. Introduction..1
    Historical Perspectives..1
    Future Expectations and Actions..3
    References...4

Chapter 2. Advanced Practice Nursing in Cancer Care.......................................5
    The Roles of Cancer Nursing..5
    Scope of Practice 6
    Predicted Cancer Care Provider Shortage..7
    Measuring Outcomes of Advanced Nursing Practice 8
    LACE Model..8
    Doctoral Education 10
    Assurance of Oncology Nursing Competencies 11
    Postgraduate Education: Future Trends...13
    Conclusion..14
    References...14

Chapter 3. Modeling Research for Practice 17
    Objectives...17
    Evidence-Based Practice 17
    Effectiveness and Efficacy Research 20
    Conduct of Research Versus Research Implementation...................................21
    Conclusion..22
    References 23

Chapter 4. Theoretical Frameworks and Philosophies of Care...........................25
    Introduction 25
    Overview of the Theories..25
    Phases of the Cancer Experience..42
    Family Caregiver Experiences...47
    Conclusion..48
    References...49

Chapter 5. Oncology Nursing Leadership and Healthcare Policy 55
    Introduction 55
    Patient Protection and Affordable Care Act 56
    The LACE Model..59

The Institute of Medicine Report on the Future of Nursing..........................59
Conclusion...63
References...63

Chapter 6. Basic Science of Genetics 65
Introduction 65
Structures of Life 65
Genetic Testing 73
Genetic Counseling 75
Genograms 76
Conclusion...79
References...79

Chapter 7. Nursing in Genetics..83
Introduction 83
Academic Programs and Continuing Education 83
Future Trends in Oncology Practice 92
Direct-to-Consumer Marketing 98
Policy and Protections...99
Law Making 101
Nurses in Politics 102
Goals of Our Government..102
Conclusion...103
References...103

Chapter 8. Systems and Safety in the Oncology Practice Environment..............107
Introduction 107
Systems, Complexity, and Healthcare Delivery 107
Patient Safety as a Theme in Healthcare Delivery..................................108
Strategies to Systematically Build Safety Into the Practice Environment.....111
Impediments to Patient Safety 117
Implications for Nursing Practice and Research 117
Conclusion...118
References...118

Chapter 9. Ethics..121
Introduction 121
Personal and Professional Ethics 122
Ethical Issues in Oncology Nursing Practice 125
Developing and Maintaining Ethical Nursing Practice 132
Conclusion...139
References...140

Chapter 10. The Reality of Gero-Oncology for Nursing in an Aging Society........145
Introduction 145
Implications of an Aging Society 146
An Agenda for the Future of Oncology Nursing......................................149
Conclusion...151
References...152

Chapter 11. Oncology Community Health 155
Introduction 155
Hospice Care...156
Palliative Care 157
Workforce Shortages 160

Conclusion 162
References 162

Chapter 12. Mental Health Issues in Cancer 165
    Introduction 165
    Clinical Screening and Outcome Measures 166
    Anxiety and Depression 167
    Cognitive Function 172
    Post-Traumatic Stress Disorder 176
    Hope 178
    Interventions 181
    Workplace Stress: Compassion Fatigue and Burnout 182
    Conclusion 186
    References 186

Chapter 13. Primary Care of the Cancer Survivor: A Collaborative Continuum-Based
    Model for Care 191
    Introduction 191
    The Continuum of Care for a Cancer Survivor: Who Is Responsible for
      Primary Care? 192
    Cancer Surveillance in Cancer Survivors 193
    Health Maintenance, Health Promotion, and Prevention Strategies for
      Cancer Survivors 198
    Conclusion 206
    References 207

Chapter 14. Reducing Cancer-Related Health Disparities: What Nurses Can Do
    to Effect Change 211
    Introduction 211
    Cancer Morbidity and Mortality in the United States 211
    Discoveries, Breakthroughs, and Innovations in Science and Cancer Care 213
    Disparities in Cancer Morbidity and Mortality Among U.S. Population Groups 213
    Health Disparities Related to Sexual Orientation and Gender Identity 217
    Nurses Call for Action 219
    Conclusion 224
    References 225

Chapter 15. Cancer Care and Informatics 229
    Introduction 229
    Overview of Health Informatics 229
    Informatics Applications for Oncology Care 235
    Informatics and Nursing Education 235
    Conclusion 236
    References 237

Chapter 16. Contemporary Issues in Oncology Nursing 245
    Introduction 245
    Future Directions 249
    Conclusion 251
    References 251

Index 253

Preface

My desire to write this book stems partially from my interest and intrigue with the history of nursing and medicine, but also from years of being present in the healthcare environment and observing how determined nurses provide leadership and improve patient outcomes in healthcare settings. Unfortunately, as well I have observed times when nurses have had opportunities to lead but sadly did not seize the opportunity. From my early traditional undergraduate nursing education forward, I learned the importance of understanding the beginnings of nursing in order to be able to understand the underpinnings necessary for the creation of a true profession, such as the nursing profession, and to avoid the trials and errors of previous generations. Few would disagree that nurses are the backbone of health care. Consistently we are rated number one in integrity among professions. Oncology nurses are intuitively bright, benevolent, empathetic, and respected by all healthcare providers. Not surprisingly, our oncology voice is often listened to by others. For example, components of our holistic, patient-centered model of care have been adapted over time by other patient care specialties and providers. Despite our many accomplishments, challenges remain and thus require that we be aware of current trends in oncology nursing. Most importantly, first we must be aware of and poised for the numerous opportunities that exist for oncology nurses and secondarily be proactive rather than reactive as we take the lead and subsequent accountability and responsibility for our actions and outcomes.

This is the first book to identify and conceptualize current trends in oncology nursing. Although not inclusive of all issues, the book provides expert content on significant trends in the care of patients with cancer and suggests a shift in the paradigm of cancer care. Some of the anticipated changes are expected, whereas others are more subtle. The first chapter provides an introduction and overview of oncology nursing. Subsequent chapters provide detailed content including trends in advanced practice nursing, research and evidence-based practice, theoretical frameworks and philosophies of care, oncology nursing leadership and healthcare policy, genetics, ethics, systems, gero-oncology, community and mental health, primary care, cancer-related health disparities, informatics, and other issues in oncology nursing.

In the future, oncology nurses will not only need to remain the experts in the care of oncology patients but also will need to expand their knowledge base in areas that are now considered standard of care for patients with cancer, such as genetics, epigentics, healthcare policy, systems, gero-oncology, mental health, primary care, and informatics. These patient-related concepts are embedded in the daily care of our patients. As oncology nurses, we must maintain a comprehensive understanding of how these concepts are related to our patients' care, safety, and outcomes. Understanding these conceptual dimensions in addition to the direct patient care provided to our patients will enable nurses and other healthcare providers to create a positive effect on the quality of care delivered, as well as improve the well-being of our patients and families. This book reflects the efforts of many highly qualified authors who have presented expert content on current trends in oncology nursing.

Judith K. Payne, PhD, RN, AOCN®

CHAPTER 1

Introduction

Judith K. Payne, PhD, RN, AOCN®

> *No man can know where he is going unless he knows exactly where he has been and exactly how he arrived at this present place.*
> —Maya Angelou

> *Courage is the first of human qualities because it is the quality which guarantees the others.*
> —Aristotle

Oncology nursing emulates the best of nursing today. Where else do nurses provide such benevolent care for the soul of a human being, the soul of their patients? We thoughtfully assess and evaluate our patients, select and implement interventions based on evidence when possible, use our presence to provide thoughtful care throughout the cancer experience—from diagnosis to treatment, remission, recurrence, cure, and survival. Cancer care is complex and requires an understanding of multiple physiologic and psychological responses to the disease process and numerous treatment modalities. In addition, numerous factors, such as age, gender, socioeconomic status, ethnicity, and race, can influence incidence rates of cancer, response to treatment, and survival outcomes. Oncology nurses scientifically and intuitively know that sometimes process is as important as outcome.

Historical Perspectives

History can be defined as a study of events from our past leading up to the present time. However, the study of history focuses on not just the chronology of events but also the impact and influence those events continue to have throughout time (Egenes, 2009). Over time, healthcare events occur and trends emerge. These historical trends, in turn, can influence or sway the fortune of individuals and groups (Egenes, 2009). The development and evolution of the nursing profession is intricately and powerfully connected to historical influences over the years.

Nursing has often been called the oldest of arts and the youngest of professions (Donahue, 2010). Although the origins of nursing predate the mid-19th century, the history of professional nursing traditionally begins with Florence Nightingale. However, the hospital schools established in the United States differed from the Nightingale schools in Europe in one very important respect: they were not endowed as they were in Nightingale's era and thus had no independent financial backing (Ashley, 1976). As a way to resolve this economic challenge, the hospital-based schools agreed to provide nursing service in exchange for the hospitals offering clinical experience. This type of apprenticeship arrangement was primarily an economical relationship prompting hospitals to establish schools on their own initiative; thus, the hospital was in charge and the student nurse was the apprentice who provided free labor to the hospital in return for informal training (Ashley, 1976).

The first permanent school of nursing in the United States is reported to be the nurse training school of the Women's Hospital of Philadelphia, which was established in 1872 (Egenes, 2009). Following the Nightingale model, the school had a set curriculum, paid instructors, equipment for the development of skills, provisions for experiences in other hospitals, and a nurses' library. In spite of resistance from early physicians, in 1873, three notable nurse training schools were established: the Bellevue Hospital Training School of New York, the Connecticut Training School in New Haven, and the Boston Training School in Massachusetts General Hospital (Egenes, 2009). Notwithstanding an intriguing history of obstacles and resistance from the medical community, nursing as a profession has made significant progress. Over past decades, standardization and accreditation of nursing schools has expanded, and as the body of knowledge and science has increased, so has the complexity of patient care.

In nursing, like other healthcare disciplines, much of patient care has evolved to be specialty based. In some areas of health care, specialization in nursing practice began as early as the 1940s; however, it was not until the 1970s and 1980s that specialization of nursing practice flourished and specialty certifications became common. The most notable exception was in pediatric oncology nursing, which became a subspecialty in the early 1940s. These nurses initially worked with tumor specialists and became self-taught in cancer nursing practices. During the early years, pediatric oncology nurses primarily worked to ensure patients were comfortable. By the 1960s, pediatric oncology nurses were practicing advanced clinical skills, and pediatric nursing was the first specialty to develop standards for cancer care.

In adult oncology practices before the 1950s, cancer treatment primarily involved surgery. In 1971, the National Cancer Act was adopted to reduce the incidence of cancer and cancer deaths. Cancer care become more comprehensive, and nurses assumed broader roles in the specialty care of patients. Recognizing the need to provide better care to patients with cancer and to foster professional development of nurses taking care of patients with cancer, a group of pioneer oncology nurses got together and developed a charter for the first oncology nursing professional organization. The Oncology Nursing Society (ONS) was founded in 1975, and in 1979, ONS released its standards for nursing practice. ONS administered its first certification examination in 1986. These historical events were the foundation of oncology nursing practice as we know it today.

The history of nursing demonstrates a pattern of recurrent issues that the profession has been prodded to address over time. Some of these issues include professional standards, autonomy of practice, scope of practice, and control of professional practice. Through the years, the profession has dealt with nursing shortages, new categories of healthcare providers, ethical issues, and changes in healthcare delivery systems. In retrospect, history has shown that not all the concerns facing nursing have been successfully resolved in a clear and proactive manner. However, past decades have brought new insights into the way our profession can better meet these challenges. Only by understanding the challenges of the past will we be able to find solutions for today.

The history of nursing has distinctly been linked to a tradition of caring (Reverby, 1987). Traditionally, nurses have felt a responsibility to reach out to those in need and to advocate on their behalf. However, Reverby (1987) also contended that nursing's core value of caring may contribute to the dilemma of nursing in the United States, in part because nurses have often equated the "mandate to care" with properly fulfilling the role of a professional nurse. In this context, nurses continue to deal with the dilemma of altruism versus autonomy in their practice. Accordingly, nurses face challenges to fulfill this mandate in a society that has typically refused to value caring (Reverby, 1987). Therefore, it is our responsibility to create a political awareness for the basis of caring and to find new ways to gain the authority to implement an acceptance of caring and, in the process, gain an understanding of how to practice altruism with autonomy (Reverby, 1987). By doing what we do best, we need to focus on providing "care" while continuing our expert surveillance of patients, advances in technology and scientific discovery, and changes in societal norms, healthcare policy, and delivery systems.

An Institute of Medicine (IOM, 2011) report provided several recommendations that have the potential to transform the nursing profession. Briefly, the report's four primary recommendations were that nurses should (a) practice to the full extent of their education and training, (b) achieve higher levels of education and training through an improved education system, (c) be full partners with physicians and other healthcare professionals, and (d) develop effective workforce planning through better data collection. The report also recommended to increase the number of baccalaureate-prepared nurses from 50% to 80% and to double the number of nurses with a doctorate by 2020. It is critical to note that the report is not just about nursing per se but also is about an enhanced capacity of nurses to deliver high-quality, patient-centered care (Mason, 2011), and marks a difference in what nursing used to be and what it is going to be (Lavizzo-Mourey, 2011). However, it is important to remember that a key operative is "potential." Although nursing was clearly instrumental in creating the recommendations put forth within this monumental report, we must continue our vigilant efforts to push forward and engage in discussions with lawmakers, healthcare policy reformers, and the medical community to sustain and maintain a presence in the implementation of these provoking recommendations.

Future Expectations and Actions

Although the issues addressed in the following chapters are challenging areas that we need to continue exploring with ongoing and thoughtful discussions, the list is not inclusive. Healthcare policy is often in a state of flux as we try to balance the social and economic needs of society and the healthcare priorities we face over time. The U.S. population is aging, and with this comes an increase in age-related diseases and related syndromes. Comorbidities are common in the aging society and especially so in the oncology patient population. The number of individuals with chronic diseases such as diabetes, heart disease, hypertension, pulmonary disease, dementia, and cancer is increasing at an alarming rate. Our shift in health care needs to focus on prevention, early detection, and living with chronicity.

Healthcare providers will need to be educated in both aging concepts and chronic diseases.

According to Ashley (1976) and Donahue (2010), nursing *is* health care. Today the United States has the opportunity to transform its healthcare system. RNs can and should play a fundamental role in this transformation. However, professional organizations, the insurance industry, government, and healthcare organizations all must play a role to improve the current regulatory, business, and organizational conditions (IOM, 2011). Perhaps it is not surprising to some that more than 35 years ago, Ashley (1976) wrote, "Given recent and current criticisms of poor quality in health care, the public would do well to turn more of its attention to the developments in nursing and to the problems with which this group has to contend" (p. 132), and "It is time nursing emerged to provide the care it can provide. Society can scarcely afford the waste by ineffective utilization of the talents and abilities of professionally and technically prepared nurses" (p. 134). We are at another crossroads in our history and in our professional development. It would be wise for nurses to thoughtfully consider optimal responses to the opportunities presented in the IOM (2011) report. Indeed, no one is more qualified to chart our future direction, nursing's future, than we are. We are responsible for the direction we take and must assume the leadership and courage necessary to achieve the goals outlined in the IOM report.

References

Ashley, J.A. (1976). *Hospitals, paternalism, and the role of the nurse.* New York, NY: Teacher's College Press.

Donahue, M.P. (2010). *Nursing, the finest art: An illustrated history* (3rd ed.). St. Louis, MO: Elsevier Mosby.

Egenes, K.J. (2009). History of nursing. In G.M. Roux & J.A. Halstead (Eds.), *Issues and trends in nursing: Essential knowledge for today and tomorrow* (pp. 1–26). Burlington, MA: Jones and Bartlett.

Institute of Medicine. (2011). *The future of nursing: Leading change, advancing health.* Washington, DC: National Academies Press.

Lavizzo-Mourey, R. (2011). Foreword. In D.J. Mason, S.L. Isaacs, & D.C. Colby (Eds.), *Robert Wood Johnson Foundation series on health policy: The nursing profession: Development, challenges, and opportunities* (pp. ix–x). Princeton, NJ: Robert Wood Johnson Foundation.

Mason, D.J. (2011). Review of the nursing field. In D.J. Mason, S.L. Isaacs, & D.C. Colby (Eds.), *Robert Wood Johnson Foundation series on health policy: The nursing profession: Development, challenges, and opportunities* (pp. 3–71). Princeton, NJ: Robert Wood Johnson Foundation.

Reverby, S.M. (1987). *Ordered to care: The dilemma of American nursing, 1850–1945.* New York, NY: Cambridge University Press.

CHAPTER 2

Advanced Practice Nursing in Cancer Care

Margaret Quinn Rosenzweig, PhD, FNP-BC, AOCNP®

The Roles of Cancer Nursing

The scope of oncology nursing practice has changed dramatically in the past several decades. At the inpatient or outpatient RN level, the cancer nurse's role has evolved. Specific knowledge is necessary for fully collaborative nursing participation in this highly complex specialization. RNs ideally work as partners with oncologists and other cancer care providers in the complex care of patients with cancer and their families. This role remains vital for the optimal care of patients. However, when addressing the issues of scope of practice and role change, the oncology advanced practice registered nurse (APRN) is realizing a tremendous increase in demand and an almost constant role evolution. Changes in role, scope of practice, and demand have implications for licensure, education, and competency at entry to practice. Therefore, this chapter will focus on issues relevant specifically to APRNs in cancer care.

APRNs are nurses who are academically prepared beyond the RN level. The Oncology Nursing Society (ONS) recognizes two APRN roles in cancer care, the clinical nurse specialist (CNS) and the nurse practitioner (NP) (Cunningham, 2004). Historically, the predominant advanced practice role in cancer care was the CNS. This role adds to cancer care's quality and cost-effectiveness through three spheres of influence: the patient, the nurse and nursing practice, and the organization or system. The CNS influences quality outcomes for patients through the support of nursing and the strengthening of the healthcare organization to support the efforts of nursing (National Association of Clinical Nurse Specialists [NACNS], n.d.). An estimated 72,521 RNs have the education and credentials to practice as a CNS (NACNS, n.d.). Healthcare changes realized in the 1980s left the CNS role vulnerable because these professionals were not providing direct reimbursable care. Many oncology CNSs faced role modifications and potential position elimination. Unfortunately, the regulations that apply to the CNS regarding the ability to directly bill for services vary according to state regulations.

NPs are RNs with advanced education who provide a broad range of healthcare services focusing primarily on patient healthcare needs with quality and cost-effectiveness. (See American Academy of Nurse Practitioners [AANP], 2010b and 2010c and Newhouse et al., 2011 for reviews.) The use of NPs, alone or in collaboration with physicians, has a long history of equivocal or superior patient outcomes in primary and specialty care (Gershengorn et al., 2011; Hayes, 2007; Hoffman, Tasota, Scharfenberg, Zullo, & Donahue, 2003).

Patient education, communication, and adherence to evidence-based practice guidelines are particular strengths of NPs (Bryant-Lukosius & Dicenso, 2004; Murphy-Ende, 2002). The success of the NP in many aspects of general patient care led to the utilization of NPs in cancer care (Bishop, 2009; Nevidjon et al., 2010; Rosenzweig et al., 2012).

Specifically in cancer care, improved outcomes in quality of life and increased productivity with NPs have been documented in hematology/oncology practices (Akscin, Barr, & Towle, 2007; Cunningham, 2004; Murphy-Ende, 2002; Nevidjon et al., 2010; Young, 2005).

NPs are prevalent in cancer care, and their numbers are expected to increase. As of 2005, nearly 10,500 oncologists were practicing in the United States; 81% were medical oncologists or hematologist-oncologists, and 5% were gynecologic oncologists. Of these, 56% worked with NPs or physician assistants (Center for Workforce Studies, 2007; Polansky, Ross, & Coniglio, 2010). Of the 140,000 practicing NPs in the United States, between 4,000 and 6,000 are working in oncology, with an expected twofold increase by 2015 (AANP, 2010a; Britell, 2010).

Scope of Practice

The Institute of Medicine (IOM, 2011) report on the future of nursing commented that nurses must continue to be elevated as important providers in the constant struggle to deliver affordable, quality cancer care to all Americans. The report recommended that nurses must work to their maximum licensure capacity. Licensure capacity can differ dramatically according to state. Individual states' nursing practice acts predominately regulate APRN scope of practice, and state boards of nursing or other state regulatory agencies govern nursing practice. Additional influences to the advanced practice role and scope of practice are institutional policies, specialty organizations, and the individual APRN's sense and comfort with his or her individual scope of practice. Regulations vary by state. For example, in some states, the CNS role is not recognized as an advanced practice role, and in other states the CNS functions in a similar clinical role to the NP. Myriad laws and regulations create confusion on the part of the public and may undermine the credibility of all APRN roles (Advanced Practice Registered Nurse [APRN] Consensus Work Group & the National Council of State Boards of Nursing [NCSBN] APRN Advisory Committee, 2008). For the purpose of the discussion of the APRN role in oncology, this chapter will refer to the APRN in oncology, NP or CNS, who is providing and being reimbursed for direct patient care.

Not surprisingly, despite the IOM (2011) report, some oppose the expanded role of nursing in overall healthcare delivery. Some state boards of medicine argue that APRNs are not adequately educated to provide independent and safe care. In support of this premise, the American Medical Association (AMA, 2009) cited studies of APRNs self-reporting lack of preparation at entry to practice, but failed to cite specific evidence indicating poor outcomes as the result of NP practice. Although AMA consistently notes that they are concerned about patient safety and welfare, the issue of competitive self-interest makes the argument somewhat dubious. A recent editorial in the *New England Journal of Medicine* written collaboratively by a nurse, physician, and policy expert stated, "Fighting the expansion of nurse practitioners' scope of practice is no longer a defensible strategy. The challenge will be for all health care professionals to embrace these changes and come together to improve U.S. health care" (Fairman, Rowe, Hasmiller, & Shalala, 2011, p. 195).

By 2006, NPs in all 50 states had some degree of prescriptive authority, with variable rates of requisite physician oversight and ability to prescribe controlled substances. In order to prescribe controlled substances, APRNs must register with the U.S. Drug Enforcement Administration (DEA) to receive a DEA number for the prescription of controlled substances. A DEA number will not be issued to APRNs in states that do not allow APRNs to prescribe controlled substances (U.S. Department of Justice, n.d.).

There is wide state-to-state variability in APRN reimbursement. Reimbursement largely depends on state law. Medicare from the federal level has provisions to reimburse NPs, but individual states still have great influence in the delivery of this reimbursement. Third-party reimbursement for APRNs is also largely dependent on state law (Safriet, 1992).

The Pearson Report, an annual summary of NP licensure and regulation, noted that as of 2010, 24 states allowed completely autonomous APRN diagnosis and practice, and 16 states allowed diagnosis and practice with physician oversight for prescriptive privileges (Pearson, 2011). The somewhat arbitrary rules for physician oversight and prescriptive authority and the territorial bickering over APRN scope of practice without an evidentiary foundation only undermine the ability of APRNs to practice to the full extent of their licensure.

Predicted Cancer Care Provider Shortage

The nation is facing a shortage of cancer care providers needed to provide high-quality care. The current oncology workforce of physicians, NPs, and general RNs is without proportionate replacement for expected clinician attrition (Erikson, Salsberg, Forte, Bruinooge, & Goldstein, 2007; Patlak & Levit, 2009; Warren, Mariotto, Meekins, Topor, & Brown, 2008). More than half of currently practicing oncologists are 50 years old or older and are likely to retire by 2020. While current oncologists are retiring rapidly, the rate of new oncologists entering the workforce is not proportionate to projected need (Erikson et al., 2007). Patient factors are also contributing to a potential workforce shortage. The number of people diagnosed and living with cancer will rise by 81% by 2020 due to an aging population, more complex cancer treatments, and prolonged survival among individuals with cancer (Erikson et al., 2007; Patlak & Levit, 2009; Warren et al., 2008). Subsequently, cancer care visit demands are projected to grow at a more rapid pace than the number of visits oncologists can provide (Erikson et al., 2007; Patlak & Levit, 2009; Warren et al., 2008).

The American Society of Clinical Oncology (2008) Workforce Strategic Plan and the IOM (2009) report *Ensuring Quality Cancer Care Through the Oncology Workforce* urged the redesign of current work practices and the development of a workforce to ensure continuous delivery of high-quality cancer care. Part of this redesign will include physicians no longer providing as much direct care but directing teams of providers, including NPs (Erikson et al., 2007). Restrategizing oncology care delivery through increasing the numbers and expanding the roles of nonphysician practitioners, such as NPs, is considered to be critically important to meet the current and future cancer care needs of the U.S. population.

Measuring Outcomes of Advanced Nursing Practice

Although APRNs may be called upon to mitigate the impending oncologist work-force shortage, it is also important that outcomes of oncology advanced nursing practice be measured and recognized not as a physician replacement but as a unique and valuable entity of the cancer care delivery team. The outcomes can be evaluated by traditional measures of productivity such as patients seen, procedures performed, and costs saved. However, the critically important measurement should be patient-centered outcomes. The measurement of the APRN's influence on oncology patient-centered outcomes is slowly expanding. While productivity measured by patients seen and procedures performed can be quantified, patient-centered outcomes are more difficult to measure. Methods are available that APRNs can use to measure the impact of their practice on specific patient-centered outcomes.

It is not enough for APRNs to hear "the patients love you," or "you spend so much more time than the doctor"; oncology APRNs must quantify these accolades into empiric evidence of quality improvement or cost savings. The methodology for measuring specific outcomes must be outlined. For example, a cancer practice may determine that emergency department visits by patients recently discharged from the oncology inpatient unit is an identified problem. The oncology APRN may then intervene to provide additional discharge information and anticipatory guidance, which could result in a subsequent decrease in emergency department visits by patients recently discharged. APRNs must quantify the content (patient education) and dose (time spent in delivery) that they are uniquely providing in order to document and sustain a particular positive patient-centered outcome. Previous research has documented that the unique components of APRN interventions are health education, symptom management, anticipatory guidance, and emotional support. Although traditional outcome variables of disease progression and survival will sometimes improve with APRN interventions, these variables alone will not quantify all the benefits that oncology APRNs provide (McCorkle et al., 2000, 2008; Temel et al., 2010). Additionally, although oncology outcomes improve with APRN practice, the exact mechanisms by which they improve have not been identified. The measurement of feelings of support, knowledge, and trust and the consistent interpersonal relationship that may result from the APRN role have not been quantified in order to better capture the "ingredient" for improved outcomes. These types of investigations may be conducted with the assistance of a research partnership through a local university or a hospital-based expert in quality improvement.

LACE Model

More than 250,000 nurses are self-described as APRNs in the United States (U.S. Department of Health and Human Services Health Resources and Services Administration, 2010). Currently, however, there is no uniformity in the APRN role across states. Confusion among the public weakens the APRN position in the public policy arena and healthcare community and limits access to APRNs across states and settings. The Consensus Model for Advanced Practice Registered Nurses has been operationalized through the Licensure, Accreditation, Certification and Education (LACE) Model, a plan to regulate the licensure of APRNs in a nationally uniform manner, through accreditation, certification, and education (APRN Consensus Work Group & NCSBN APRN Advisory Committee, 2008).

This model has been endorsed by major nursing organizations, such as the AANP, AANP Certification Program, NACNS, Oncology Nursing Certification Corporation (ONCC), and ONS, and is scheduled for 2015 implementation. Under this regulatory model, four specific APRN roles are recognized: certified registered nurse anesthetist (CRNA), certified nurse-midwife (CNM), clinical nurse specialist (CNS), and certified nurse practitioner (CNP). Although each specialty will have specific content according to each domain, they must all contain the "three Ps"—pathophysiology, pharmacology, and physical diagnosis for core courses (APRN Consensus Work Group & NCSBN APRN Advisory Committee, 2008).

Licensure

Scope of practice and prescriptive privileging is a professional issue for all APRNs. This is increasingly complex according to state law. Each state holds nursing under different professional umbrellas with a multitude of professional regulations. The APRN is responsible for knowing the state regulations where he or she practices in order to ensure that practice and prescriptive privileges are within the confines of the state law. Additionally, the oncology APRN must then become politically astute and active. The APRN must work within state nursing organizations to preserve the autonomy already established and continue to work toward maximum collaboration and respect in order to provide optimal cancer care to patients and families. The LACE model is attempting to standardize the licensure of APRNs through certification examinations in specific APRN roles.

LACE and Certification

The need for licensure for APRNs to practice may vary state to state. However, according to the new APRN model, graduates of all APRN education programs must be eligible for national certification and must sit for a certification examination required and recognized by state licensing bodies. Certification examinations will assess the nationally recognized competencies of the specific APRN core role (NP or CNS) and at least one population-focus area of practice. APRN certification will require a continued competency mechanism. In the future, all APRNs will be required to sit for national certification prior to becoming licensed, regardless of the state in which they practice. NPs must sit for the certification program of their educational program's population focus. Until 2015, if an APRN is practicing in a state that does not require state licensure for practice, he or she is still strongly encouraged to obtain national certification from one of the certification entities recognized by state boards. This will allow maximum professional flexibility.

LACE and Specialty Care

The LACE model encourages APRNs practicing in specialty care to become certified in that specialty as well as in a focused population. The oncology certification examinations for adult patients with cancer include ONCC's Advanced Oncology Certified Nurse Practitioner (AOCNP®) and the Advanced Oncology Certified Clinical Nurse Specialist (AOCNS®) tests.

Of the more than 32,000 oncology nurses who are certified through ONCC, approximately 870 NPs currently hold the AOCNP® credential and 450 CNSs are certified with an AOCNS® credential. Additionally, approximately 995 APRNs hold the Advanced Oncology Certified Nurse (AOCN®) certification (P. Asfahani, personal communication, January 20, 2012). (The AOCN® examination is no longer administered, but NPs and CNSs can maintain the credential through professional development.)

LACE and Education

Educational programs may concurrently prepare individuals in a specialty providing they meet all of the other requirements for APRN educational programs, including preparation in the APRN core, role, and population core competencies. An issue that is not resolved with the LACE model that may have implications for advanced practice nursing in oncology is education and scope of practice. Increasingly, states are requesting that APRNs seek practice privileges only in the area of practice of their specific education. For example, some hospitals will not grant privileges for NPs if they are graduates of a family or adult primary care APRN program, citing lack of adequate preparation for the acute care setting. This leaves oncology nursing in a quandary. Cancer nursing care can be provided in the outpatient clinic, but a primary care education may not be adequate for the level of acuity of many patients with cancer. Conversely, an acute care educational focus may be inappropriate to understand the concomitant chronic care or health promotion needs of most patients with cancer. No population-specific education specifically matches oncology, and many young students may not be certain of the type of oncology nursing they may want to practice in the future. This new rule may limit the scope of practice for individual oncology nursing. This issue will continue to require discussion.

Doctoral Education

An additional issue for nurses considering the APRN role is the consideration of doctoral education either with the APRN education or as an additional degree. In 2004, the American Association of Colleges of Nursing (AACN) made the controversial recommendation that advanced nursing practice education be moved from the master's level to the doctorate level by 2015 (AACN, 2004). Doctoral programs in nursing fall into two principal categories: research focus and practice focus. The two doctoral degrees that are most commonly sought for oncology APRNs are doctor of philosophy (PhD) or doctor of nursing practice (DNP).

The PhD degree is a program of study designed to prepare the student with the ability to conduct original research and contribute to the science of nursing care for patients with cancer and their families. These programs are designed to prepare nurse scientists and focus on research theory and methodology. Completion of these programs requires original research and dissemination of research and scholarly work. The DNP curriculum focuses on preparing the nurse as an expert clinician, with the tools for analysis of patient or institutional data in order to improve patient care and implement evidence-based practice. These programs focus on the APRN bringing evidence into the clinical setting. Although both degrees can ultimately influence patient care, the research distinction is important. The DNP focuses on preparing the clinical expert in a specific setting with an ability to use literature to improve patient care, to analyze practice for possible areas of improvement, and to collect and implement patient data to improve care delivery.

The DNP role is still fairly new. Although "clinical doctorates" have long been available, the first DNP programs were established as post-MSN programs, preparing APRNs with the tools necessary to put evidence into practice and provide clinical leadership. AACN's position statement on DNP practice noted that

> Nurses prepared at the doctoral level with a blend of clinical, organizational, economic and leadership skills are most likely to be able to critique nursing and other clinical scientific findings and design programs of care delivery that are locally acceptable, economically feasible, and which significantly impact health care outcomes. (AACN, 2004, p. 3)

The DNP degree is now offered nationwide as a post-MSN program or integrated within the post-baccalaureate APRN curriculum. Some nursing professionals are concerned that the role definition for practice beyond clinical care for this newly prepared clinician is poorly defined, leaving vulnerability for the APRN to not fully use the nonclinical skills obtained through the completion of a capstone project. Nursing must continue to measure long-term outcomes from the utilization of DNPs within the clinical setting (AACN, 2009). Outcomes such as quality indicators, safety, and cost are quantifiable, well-accepted outcomes that can begin to quantify the benefit of the DNP role in general or specialty practice.

The 2015 recommendation from ANCC has implications in licensure, certification, and education. The DNP degree will truly become mandatory when the DNP degree only (no MSN) is accepted for certification examination eligibility. With the implementation of the LACE model, all state boards of nursing will require NP certification for licensure. This change in the eligibility for certification examinations will essentially mandate this degree for all NPs. If NP programs evolve from MSN to DNP programs, the core elements of the education must be kept intact so that the educational programs are in congruence with state laws and accreditation criteria for NP educational programs.

Assurance of Oncology Nursing Competencies

To begin to better define the role and standardize knowledge and skill preparation into oncology practice, ONS (2007, 2008) published specific competencies for entry-level NPs and CNSs.

Nurse Practitioner Competencies

The ONS (2007) NP competencies build on core competencies for all NPs to meet the unique needs of patients with a past, current, or potential diagnosis of cancer, including

- Assessing all aspects of the patient's health status, including health promotion, health protection, and disease prevention

- Diagnosing health status, including critical thinking, differential diagnosis, and integration and interpretation of various forms of data
- Planning and implementing interventions to return the patient to a stable state to optimize health
- Imparting knowledge and skills for patient self-care.

The ONS (2007) NP competencies assume that NPs have completed graduate course work and clinical experiences to

> Provide advanced nursing care to meet the specialized physiologic and psychological needs of patients throughout the continuum of care, including cancer prevention and detection, cancer diagnosis and treatment, rehabilitation, survivorship, and end-of-life care. (ONS, 2007, p. 6)

Clinical Nurse Specialist Competencies

ONS (2008) developed CNS competencies using the same iterative process as the NP competencies. The competencies delineate the knowledge and skills necessary for the provision of expert clinical care for the advocacy of expert patient care for patients and families "with complex cancer-related problems and diagnoses" (ONS, 2008, p. 6). The CNS also works to promote cost-efficient, well-organized and evidence-based cancer care. The CNS competencies are broadly categorized into the three core spheres of influence in CNS curriculum (ONS, 2008):
- Patient/client sphere of influence
- Nurse and nursing practice sphere of influence
- Organization/systems sphere of influence.

Oncology Nursing Society's Bridging the Gap Study Findings

Providing the specific oncology education necessary to meet the ONS APRN competencies in oncology is a separate but equally important consideration. For APRNs entering oncology, additional professional education is necessary for the provision of safe and appropriate care of patients with cancer and their loved ones across the cancer care trajectory (Nevidjon et al., 2010). Currently, APRNs, specifically NPs without previous cancer care experience, enter oncology positions that require a high degree of autonomy and decision making without any specific cancer training or education. Nevidjon et al. (2010) found that traditional oncology nursing orientations that include topics such as chemotherapy administration are inadequate for the oncology NP's unique role.

ONS surveyed NPs working in cancer care to assess their learning needs at entry to practice. Of the 607 oncology NPs contacted, 17% (n = 104) responded (Rosenzweig et al., 2010). In the first year of practice, 90% rated themselves as "prepared" or "very prepared" in the generic NP practices of obtaining patient history, performing physical examination, and documenting findings, but in the oncology-specific categories, many rated themselves as "not at all" or only "somewhat" prepared in clinical issues of chemotherapy/biotherapy competency, recognizing and managing oncologic emergencies, and recognizing and managing drug toxicities. The primary source of oncology education for NPs new to practice was almost exclusively collaborating/supervising physicians. As of yet, no flexible curriculum exists to provide this specialized knowledge for the working NP new to cancer care (Rosenzweig et al., 2010).

Postgraduate Education: Future Trends

In 2010, two concurrent events occurred with regard to the nursing profession. First, the Affordable Care Act of 2010 was passed by the U.S. Congress, potentially allowing greater access to health care for many patients who had been previously denied services because of the inability to pay or preexisting conditions (AACN, 2010). The concern about adequate numbers of medical providers was deepened with the potential for more patients having access to medical care, including cancer care. Some of the proposals and components of the Affordable Care Act are yet to be operationalized but offer great potential for oncology APRNs. For example, nurse-managed clinics will be encouraged and funded through the Affordable Care Act (AACN, 2010). Although we traditionally think of these clinics as designated for primary care, cancer care NPs specializing in rehabilitation or survivorship may be eligible for this novel funding.

The second major initiative that was very important to nursing in 2010 was the Robert Wood Johnson Foundation and IOM report on the future of nursing, presenting their recommendations for the direction and role of nursing in a transformed healthcare system (IOM, 2011). The report highlighted the wonderfully adept "fit" of nursing, particularly advanced practice nursing, to fill the growing needs for quality, continuity of care, and accessibility.

The IOM (2011) report highlighted four key messages:

- Nurses should practice to the full extent of their education and training.
- Nurses should achieve higher levels of education and training through an improved education system that promotes seamless academic progression.
- Nurses should be full partners with physicians and other healthcare professionals in redesigning health care in the United States.
- Effective workforce planning and policy making require better data collection and information infrastructure.

In order to meet these goals, the IOM report states that education curricula in academic settings such as nursing must be reformed. Patient-centered outcomes must be at the center of care and nursing education must ensure the attainment of requisite competencies to deliver high-quality care (IOM, 2011).

An additional IOM report on the provision of cancer care titled *Ensuring Quality Cancer Care Through the Oncology Workforce: Sustaining Care in the 21st Century* specifically addressed the potential oncology nurse workforce shortage issue (Patlak & Levit, 2009). IOM suggested two remedies for the oncology nursing and NP shortages: (a) include meaningful cancer care curricula in oncology NP programs, or (b) on-the-job training for NPs in a program that provides didactic and clinical oncology fellowship education in a cancer center, such as the model program at the University of Texas MD Anderson Cancer Center (n.d.). These solutions are problematic for today's NP education and workforce. Adding meaningful oncology content in established NP programs is difficult due to curricula that are already full to capacity with required content for national educational accreditation. Specialty education in NP curricula is now discouraged, with educational trends moving toward more general, population-based education and away from disease-focused content. IOM's second suggestion for on-the-job cancer care training through NP fellowship programs is modeled on the traditional medical oncology fellowship. Although a fellowship program may be educationally optimal, it is often not feasible given that NPs traditionally transition to the advanced practice role in middle age or mid-career with familial and financial obligations limiting their professional flexibility.

Conclusion

The role of the APRN, specifically the NP, has grown rapidly in the past several years. Currently, a great deal of confusion exists regarding APRN education, scope of practice, and certification. The LACE model will achieve a great deal toward standardizing education and clinical preparedness, as well as reducing the overall ambiguity of the APRN role. Although some aspects of this model's application to oncology nurses are still unclear, the trend toward standardization of the role will only enhance its validity.

APRNs must continue to stay politically active so that barriers to practice are reduced or eliminated. Documentation of patient outcomes will continue to support and enhance the viability of the APRN role for oncology. APRNs in oncology should work toward oncology-specific certification in order to demonstrate clinical competency. Additionally, APRNs have a responsibility to work toward the education of the new generation of APRNs entering oncology practice. Strengthening the newest APRNs in oncology will continue to ensure safe, quality care for all patients with cancer and their families.

References

Akscin, J., Barr, T., & Towle, E. (2007). Benchmarking practice operations: Results from a survey of office-based oncology practices. *Journal of Oncology Practice, 3*, 9–12. doi:10.1200/JOP.0712504

American Academy of Nurse Practitioners. (2010a). Frequently asked questions: Why choose a nurse practitioner as your healthcare provider? Retrieved from http://www.aanp.org/NR/rdonlyres/A1D9B4BD-AC5E-45BF-9EB0-DEFCA1123204/4710/2011FAQswhatisanNPupdated.pdf

American Academy of Nurse Practitioners. (2010b). Nurse practitioner cost-effectiveness. Retrieved from http://www.aanp.org/NR/rdonlyres/197C9C42-4BC1-42A5-911E-85FA759B0308/0/CostEffectiveness4pages.pdf

American Academy of Nurse Practitioners. (2010c). Quality of nurse practitioner practice. Retrieved from http://www.aanp.org/NR/rdonlyres/34E7FF57-E071-4014-B554-FF02B82FF2F2/0/QualityofNPPractice4pages.pdf

American Association of Colleges of Nursing. (2004, October). Position statement on the practice doctorate in nursing. Retrieved from http://www.aacn.nche.edu/dnp/dnppositionstatement.htm

American Association of Colleges of Nursing. (2009, October 5). Frequently asked questions: Position statement on the practice doctorate in nursing. Retrieved from http://apps.aacn.nche.edu/DNP/DNPFAQ.htm

American Association of Colleges of Nursing. (2010). Patient protection and affordable care act—Public law no.: 111-148. Nursing education and practice provisions. Retrieved from http://www.aacn.nche.edu/government-affairs/HCRreview.pdf

American Medical Association. (2009, October). AMA scope of practice data series: A resource compendium for state medical associations and national medical specialty societies—Nurse practitioners. Retrieved from http://aanp.org/AANPCMS2/publicpages/08-0424%20SOP%20Nurse%20Revised%2010-09.pdf

American Society of Clinical Oncology. (2008). ASCO 2008–2013 workforce strategic plan to ensure continuing access to quality cancer care. Retrieved from http://www.asco.org/ASCO/Downloads/Research%20Policy/Workforce%20Page/ASCO%20Workforce%20Strategic%20Plan.pdf

APRN Consensus Work Group & National Council of State Boards of Nursing APRN Advisory Committee. (2008, July 7). Consensus model for APRN regulation: Liscensure, accreditation, certification, and education. Retrieved from http://www.aacn.nche.edu/education-resources/APRNReport.pdf

Bishop, C.S. (2009). The critical role of oncology nurse practitioners in cancer care: Future implications. *Oncology Nursing Forum, 36*, 267–269. doi:10.1188/09.ONF.267-269

Britell, J.C. (2010). Role of advanced nurse practitioners and physician assistants in Washington State. *Journal of Oncology Practice, 6*, 37–38. doi:10.1200/JOP.091068

Bryant-Lukosius, D., & Dicenso, A. (2004). A framework for the introduction and evaluation of advanced practice nursing roles. *Journal of Advanced Nursing, 48,* 530–540. doi:10.1111/j.1365 -2648.2004.03235.x

Center for Workforce Studies. (2007, March). *Forecasting the supply of and demand for oncologists: A report to the American Society of Clinical Oncology (ASCO) from the AAMC Center for Workforce Studies.* Retrieved from http://www.asco.org/ASCO/Downloads/cancer%20research/oncology%20 workforce%20report%20FINAL.pdf

Cunningham, R.S. (2004). Advanced practice nursing outcomes: A review of selected empirical literature. *Oncology Nursing Forum, 31,* 219–232. doi:10.1188/04.ONF.219-232

Erikson, C., Salsberg, E., Forte, G., Bruinooge, S., & Goldstein, M. (2007). Future supply and demand for oncologists: Challenges to assuring access to oncology services. *Journal of Oncology Practice, 3,* 79–86. doi:10.1200/JOP.0723601

Fairman, J.A., Rowe, J.W., Hasmiller, S., & Shalala, D.E. (2011). Perspective: Broadening the scope of nursing practice. *New England Journal of Medicine, 364,* 193–196. doi:10.1056/NEJMp1012121

Gershengorn, H.B., Wunsch, H., Wahab, R., Leaf, D.E., Brodie, D., Li, G., & Factor, P. (2011). Impact of nonphysician staffing on outcomes in a medical ICU. *Chest, 139,* 1347–1353. doi:10.1378/ chest.10-2648

Hayes, E. (2007). Nurse practitioners and managed care: Patient satisfaction and intention to adhere to nurse practitioner plan of care. *Journal of the American Academy of Nurse Practitioners, 19,* 418–426. doi:10.1111/j.1745-7599.2007.00245.x

Hoffman, L.A., Tasota, F.J., Scharfenberg, C., Zullo, T.G., & Donahue, M.P. (2003). Management of patients in the intensive care unit: Comparison via work sampling analysis of an acute care nurse practitioner and physicians in training. *American Journal of Critical Care, 12,* 436–443. Retrieved from http://ajcc.aacnjournals.org/content/12/5/436.long

Institute of Medicine. (2009, April 24). *Ensuring quality cancer care through the oncology workforce: Sustaining care in the 21st century.* Retrieved from http://www.iom.edu/Reports/2009/Ensuring -Quality-Cancer-Care-through-the-Oncology-Workforce-Sustaining-Care-in-the-21st-Century -Workshop-Summary.aspx

Institute of Medicine. (2011). *The future of nursing: Leading change, advancing health.* Retrieved from http://www.nap.edu/catalog.php?record_id=12956

McCorkle, R., Dowd, M., Ercolano, E., Schulman-Green, D., Williams, A.L., Siefert, M.L., ... Schwartz, P. (2008). Effects of a nursing intervention on quality of life outcomes in post-surgical women with gynecological cancers. *Psycho-Oncology, 10,* 1002–1012. doi:10.1002/pon.1365

McCorkle, R., Strumpf, N.E., Nuamah, I.F., Adler, D.C., Cooley, M.E., Jepson, C., ... Torosian, M. (2000). A specialized home care intervention improves survival among older post-surgical cancer patients. *Journal of the American Geriatrics Society, 48,* 1707–1713.

Murphy-Ende, K. (2002). Advanced practice nursing: Reflections on the past, issues for the future. *Oncology Nursing Forum, 29,* 106–112. doi:10.1188/02.ONF.106-112

National Association of Clinical Nurse Specialists. (n.d.). Advanced practice registered nurses: The clinical nurse specialists (CNS). Retrieved from http://www.nacns.org/docs/APRN-Factsheet .pdf

Nevidjon, B., Rieger, P., Murphy, C., Rosenzweig, M., McCorkle, M., & Baileys, K. (2010). Filling the gap: Development of the oncology nurse practitioner workforce. *Journal of Oncology Practice, 6,* 2–6. doi:10.1200/JOP.091072

Newhouse, R., Bass, E.B., Steinwachs, D.M., Stanik-Hutt, J., Zangaro, G., Heindel, L., ... Fountain, L. (2011). Advanced practice nurse outcomes 1990–2008: A systematic review. *Nursing Economics, 29*(5), 1–22. Retrieved from https://www.nursingeconomics.net/ce/2013/article3001021.pdf

Oncology Nursing Society. (2007). Oncology nurse practitioner competencies. Retrieved from http://www.ons.org/media/ons/docs/publications/npcompentencies.pdf

Oncology Nursing Society. (2008). Oncology clinical nurse specialist competencies. Retrieved from http://www.ons.org/media/ons/docs/publications/cnscomps.pdf

Patlak, M., & Levit, L. (2009). *Ensuring quality cancer care through the oncology workforce: Sustaining care in the 21st century: Workshop summary.* Retrieved from http://www.nap.edu/catalog/12613.html

Pearson, L. (2011). *The Pearson report.* Retrieved from http://www.pearsonreport.com

Polansky, M., Ross, A.C., & Coniglio, D. (2010). Physician assistant perspective on the ASCO workforce study regarding the use of physician assistants and nurse practitioners. *Journal of Oncology Practice, 6,* 31–33. doi:10.1200/JOP.091063

Rosenzweig, M., Giblin, J., Mickle, M., Morse, P., Sheehy, S., & Sommer, V. (2010). Knowledge needs of nurse practitioners new to oncology care [Abstract]. *Journal of Clinical Oncology, 28*(Suppl. 15), e16532. Retrieved from http://meeting.ascopubs.org/cgi/content/abstract/28/15_suppl/e16532?sid=d53ffd6e-ec77-4c60-9b58-45e77fda5c0c

Rosenzweig, M., Giblin, J., Morse, P., Sheehy, S., Sommer, V., & Bridging the Gap Working Group. (2012). Bridging the gap: A descriptive study of knowledge and skill needs in the first year of oncology nurse practitioner practice. *Oncology Nursing Forum, 39,* 195–201. doi:10.1188/12.ONF.195-201

Safriet, B.J. (1992). Health care dollars and regulatory sense: The role of advanced practice nursing. *Yale Journal on Regulation, 9,* 417.

Temel, J.S., Greer, J.A., Muzikansky, A., Gallagher, E.R., Adame, S., Jackson, V.A., ... Lynch, T.J. (2010). Early palliative care for patients with metastatic non-small-cell lung cancer. *New England Journal of Medicine, 363,* 733–742. doi:10.1056/NEJMoa1000678

University of Texas MD Anderson Cancer Center. (n.d.). Post graduate fellowship in oncology nursing. Retrieved from http://www.mdanderson.org/education-and-research/education-and-training/schools-and-programs/nursing-education/post-graduate-fellowship-in-oncology-nursing/index.html

U.S. Department of Health and Human Services Health Resources and Services Administration. (2010, September). The registered nurse population: Initial findings from the 2008 National Sample Survey of Registered Nurses. Retrieved from http://bhpr.hrsa.gov/healthworkforce/rnsurveys/rnsurveyfinal.pdf

U.S. Department of Justice Office of Diversion Control. (n.d.). Registration applications. Retrieved from http://www.deadiversion.usdoj.gov/drugreg/reg_apps/onlineforms_new.htm

Warren, J., Mariotto, A., Meekins, A., Topor, M., & Brown, M. (2008). Current and future utilization of services from medical oncologists. *Journal of Clinical Oncology, 26,* 3242–3247. doi:10.1200/JCO.2007.14.6357

Young, T. (2005). Utilizing oncology nurse practitioners: A model strategy. *Community Oncology, 2,* 218–224. Retrieved from http://www.communityoncology.net/co/journal/articles/0203218.pdf

CHAPTER 3

Modeling Research for Practice

Leah L. Shever, PhD, RN

Objectives

This chapter will provide an overview of evidence-based practice (EBP), describe the EBP process, differentiate between research and implementation of research findings in practice, and compare efficacy and effectiveness research. After reading this chapter, the learner will be able to

- Understand EBP and the role of research in EBP
- Understand the initial steps of research and implementation of research findings and how they are similar
- Describe the differences between research and use of research in practice
- Describe the differences between efficacy and effectiveness research.

Evidence-Based Practice

Healthcare providers strive to provide the highest quality of care possible for patients and families. But how does one judge whether care is high quality? In order to determine the quality of care provided, the care must be evaluated, or studied, for its impact. Studying care provided in a scientific method produces results (evidence) that help determine whether the impact of that care improves patient outcomes. When the evidence from studies is used in practice, it is referred to as the *implementation of research findings into practice*, or *EBP*. Therefore, EBP involves both conducting research and implementing research into practice.

EBP can be defined as "applying the best available research results (evidence) when making decisions about health care. Healthcare professionals who perform evidence-based practice use research evidence along with clinical expertise and patient preferences" (Agency for Healthcare Research and Quality, n.d.). Figure 3-1 is a simplistic depiction explaining the whole cycle of the EBP process. It includes both the conduct of research (studying the phenomenon of interest) and the use of research in practice (implementation of research findings) (Nieva et al., 2005; Sudsawad, 2007; Titler et al., 2001). Both the conduct of research and the implemen-

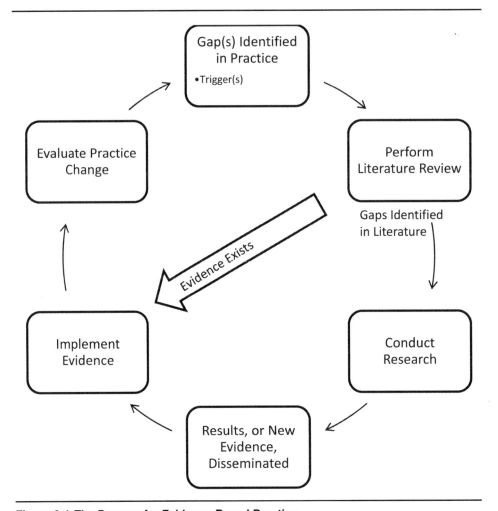

Figure 3-1. The Process for Evidence-Based Practice

tation of research findings start with the identification of gaps, or triggers, in clinical practice (Titler et al., 2001). Gaps are identified through a number of mechanisms. They may be highlighted when a problem or issue, such as a serious patient safety event, occurs, or they can also be triggered by new knowledge or philosophy being put forth by a professional organization, a department, or an institution. Often, a gap is highlighted by someone asking the questions "Why do we do this?" or "Is there a better way to do this?"

Regardless of how the gap is identified, it is important to be clear about the problem to be solved. A clear grasp of the problem, what population it impacts, and the desired outcomes will help guide the literature review. For example, the fall prevention committee at a hospital might be interested in how mobility impacts falls. To further define the problem, the committee members may identify that they are interested in adult inpatients only, that mobility may be defined in a number of different ways (e.g., strength and balance training, ambulation, sitting up in chair), and that the outcomes of interest are going to be falls and injuries from falls. One method commonly employed to clearly state the problem is the problem/population, intervention, comparison(s), outcome(s) (PICO) statement (McKibbon & Marks, 2001; National Nursing Practice Network, 2009). Using the same example, the PICO statement might look like this:

P—Adult patients in the hospital are falling too frequently.

I—Mobility

C—Current practice

O—Falls and falls with injury while in the hospital

After the gap has been identified and the problem statement is clearly established, the review of existing literature begins. The problem, or PICO, statement should help guide the search for articles. To find relevant literature or research, searches are conducted with the help of robust bibliographic databases such as PubMed (www.ncbi.nlm.nih.gov/pubmed) or CINAHL® (the Cumulative Index to Nursing and Allied Health Literature). Words or phrases in the problem statement can be used to find relevant research. These words or phrases are referred to as *search terms* or *keywords* and describe the phenomenon of interest (Burns & Grove, 2001). It is helpful to save the databases searched, the search terms used, and any limits that were applied so that the process can be described and replicated later. Figure 3-2 is a tool that can be used to track key elements of literature searches.

Once research articles, guidelines, systematic reviews, and other sources of evidence have been identified for review, they are critiqued to judge the quality and applicability of the evidence. Resources are available to assist with the critique of evidence such as the Appraisal of Guidelines for Research and Evaluation (AGREE) tool (AGREE Research Trust, 2009) to critique guidelines and the Preferred Reporting for Systematic Reviews and Meta-Analyses (PRISMA) (Moher, Liberati, Tetzlaff, Altman, & PRISMA Group, 2009) for critiquing meta-analyses, and additional literature to guide critiques of quantitative and qualitative research articles (Burns & Grove, 2001; Coughlan, Cronin, & Ryan, 2007; Ryan, Coughlan, & Cronin, 2007). When judging a research study for its potential use in practice, another important aspect to consider is the feasibility to replicate in practice. If a study intervention is so complex or resource intensive that it could never be implemented in a real-world setting, then the critique should include that as a limitation of the study.

Date	Database Used	Search Terms Used	Applied Limits
		First search term: ☐ and ☐ or Second search term: ☐ and ☐ or Third search term:	☐ English ☐ Human ☐ Date range from _____ to _____ ☐ Age range from _____ to _____ ☐ Other: _____ ☐ Other: _____ ☐ Other: _____ ☐ Other: _____

Figure 3-2. Literature Searches Tracking Tool

The sources of evidence (e.g., guidelines, systematic reviews, research articles) are individually critiqued and synthesized and evaluated as a body of evidence. The synthesis of all of the evidence sources should be evaluated to determine whether a change in practice is needed. Often, a synthesis table is used to capture the critique of the individual evidence sources, making it easier to see the settings, populations, and key findings, across all studies and sources. Based on the review of all of the critiqued literature, a judgment is made regarding whether sufficient evidence exists to make a change in practice or whether gaps are still present. The judgment is based on both the quality and quantity of evidence, weighing the risks and benefits of the proposed practice change.

When enough high-quality evidence demonstrates that the benefits of a practice change outweigh the risks, it is appropriate to implement the research findings into practice (see Figure 3-1). After implementation of the research findings, the change is evaluated to determine if it led to the desired results. The process of implementing evidence-based changes and evaluating the impact is an ongoing cycle and aligns with continuous quality-improvement processes where care and care changes are systematically evaluated.

When the review and synthesis of the literature does not produce enough robust evidence, the findings are not consistent, the study populations are not congruent with the patient population of interest, or the interventions are not feasible for use in practice, a gap in the literature may exist, and therefore further research is called for (see Figure 3-1). The next step of conducting research is a longer process but still influenced by the review of related literature. At times, the synthesis table becomes a gap table because it identifies the available research and therefore what themes are and are not present related to a specific topic or phenomenon.

The PICO statement can be modified into research questions, hypotheses, or aims for a research study. The numerous steps to conducting a robust research study are beyond the scope of this chapter. However, it is important to understand that research questions are often triggered by clinical questions and that the first steps for both conducting research and implementing research findings are to define the problem statement and to review the relevant existing literature and research.

Effectiveness and Efficacy Research

The feasibility of implementing interventions or processes of care used in a research study into a practice setting is one criterion that nurses can use to determine if a study's findings are valid before making a practice change. As stated previously, if the research interventions or processes are too complex or resource intensive for the real-world setting, those same processes are very difficult to replicate. As a result of not being able to replicate the research processes, it is possible that the same desired outcomes will not be achieved. Therefore, research studies with design and methods comparable to real-life settings and processes lend themselves better to implementation of results.

This type of research conducted in real-world settings where an intervention's impact is examined in association with multiple other factors that affect patient outcomes is referred to as *effectiveness research* (Brown, 2002; Sidani & Epstein, 2003; Sidani, Epstein, & Moritz, 2003; Titler, Dochterman, & Reed, 2004; Whittemore & Grey, 2002). In contrast, efficacy research attempts to control the environment and other outside factors that may influence an outcome of interest, thereby determining the impact of a treatment in isolation. More specifically, efficacy research attempts to limit or eliminate (i.e., control for) the effect of multiple factors and focus only on the intervention of interest. The study design and methods control for as many extraneous variables as possible in order to isolate the efficacy, or potential benefits, of the treatment or intervention being studied (Brown, 2002; Shwartz & Ash, 2003; Sidani & Epstein, 2003; Sidani et al., 2003; Whittemore & Grey, 2002). Randomized clinical trials are a type of efficacy research where subjects are selected on strict inclusion and exclusion criteria and randomly assigned to either a treatment or control (i.e., no treatment) group.

Efficacy research provides a good understanding of a treatment effect when that treatment is provided in isolation. However, many issues are associated with efficacy research, especially within nursing. One issue is that this research is difficult to conduct. For example, randomizing patients to nursing treatments in a hospital setting is very difficult to do. Also, it is rare that a nursing treatment is ever provided in isolation for a patient. More commonly, nursing treatments work in harmony with other interventions (e.g., medical procedures, medications, physical therapy sessions) to achieve desired patient outcomes.

In addition, the controlled environment rarely mimics what happens in real life. Therefore, some efficacy research is very limited in its applicability because the treatment may have worked well in isolation but was never tested in the true settings in which it would be implemented. To avoid this limitation, the goal of effectiveness research is to test the treatment's effect in the environment where it will be used along with other factors that commonly occur in practice. This type of research is easier to generalize to patient care settings. The ability to generalize findings from efficacy studies is limited; therefore, effectiveness research is very useful when trying to improve patient outcomes in clinical settings (Sidani et al., 2003).

Whether the research is qualitative or quantitative, effectiveness or efficacy, investigators should disseminate results via manuscripts and presentations. As the findings are disseminated, they can be considered for practice implementation (see Figure 3-1). As stated earlier, new findings from a research study may identify a gap in current practice that needs to be examined, which starts the EBP process all over again. Findings from research studies are a necessary component to EBP—they are the evidence in EBP. Therefore, the conduct of research, which produces research findings, is an important part of the EBP process.

Conduct of Research Versus Research Implementation

The first part of this chapter described the process for EBP and highlighted the fact that the conduct of research is part of the larger EBP process. The first steps of conducting research and implementing research into practice are very similar as described earlier and as depicted in Figure 3-1. However, that does not mean that the conduct of research is synonymous with EBP nor with implementation of research findings. Many important distinctions exist between the conduct of research and the implementation of research findings (see Table 3-1), starting with the purpose.

The purpose of conducting research is to generate new knowledge, whereas the purpose of implementing research findings is to put existing knowledge into practice. Although both the conduct of research and the implementation of research findings involve a review and synthesis of the literature, the end results of the liter-

Table 3-1. Comparison of the Conduct of Research and the Implementation of Research

Comparison Criteria	Conduct of Research	Implementation of Research Findings
Purpose	Nurse scientists want to generate new knowledge. Purpose is often shared in the form of research questions, aims, or hypotheses.	Nurses want to put existing knowledge into practice to achieve desired results. Purpose is communicated in PICO statement or problem and purpose statement.
End result of literature synthesis	Identification of a gap in knowledge leads to research questions.	Enough information is generated to decide whether to make a change in practice.
Human participants	An institutional review board (IRB) review is required to protect potential participants. Participation may or may not benefit the participants.	IRB approval is typically not needed unless the researchers plan to publish or present the findings. Interventions are implemented expressly to benefit the patient.
Personnel	PhD-prepared researchers typically lead the study.	Advanced practice nurses typically lead the study.
Protocols and guidelines	Standards and protocols are strict and rigorous; deviating from them can jeopardize the integrity of the study.	Standards and guidelines are adapted to the environment and user to increase ease of implementation.
Evaluation	Data analysis is aligned with methods.	Evaluation is often trends or statistical control charts.

ature synthesis differ. When trying to implement research findings, the end result of the literature synthesis is having adequate information to make a decision as to whether a practice change is needed. The end result of a literature synthesis for the conduct of research is the identification of a gap in current literature.

Another key difference is the role of the patients or participants. When implementing research findings, the patient is the primary beneficiary. One of the key decision points for implementation of research findings is weighing the risks against the benefits for the patients (Titler et al., 2001). When conducting research, it may be unclear whether the treatment being researched will benefit the participant.

Protocols or guidelines for conducting research are usually rigid, and deviating from them can negatively affect the quality of a study. When implementing research into practice, it is possible to modify the processes of care to fit the environment if the key concepts are maintained. The ability to adapt the processes of care can make it easier to implement in practice (Rogers, 2003).

Conclusion

Identifying a problem, collecting relevant evidence, critiquing the evidence, and synthesizing the evidence are the initial steps in both the conduct of research and the implementation of research findings. It is not until the literature has been synthesized that it becomes clear whether more research is needed or whether sufficient evidence is available to make a change in practice. The conduct and implementation of research are important components of EBP; however, they are related but distinct processes.

References

Agency for Healthcare Research and Quality. (n.d.). Effective health care program: Glossary of terms. Retrieved from http://www.effectivehealthcare.ahrq.gov/index.cfm/glossary-of-terms/?pageaction=showterm&termid=24

AGREE Research Trust. (2009). Appraisal of guidelines for research and evaluation II: AGREE II Instrument. Retrieved from http://www.agreetrust.org

Brown, S.J. (2002). Nursing intervention studies: A descriptive analysis of issues important to clinicians. *Research in Nursing and Health, 25,* 317–327. doi:10.1002/nur.10039

Burns, N., & Grove, S. (2001). *The practice of nursing research: Conduct, critique and utilization* (4th ed.). Philadelphia, PA: Saunders.

Coughlan, M., Cronin, P., & Ryan, F. (2007). Step-by-step guide to critiquing research. Part 1: Quantitative research. *British Journal of Nursing, 16,* 658–663.

McKibbon, K.A., & Marks, S. (2001). Posing clinical questions: Framing the question for scientific inquiry. *AACN Clinical Issues, 12,* 477–481.

Moher, D., Liberati, A., Tetzlaff, J., Altman, D.G., & PRISMA Group. (2009). Preferred reporting items for systematic reviews and meta-analyses: The PRISMA statement. *Journal of Clinical Epidemiology, 62,* 1006–1012. doi:10.1016/j.jclinepi.2009.06.005

National Nursing Practice Network. (2009). P-I-C-O tutorial. Retrieved from http://www.nnpnetwork.org

Nieva, V.F., Murphy, R., Ridley, N., Donaldson, N., Combes, J., Mitchell, P., … Carpenter, D. (2005). From science to service: A framework for the transfer of patient safety research into practice. In K. Henriksen, J.B. Battles, E.S. Marks, & D.I. Lewin (Eds.), *Advances in patient safety: From research to implementation* (Vol. 2, pp. 441–453). Rockville, MD: Agency for Healthcare Research and Quality.

Rogers, E.M. (2003). *Diffusion of innovations* (5th ed.). New York, NY: Free Press.

Ryan, F., Coughlan, M., & Cronin, P. (2007). Step-by-step guide to critiquing research. Part 2: Qualitative research. *British Journal of Nursing, 16,* 738–744.

Shwartz, M., & Ash, A.S. (2003). Estimating the effect of an intervention from observational data. In L.I. Iezzoni (Ed.), *Risk adjustment for measuring health care outcomes* (3rd ed., pp. 275–295). Chicago, IL: Health Administration Press.

Sidani, S., & Epstein, D.R. (2003). Enhancing the evaluation of nursing care effectiveness. *Canadian Journal of Nursing Research, 35*(3), 26–38.

Sidani, S., Epstein, D.R., & Moritz, P. (2003). An alternative paradigm for clinical nursing research: An exemplar. *Research in Nursing and Health, 26,* 244–255. doi:10.1002/nur.10086

Sudsawad, P. (2007). CIHR research cycle superimposed by the six opportunities to facilitate KT. Knowledge translation: Introduction to models, strategies, and measures. Retrieved from http://198.214.141.98/kt/products/ktintro/ktmodels.html#fig1

Titler, M., Dochterman, J., & Reed, D. (2004). *Guideline for conducting effectiveness research in nursing and other health services.* Iowa City, IA: The University of Iowa, College of Nursing, Center for Nursing Classification and Clinical Effectiveness.

Titler, M.G., Kleiber, C., Steelman, V.J., Rakel, B.A., Budreau, G., Everett, L.Q., … Goode, C.J. (2001). The Iowa model of evidence-based practice to promote quality care. *Critical Care Nursing Clinics of North America, 13,* 497–509.

Whittemore, R., & Grey, M. (2002). The systematic development of nursing interventions. *Journal of Nursing Scholarship, 34,* 115–120. doi:10.1111/j.1547-5069.2002.00115.x

Theoretical Frameworks and Philosophies of Care

Marilyn J. Hammer, PhD, DC, RN
Frances Cartwright-Alcarese, PhD, RN, AOCN®
Wendy C. Budin, PhD, RN-BC, FAAN

Introduction

The underlying theories that drive nursing practice are an essential part of excellence in patient care. As Meleis (2007) eloquently stated, "Caring for patients, families, and communities is predicated on theories and research that provide the framework and the evidence" (p. ix). Oncology nursing, in particular, is driven by a number of theories and conceptual models that target the many components of this multifaceted and complex practice. Philosophies of care underscore the theoretical frameworks driving oncology nursing practice. This chapter will discuss the role of the oncology nurse from the perspective of theory-driven (or in some cases, concept-driven) practice. The full scope of the patient and family caregiver experience from diagnosis through long-term follow-up or end-of-life care is discussed. Table 4-1 outlines the phases, related processes, and corresponding theories, concepts, and models driving oncology nursing practice.

Overview of the Theories

The theories and concepts that can be used to drive nursing practice are as numerous as oncology nursing practice is varied and complex. The concepts, theories, and models underlying practice highlighted in this chapter include but are not limited to some of the more commonly used and evidence-based. Some are true theories, whereas others are actually concepts in practice. It is important to make a distinction between concepts, theories, and models.

Concepts are the building blocks from which theories are constructed; definitions of concepts differ based on the framework of the theory of which they are a part. More specifically, "a concept is a word that expresses an abstraction formed by generalization from particulars (inductive logic)" (Hoskins, 1998, p. 17). A concept or statement may have different meanings depending upon the lens through which an

Table 4-1. Underlying Theories, Concepts, and Models Driving Oncology Nursing Practice

Phase	Process	Biobehavioral and systems biology	Clinical reasoning and decision making	Patient navigation	Caring	Patient-provider relationships and communication	Symptom experience	Culture	Resilience	Self-help	Integrative health care	Survivorship	Uncertainty in illness	Unitary human beings
Screening and diagnosis	Onset/underlying physiology; fear, anxiety, disbelief	X	X		X	X		X	X	X	X		X	X
Treatment decisions	Type of malignancy; stage and grades; treatment options	X	X	X	X	X		X	X	X	X		X	X
Treatment planning	Healthcare team; patient and family	X	X	X	X	X		X	X	X	X		X	X
Treatment administration	Lifestyle adjustment	X	X	X	X	X	X	X	X	X	X		X	X
Outcome assessment	Underlying physiology: fear, anxiety	X	X		X	X	X	X	X	X	X		X	X
Outcome planning: Remission or return to treatment decisions	Remission: Discharge planning, separation anxiety from health-care team. No remission: Treatment decisions, fear, anxiety	X	X		X	X	X	X	X	X	X	X	X	X

(Continued on next page)

Table 4-1. Underlying Theories, Concepts, and Models Driving Oncology Nursing Practice *(Continued)*

Phase	Process	Biobehavioral and systems biology	Clinical reasoning and decision making	Patient navigation	Caring	Patient-provider relationships and communication	Symptom experience	Culture	Resilience	Self-help	Integrative health care	Survivorship	Uncertainty in illness	Unitary human beings
Remission and follow-up	Periodic reassessments; underlying fear of recurrence	X	X		X	X	X	X	X	X	X	X	X	X
Long-term care and chronicity	Self-management; continued assessments	X	X	X	X	X	X	X	X	X	X	X	X	X
Palliative care	Comfort-measures throughout	X	X	X	X	X	X	X	X	X	X	X	X	X
Hospice care	Terminal prognosis	X			X	X	X	X			X			X
Family/caregiver experiences	Lifestyle adjustment; chronic fear and anxiety, coping mechanisms				X			X	X	X	X		X	X

individual perceives or interprets it. The relationships between or among concepts define, generate, and develop the theory. "Theory is more than the mere description of events. It's an internally consistent body of relational statements about phenomena which is useful for prediction and control" (Chinn & Jacobs, 1997, p. 452). "The theoretical framework within which a given problem is lodged is of crucial importance in every stage of the research. It identifies the variables needed to explain the phenomenon and suggests the nature of the relationships among the variables" (Hoskins, 1998, p. 3). "Nursing theories promote our understanding of the human response to illness" (Haylock, 2010, p. 185).

Theory contains the interrelationships between known facts and research evidence. It is also based on what is assumed true from scientific and theoretical publications. Theory serves to explain, predict, and give direction to research through a priori prediction of the variables needed for analyses. It also assists in the selection process for utilization of the most appropriate variables that will guide the design of the study. This provides a framework of the variables in which to compare and integrate the findings in relation to other research. Theory also drives the formation of the hypotheses and subsequent interpretation of the findings. Finally, theory provides a framework for linking the variables—they must have empirical or theoretical support for coexistence and testing. Logic is applied in defining the definitions between variables. For example, if A is related to B, and B is related to C, then it may be assumed that A is likely related to C (Hoskins, 1998).

The operational definition within a theory tells how the concepts are measured or linked to specific aspects of biobehavioral or systems biology frameworks and suggests how hypotheses can be tested. Theories then are useful to make scientific findings meaningful and to develop operational definitions; they provide direction to the development and refinement of research, education, and practice. A model, on the other hand, provides a systematic illustration of some phenomenon through a visual of related concepts that describe a specific theory. Hypotheses can continue to be developed to test and refine the theory. Thus, a model can be viewed as an illustration that adds clarity to the symbolic representation of a theory or conceptual framework. Because theories can be very complex, a visual representation can illustrate abstract concepts so that their meaning is clear to everyone.

The major concepts, theories, and models driving oncology nursing practice discussed in this chapter include biobehavioral and systems biology, clinical reasoning and clinical decision making, patient navigation, caring, patient-provider relationships and communication, symptom experience, culture, resilience, self-help, integrative health care, survivorship, Mishel's Model of Uncertainty in Illness, and Rogers' Science of Unitary Human Beings as an umbrella theory for all aspects of the cancer experience. In addition, many other theories and conceptual frameworks are discussed pertaining to various aspects of the cancer experience. Some of these include the diffusion of innovations theoretical model, stress and coping, cognitive behavioral theory, Leininger's theory of transcultural nursing, theories of reasoned action and planned behavior, modeling and remodeling theory, and Roy's adaptation model. All of these theories, concepts, and models help drive oncology nursing practice. By applying biobehavioral and systems biology frameworks in a unique way, nurses use critical reasoning and clinical decision making to derive theory that guides nursing practice. Evidence-based nursing practice can only be advanced by nurses—novices and experts alike—who understand established theories and are able to interpret phenomena by applying superior critical thinking skills.

Biobehavioral and Systems Biology

In oncology, biobehavioral and systems biology are valuable frameworks for understanding the physiologic mechanisms contributing to cancer formation, progression, and outcomes. Systems biology incorporates numerous scientific disciplines with an overarching focus of the underlying genetic, epigenetic, proteomic, metabolomic, physiologic, and biologic processes that drive human function (Founds, 2009; Khalil & Hill, 2005). A unique and salient aspect of the systems biology theory is its holistic focus (Founds, 2009). The holistic aspect is captured through four major focal points that are incorporated into patient care: prediction, prevention, personalization, and participation (Schallom, Thimmesch, & Pierce, 2011). The predictive area evaluates the underlying genetic/epigenetic and biophysiologic functioning of the disease process in conjunction with the patient's health status and environmental influences. Prevention is the long-term plan incorporating current health conditions and underlying genetic predisposition. Personalization then takes into account all of these factors in creating a health plan that is individualized. Participation denotes the patient's active involvement in the process (Schallom et al., 2011).

Creating the individualized health plan cannot be successfully achieved without a complete understanding of the disease process. Because of the nonlinear nature of malignancies, systems biology incorporates mathematical and computational models to best understand cancer formation to optimize treatments that can arrest this process (Wang, 2010). These methods help capture and quantify the vast amount of information in large biologic datasets created through oncology research studies. More importantly, these computational methods help determine which treatments will be most effective for each individual because numerous variables can alter a patient's response to treatment (Wang, 2010). In effect, systems biology helps expedite the translation of research from in vitro stages in the lab to in vivo (in the living patient) (Khalil & Hill, 2005) and predict optimal treatment choices based on individual factors (Wang, 2010).

From a nursing perspective, using the systems biology approach requires an understanding of the underlying biophysiologic mechanisms of the disease process and measures that need to be taken for optimizing treatment outcome as described within the focal points of prediction, prevention, personalization, and participation (Schallom et al., 2011). For example, patients undergoing therapies for cancer tend to become immunocompromised. Adhering to strict infection control guidelines can minimize patient risk for infections. Prediction would include an understanding of the underlying mechanisms and sequelae of living in an immunocompromised state. Prevention would include infection prevention measures by the patient and those in contact with the patient, including the healthcare team. Personalization would incorporate other factors such as age and comorbidities that could increase infection risk in whichever environment the patient is living. Personalization would also involve creating a strategic long-term plan for infection prevention based on the patient's specific status. Similarly, focusing on best nutritional approaches, medication adherence, and psychosocial needs can promote better outcomes while under the direct care of the healthcare team. Participation would include patient education to help promote continuation of these behaviors in the home. From this perspective, systems biology then blends into the biobehavioral model.

Behavior can influence malignancy onset, progression, and outcome but is by no means a clear cause nor does it prevent cancer. Indeed, many individuals who maintain a lifestyle considered unhealthy (e.g., relatively sedentary; tobacco use; diets with significant amounts of high-sugar, high-fat foods, red meats, processed foods, alcohol, and other carcinogen-promoting consumables) live long, cancer-free lives. Conversely, some individuals who adopt "healthy" lifestyles (e.g., highly physically active/ regular exercise; no tobacco use; diets predominately consisting of health-promoting foods such as vegetables and fruits, low-fat organic meats, and fish, with modest or no alcohol consumption) develop cancer. Underlying genetic predisposition may be a contributor (Hochedlinger & Plath, 2009; Wilson, 2008). Stress and adaptation to stress are other influencing factors (Godbout & Glaser, 2006). Some studies suggest that psychological stress can be a direct underlying factor leading to the onset of a malignancy or progression or recurrence, but solid evidence is lacking (Cohen, Janicki-Deverts, & Miller, 2007). Additionally, how patients perceive their personal influence on their cancer diagnosis can affect how they respond throughout treatment and post-treatment (Bergner, 2011).

Patients' perceptions of their personal influence on their cancer diagnosis are one aspect; however, how to help individuals change behaviors associated with a cancer diagnosis is another aspect to be considered. One of the few direct causal links between a personal behavior and cancer formation is smoking (Koul & Arora, 2010). Yet despite this universal knowledge, more than 20% of the adult U.S. population and almost 20% of high school students smoke (National Cancer Institute, 2011). Many smokers who acquire lung cancer report a sense of guilt or regret over their diagnosis, and both smokers and nonsmokers with lung cancer face social stigmatism (sometimes directly from their healthcare providers) (Raleigh, 2010). How these feelings translate to health outcomes is less clear and warrants examination.

One area that is clear and where nurses can intervene is promoting smoking prevention and cessation. African Americans, in particular, suffer health-related consequences from smoking (Webb, de Ybarra, Baker, Reis, & Carey, 2010). With rates well above the national proportion of smokers for all races, more than 25% of African American men are smokers (American Heart Association, 2012). Studies further show that nicotine dependency and difficulty with quitting smoking is greater among both male and female African American smokers compared to other ethnic groups (Webb et al., 2010). Webb et al. (2010) found cognitive-behavioral therapy a promising intervention for helping African American smokers to quit.

The biobehavioral model is also often used for cancer symptom management. For example, Budin, Cartwright-Alcarese, and Hoskins (2008) used a theoretical framework based upon the biobehavioral model, including stress and coping to guide the development of the interventions and selection of outcome measures in their randomized clinical trial of phase-specific evidence-based psychoeducation via video and telephone counseling interventions to enhance emotional, physical, and social adjustment in patients with breast cancer and their partners. Physical adjustment included symptom experience. Patients who received a combination of psychoeducation via video combined with telephone counseling showed a decrease in symptom severity and distress over time as compared to those in the standard care disease management group.

Exercise for cancer-related fatigue or for weight reduction is an example of a biobehavioral intervention that is often nurse-directed (Al-Majid & Gray, 2009). Biobehavioral and systems biology are underpinning theories that direct much of holistic nursing care throughout the cancer experience.

Clinical Reasoning and Clinical Decision Making

A highly important component of excellence in nursing is the skill of critical thinking. Particularly in oncology, the nurse's ability to effectively evaluate, assimilate, and make autonomous decisions is essential to patient care. The conceptual models of clinical reasoning and clinical decision making can aid in this process. Clinical reasoning incorporates knowledge, experience, judgment, and various levels of cognitive processes in delivering care to patients (Simmons, 2010). For example, a patient who has undergone ablative chemotherapy followed by a stem cell reinfusion and develops neutropenic fever would require the nurse's ability to know that the condition is life threatening requiring immediate blood cultures and start of broad-spectrum antibiotics. The nurse would also understand that as soon as the blood culture results are available, a specific antibiotic should be started. Order sets based on evidence-based guidelines ensure that the nurse can do this independently to avoid delay. With an understanding of the mechanisms and potential outcomes, the nure can use the clinical reasoning process to guide decisions.

Dovetailing clinical reasoning is clinical decision making. Decision making begins with a problem that needs a resolution coupled with a degree of uncertainty as to how to resolve the problem (Muir, 2004). If knowledge and experience are key elements in decision making, then where does this leave the novice nurse who may have recent textbook knowledge, yet little clinical experience? Because the novice nurse lacks experience, the increased likelihood of making errors is an issue to consider (Saintsing, Gibson, & Pennington, 2011). Some suggestions for decreasing errors and increasing accurate decision making involve enhancing critical thinking skills in nursing school curricula, coupled with providing technology-based tools in the clinical setting for easy access to information that the nurse might not have yet committed to memory (Saintsing et al., 2011). Additionally, working with more experienced nurses and consulting with them when a decision is unclear are paramount for optimal and safe patient care. Over time, increased knowledge and experience promote effective decision-making processes.

Standards that represent the evidence-based supportive literature as well as accountabilities of each member of the interdisciplinary healthcare team provide a framework to generate policies and procedures, protocols, guidelines, and care pathways. National guidelines and patient care documents also promote evidence-based options in decision making that reflect the most current standard of care. These documents are developed by panels of experts in the field of oncology (American Society of Clinical Oncology [ASCO], 2005–2011; National Comprehensive Cancer Network [NCCN], 2011; Oncology Nursing Society [ONS], n.d.; Society for Integrative Oncology [SIO], 2009).

It is also vital for patients to participate in the informed decision-making process. Evidence-based practice guidelines (ASCO, 2005–2011; NCCN, 2011; ONS, n.d.; SIO, 2009) can assist the healthcare provider in offering treatment options; these guidelines also consider the quality of life and supportive care so that patients have information to make informed decisions (Peppercorn et al., 2011). Many factors influence patient decisions about their health care and the theories of reasoned action and planned behavior have an underlying role in decision making. These theories take into consideration that individuals are rational, make use of information before making a decision, and evaluate the implications of their decisions prior to taking action (Gullatte, 2006). Understanding these driving forces can direct the nurse in helping and supporting patients through their decision-making processes.

Patient Navigation

Although most institutions providing treatment for patients with cancer boast excellence in their patient care, gaps in transition from one phase of treatment to another sometimes leave patients feeling lost and vulnerable. The patient navigation model is a psychosocial approach to ensuring patient needs are met through every phase of the diagnosis, treatment, and recovery. The components of patient navigation include providing support, assistance with finding resources, assistance with practical issues, and community support systems (Pedersen & Hack, 2011). Patient navigation programs often involve identified members of the healthcare team designated as patient navigators to help patients through the healthcare system. Other tools can also be used to help facilitate navigation. One institution developed a Breast Cancer Navigation Kit for patients. The kit included informational sections on what breast cancer is, coping and well-being strategies, what to do when treatment ends, and specific practical information (Skrutkowski, Saucier, & Meterissian, 2011). The pilot use of the kit was found to be effective, with the notation that direct contact with members of the healthcare team was still essential (Skrutkowski et al., 2011). The patient navigation model has been used in many facets of oncology care, including community-based efforts to improve cancer screenings among populations who often have limited access to care. The Avon Foundation, for example, instituted an Education and Outreach Initiative Community Patient Navigation Program to increase mammography screening among African American women in the United States (Mason et al., 2011). In this program, community-based patient navigators hosted recruitment events, referred participants to nurse practitioners who aided with eligibility for low-cost or free mammograms, and conducted follow-up telephone calls to encourage adherence to mammography appointments (Mason et al., 2011). Similarly, patient navigation programs have been instituted to improve cancer screenings specifically among Hispanic individuals. Patient navigation systems have helped U.S. Hispanic populations improve both mammography and colonoscopy screenings in addition to helping them receive timely treatment in the situations when cancer was diagnosed (Robie, Alexandru, & Bota, 2011). Patient navigators can not only help provide access to timely care and disseminate information, but they can also help minimize anxiety and feelings of helplessness throughout the process.

Caring

Caring is inherent to nursing and has often been perceived as the essence of nursing (Bassett, 2002). Particularly in oncology, nurses not only provide physical care but also are empathetic to the patient experience. Caring as a theoretical concept was described in the early 1980s using a substruction method. Substruction is a strategy used to critique a theory and methodology through analyzing the theory's components and their hypothesized relationships (Dulock & Holzemer, 1991). Caring as a theory was substructed with analysis of components comprising awareness of a need, knowledge to address the need, assessment of the relationship between the need and intended action, and evaluation of a positive change as an outcome of the action (Gaut, 1983). Although such analysis of caring is concrete, how caring is perceived and actualized can vary among individuals. Some may view good caring as expert delivery of evidence-based practice, whereas others may define good caring as provided by those who show humanistic qualities (Bassett, 2002). Bassett (2002) described four categories of caring as (a) nurses' feelings, (b) nurses' knowledge and competence, (c) nurses' actions, and (d) patient and family outcomes and nurses' rewards. These areas encompass all aspects of what can be viewed as the caring continuum from the knowledge base and physical delivery of care to the emotional support.

Defining caring also transcends cultures. For example, a study focused on patient perception of caring among patients with cancer in Beijing, China, found similar themes including professional knowledge and care delivery along with emotional support (Liu, Mok, & Wong, 2006). As caring from all vantage points is within the heart of nursing, it is an underpinning to all phases of the patient and family/caregiver experience from diagnosis through the outcome of survivorship or end of life.

Patient-Provider Relationships and Communication

Building solid relationships and lines of communication between the patient and healthcare team is essential for optimizing care for patients with cancer. Communication is initially important for obtaining a good patient history and report of the presenting issue. When the patient is faced with a physical health problem, effective communication throughout care becomes a secondary focus to treating the ailment. At the same time, one must consider that traditional healthcare education is often focused on the physical and physiologic aspects of human functioning and skill development in addressing disease processes and neglects communication skills. Healthcare providers who are unskilled at relationship building and effective communication, however, can leave patients feeling isolated and daunted. In acknowledgement of this need, communication skills have more recently become a part of curricula in the health professions within the last couple of decades (Beckman & Frankel, 2003). Furthermore, the physical, psychological, social, cultural, spiritual, and financial needs that have been identified among cancer populations might be considered in the context of the Modeling and Remodeling (MRM) Theory (as cited in Erickson, Tomlin, & Swain, 1983), holistic philosophy, and symptom clusters (Haylock, 2010). MRM theory is built on the components of knowledge, resources, and actions (Haylock, 2010). Patient-provider relationship building and communication skills are initially learned in the classroom but do not always translate to the real-world clinical setting where time constraints and unexpected issues needing immediate attention are common. Additionally, effective communication becomes critical when particularly sensitive news needs to be relayed to the patient and loved ones. Barriers to effective communication have been identified as time constraints, lack of emphasis in training, poor modeling by senior providers, disinterest in learning how to communicate, and lack of knowledge about resources in learning such skills (Orgel, McCarter, & Jacobs, 2010). Balancing the actions while maintaining good patient rapport can be facilitated through guidance and role modeling from experienced mentors as the healthcare provider gains experience and proficiency (Beckman & Frankel, 2003).

The process of building good rapport through effective communication with patients may be healthcare provider directed but must also allow for the patient to match the provider in creating an optimal working relationship. A study by Berry, Wilke, Thomas, and Fortner (2003) unveiled unbalanced provider-patient communication when discussing pain in patients with prostate or head and neck cancer. The providers tended to dominate the conversations, at times even interrupting the patients, inhibiting patients from fully disclosing pertinent information or being able to ask questions (Berry et al., 2003). One intervention that can help improve such a communication deficit is nurse-led follow-up with patients. Using a trained nurse specialist to track and follow up with patients, with the patient also having access to contact the nurse as needed, has proven to be particularly helpful in cancer pain management and other symptom-related issues (Salander, 2010).

Understanding the importance of the provider-patient relationship and good communication skills are key for optimizing nursing care—something nurses have long intuitively recognized. A qualitative study by King, Hinds, Hassey, Schum, and Lee (2002) showed that nurses identified nurse-patient communication as one of five major themes that are essential in building patient relationships. It is through these relationships that nurses can best assess patients' quality of life (King et al., 2002).

Various communication frameworks drive practice. The Patient Reported Outcomes (PRO) model, used to assess patient satisfaction and health-related outcomes, encompasses several of these attributes. Focus is placed on the individuals involved in the communication, the relationship development process, and specific components of communication activities. These include how messages are translated from one person to another, for example, feedback and feed-forward mechanisms (Feldman-Stewart & Brundage, 2009). Additionally, the PRO model takes into account the multidimensionality of relationships and their environments (Feldman-Stewart & Brundage, 2009). In nursing practice, understanding and utilizing such tools can tremendously improve a patient's experience and well-being.

Symptom Experience

Nursing research on cancer symptom management has advanced during the last decade as the concepts that define it become more precise and their relationship to each other more refined, generating theories that better explain and describe the symptom experience phenomenon. For example, in oncology nursing research, symptom experience began with a definition that included number of symptoms, severity of symptoms, and amount of distress experienced (Armstrong, 2003; Goodell & Nail, 2005), and symptom cluster was defined as "three or more symptoms that . . . occur together and are related to each other" (Dodd, Miaskowski, & Lee, 2004, p. 77). Budin et al. (2008) described the development, testing, and utility of the Breast Cancer Treatment Response Inventory (BCTRI), an instrument that captures the symptom experience of women with breast cancer. Consistent with the definitions of Armstrong (2003) and Goodell and Nail (2005), the BCTRI is a valid and reliable tool to determine and monitor numbers of symptoms, the severity of those symptoms, and the amount of distress experienced by patients with breast cancer. Data collected using the BCTRI provide information that healthcare providers can use to target interventions toward symptoms that are most troublesome or distressful. The BCTRI can be used at meaningful points in treatment, recovery, and ongoing survivorship to explore the emerging concept of symptom experience in samples that reflect socioeconomically and ethnically diverse populations. Miaskowski, Aouizerat, Dodd, and Cooper (2007) reported that when they examined symptom experience among disease subgroups, clinical characteristics were not a predictor. Miaskowski et al. (2007) posed two conceptual models to explore the fact that genetic determinants may be a predictor of those groups of patients that are at greatest or least risk of symptom severity. Brant, Beck, and Miaskowski (2010) continued to expand the conceptual model (see Figure 4-1). The researchers suggested that further explora-

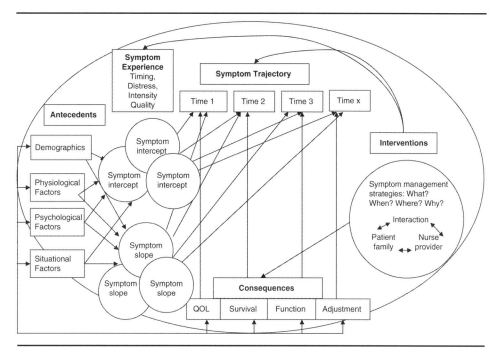

Figure 4-1. New Symptom Management Model

QOL—quality of life

Note. From "Building Dynamic Models and Theories to Advance the Science of Symptom Management Research," by J.M. Brant, S. Beck, and C. Miaskowski, 2010, *Journal of Advanced Nursing, 66*, p. 237. Copyright 2010 by John Wiley and Sons. Reprinted with permission.

tion was needed to determine whether the definition could be modified to include two or more symptoms. This is consistent with the psychology and psychiatry literature where the concept of symptom management including symptom clusters is well developed. For example, Kim, McGuire, Tulman, and Barsevick (2005) conducted a review and critique of psychology, psychiatry, general medicine, and nursing literature regarding symptom cluster research. Their findings revealed that psychology and psychiatry disciplines conducted studies to examine this concept and agreed that the number of symptoms in a cluster is not important but that the major antecedent of a symptom cluster is two or more symptoms (Kim et al., 2005). Understanding and anticipating that symptoms often occur in clusters can help in reducing the symptom experience through early interventions.

Additionally, it is important to understand underlying mechanisms that may influence the symptom experience. Hammer, Motzer, Voss, and Berry (2010) described the challenges of glycemic control in older adult hematopoietic stem cell transplant recipients. Factors including older age, history of diabetes, nutritional instability, medications such as glucocorticoids and immunosuppressants, decreased physical activity, and physiologic and psychological stress contribute to glycemic instability, which, in turn, has been found to have associations with risks for adverse outcomes including infections and mortality (Hammer et al., 2009, 2010). These factors may also contribute to symptom experiences, physiologically through inflammatory mediators (Devaraj, Venugopal, Singh, & Jialal, 2005; Mantovani, Allavena,

Sica, & Balkwill, 2008) and on other levels through the synergistic effect of coping with these instabilities and outcomes concurrently with symptoms initially induced by the malignancy and related treatments. This captures the four major points incorporated into patient care (see earlier in chapter under section "Biobehavioral and Systems Biology") including prediction (risk of glycemic instability), prevention (diet, exercise, and behavior), personalization (healthcare plan), and participation (patient partners in the healthcare plan) (Schallom et al., 2011). Understanding these relationships can help the healthcare team in symptom management through early and targeted interventions. The symptom model can serve as an underlying mechanism through which the understanding and actions can be effectively initiated.

Cultural Concerns

Patients, for the most part, are heterogeneous in nature. They enter the healthcare system coming from various backgrounds, environments, and experiences. Patients also have diverse cultural backgrounds that may vary from the predominate culture in which the healthcare facility resides. Culture also contributes to how patients receive, assimilate, and deal with health-related issues. Going through treatments for cancer can highlight such cultural differences. The diagnosis itself may be influenced by genetic determinants inherent within ethnic groups, the defining gene, and phenotype expression of the population that comprises the culture. Cultures can also be composed of populations from varying ethnic backgrounds. Being culturally competent encompasses being mindful, respectful, understanding, and, whenever possible, accommodating to the norms of the culture in which the patient lives. This can include race, gender, traditions, beliefs, customs, and values (Schim, Doorenbos, Benkert, & Miller, 2007; St. Clair & McKenry, 1999). Culture can also include sociopolitical identification such as sexual orientation and political party affiliation.

Delivering culturally competent nursing care is best described through Madeline Leininger's (2002) theory of transcultural nursing. This theory incorporates many facets of health care and culture including but not limited to the following aspects:
• Interrelationships of culture and care on well-being, health, illness, and death
• Comparative cultural care
• Holistic and multifaceted culturally based care meanings and practices
• Global cultural diversities
• Incorporation of cultural care meanings, practices, and factors influencing care by religion, politics, economics, worldview, environment, cultural values, history, language, and gender.

Leininger (2002) also noted that the "central purpose of the theory is to discover and explain diverse and universal culturally based care factors influencing health, well-being, illness, or death of individuals or groups" (p. 190). Furthermore, in order to comprehensively and effectively provide culturally competent care, the clinician must take into account the dimensions of communication, space, time, social organization, environmental controls, and biologic variations (St. Clair & McKenry, 1999).

Taking all of these factors into consideration, providing culturally competent nursing care begins with a basic understanding of the culture, including the norms and beliefs. Investigation through the literature, coworkers from the same culture, and the patient and family members themselves can provide information. Inquiring about cultural/religious dietary needs and ensuring that those needs are met during a hospital stay, for example, may be highly important to the patient (Schim et al., 2007). It is also important, however, to not stereotype cultures and be presumptive in delivering care (Kemp, 2005). To avoid such assumptions, it is extremely important for nurses to first have a solid understanding of their own cultural beliefs, values, and judgments (Maier-Lorentz, 2008). The next step is to inquire about the patient's desires regarding how he or she would prefer the care be delivered that would accomplish the goals of the care while maintaining the cultural beliefs. Points of consideration include assessing how the patient and family members view the disease and how it has impacted their lives (Kemp, 2005). This can become particularly sensitive during stages of palliative or end-of-life care. A study by Huang, Yates, and Prior (2009) evaluated nurses' perceptions and accommodations of cultural needs for patients receiving palliative care. Understanding of the individual's cultural needs came with experience, which helped to provide culturally respectful care (Huang et al., 2009). An interesting example was how patients interpret pain. From one cultural perspective, pain was a sign of life and thought of in a positive light. For another cultural perspective, pain was a result of negative behaviors in a past life (Huang et al., 2009). Taking all such considerations into account when providing care can lead to a respectful and positive experience for the patient, family members, and the healthcare team themselves.

Resilience

The essence of resilience can mean different things to different people. Resilience encompasses a dynamic perspective of individualized coping abilities in dealing with stress and adversity (Grafton, Gillespie, & Henderson, 2010). Central to the ability to cope is one's sense of an innate energy or motivating life force that is composed of a number of characteristics including coping along with adaptability, faith, hardiness, optimism, patience, self-efficacy, self-esteem, sense of humor, and tolerance (Grafton et al., 2010). In oncology, having a strong sense of resilience is extremely helpful for patients, loved ones, and even healthcare providers themselves.

Patients with cancer often display highly resilient states of being. A qualitative study evaluating resilience in patients undergoing hematopoietic stem cell transplantation revealed that hope for survival helped strengthen their courage and resilience (Coolbrandt & Grypdonck, 2010). An aid in this process was in having the patients write a positive story about their experiences. This helped them to find meaning behind the suffering that accompanied the treatment. Patients further relied on the nurses and physicians to keep them encouraged; however, the overall process of taking an active instead of passive role gave them a sense of autonomy and enhanced resilience (Coolbrandt & Grypdonck, 2010).

A resilient attitude can significantly help many other oncology populations and can be beneficial in other situations related to a cancer diagnosis. Adolescents with cancer, for example, benefit greatly from psychosocial guidance for a positive outlook (Haase, 2004). This need became so recognized that the Adolescent Resilience Model (ARM) has been established. The ARM also accounts for the various developmental phases throughout young life. Factors of the ARM include illness-related risk (uncertainty, disease and symptom distress), family protective (family atmosphere and support, resources), social protective (social integration, healthcare resources), individual risk (defensive coping), individual protective (courageous coping, derived meaning), and outcome (resilience, quality of life) (Haase, 2004).

Resilience is also an important mechanism for all age groups when facing cancer recurrence. When cancer recurs, patients can feel depressed or anxious, lose their sense of hope, and have an increased fear of death (Andersen, Shapiro, Farrar, Crespin, & Wells-Digregorio, 2005). Interestingly, one study found that patients with breast cancer recurrence were quite resilient and did not report higher levels of global distress or quality-of-life disruption; however, it did report increased levels of stress focused on the cancer itself (Andersen et al., 2005). Culture can also influence resilience. Hispanic populations have high resilience and tend to have better health outcomes compared to non-Hispanic White populations (Gallo, Penedo, Espinosa de los Monteros, & Arguelles, 2009). Even though U.S. Hispanic populations may typically have lower socioeconomic status (in some cases creating a barrier for access to good healthcare resources) compared to some non-Hispanic White counterparts with the same disease process, the Hispanic culture embraces social resources, strong family support, and religiousness during adversities, which appears to have quite a positive influence on outcomes (Gallo et al., 2009).

Within all cultures and socioeconomic levels, resilience comes from within but can clearly be enhanced by surrounding support. Autonomy is one facet that helps strengthen resilience. Oncology nurses can aid in the process of helping patients with cancer strengthen their sense of autonomy and resilience through assessing patients' initial state of being, encouraging activities such as positive story writing, and directing psychosocial services to them as needed.

Self-Help

As noted by Haylock (2010, p. 187), "Self-care actions vary according to the person's worldview, their health problem, and how they perceive potential health outcomes. Any action taken to care for oneself can be seen as a self-care action."

Promoting self-help among patients with cancer can enhance this role, and self-help can be actualized in various ways. The self-help group is one modality in which patients with cancer facilitate their own groups and use each other for a support system. Guided by nurses in the organization and fostering of relationships among group members, cancer support groups can be an invaluable tool for patients. One study showed this method to be particularly valuable for patients of varying ages who are undergoing treatments for various types of malignancies and at various stages of disease (Adamsen & Rasmussen, 2003). Of particular importance, patients identified the need to relate to others going through the same experiences—something they were unable to achieve through their family members and loved ones. Additionally, the support groups were a forum in which to learn new information and find ways through true peers of how to deal with certain situations (Adamsen & Rasmussen, 2003). Aside from the support group structure, patients can promote self-care through their daily activities. Exercise is one modality that can decrease symptom burden, enhance functional capacity, and improve overall health perceptions (Hacker, 2009).

Self-help can also come in the form of information gathering. Lazarus and Folkman's (1984) stress and coping theory poses that information is a resource that enhances coping. Many patients rely on the Internet as a resource for finding information and help. This can be challenging for individuals in lower socioeconomic situations who may not have access to computers. One innovative intervention was providing computers to low-income individuals newly diagnosed with breast cancer (Lu, Shaw, & Gustafson, 2011). Patients used the computers to contact healthcare providers for consulting with issues related to their diagnosis and treatments. The use of this tool enhanced self-efficacy, participation in health care, and provider-patient relationships (Lu et al., 2011). Encouraging self-help can enhance a patient's perception of autonomy and control over an often overwhelming situation. This form of empowerment can increase the patient experience significantly. Nurses recognizing this need can help promote such activities (Knobf & Sun, 2005).

Integrative Health Care

Unique to the science of nursing is that care encompasses the physical, psychological, social, cultural, spiritual, and financial domains. Because biobehavioral and systems biology theories and models include biologic, physical, psychological, social, cultural, spiritual, and financial needs, they provide a framework to capture how these dimensions vary throughout the cancer trajectory based on personal priorities and disease concerns. For example, during the diagnostic period, survival is a major concern, whereas in ongoing recovery, other concerns will take precedence. It is only by considering the holistic needs of the individual that the other elements can be included.

Integrative health care includes but is not limited to the use of mind-body strategies, fitness, meditation, massage/touch therapies, yoga, music, acupuncture, relaxation techniques, and homeopathy to promote well-being or treat health conditions. Results of randomized clinical trials that have examined integrative healthcare therapies collectively demonstrate these practices to be effective for physical, psychological, social, cultural, and spiritual aspects of caring (Cassileth & Gubili, 2008; Deng et al., 2009; SIO, 2009). The Consortium of Academic Health Centers for Integrative Medicine (2009) defines *integrative medicine* as "the practice of medicine that reaffirms the importance of the relationship between practitioner and patient, focuses on the whole person, is informed by evidence, and makes use of all appropriate therapeutic approaches, healthcare professionals, and disciplines to achieve optimal health and healing" (para. 5). SIO (2009) developed evidence-based practice guidelines that include risk-benefit recommendations. The role of integrative health interventions to address prevention, control, and quality of life is in its nascence in nursing research. Rigorous randomized controlled trials need to be developed and implemented using theoretical frameworks that will capture the personal and disease-related concepts that impact physical, psychological, social, spiritual, and financial outcomes.

MRM theory (proposed by Erickson et al., 1983) "offers a way to holistically approach health, wellness, and healing among cancer survivors, laying the groundwork for crafting interventions and services for various populations" (Haylock, 2010, p. 185). Mullen's model of survivorship is comprised of distinct stages that can be linked to MRM Theory's basic assumptions. "MRM is a theory that can encompass the complex and intertwining dimensions associated with the processes of living with advanced cancer" (Haylock, 2010, p. 186).

Survivorship

The National Coalition for Cancer Survivorship (NCCS, n.d.) regards patients with cancer as survivors from the moment of diagnosis, as they are in the present moment living with the malignancy. Survivorship, however, is sometimes thought of within the context of post-treatment remission, such as with bone marrow transplantation (National Marrow Donor Program [NMDP], 2011). Post-treatment survivorship includes a focus on disease-specific concerns (continuous follow-up evaluations to screen for cancer recurrence or new onset of malignancy), as well as long-term symptom management and life considerations (e.g., fertility issues, nutritional considerations) (Gage et al., 2011). Patients who survive five or more years are considered long-term survivors and can experience a number of physical and psychosocial issues, including continued symptoms, psychological distress, challenges with sexual intimacy, social relationship problems, financial difficulties, and an overall decreased quality of life compared to their prediagnosis life (Foster, Wright, Hill, Hopkinson, & Roffe, 2009). Various other factors can also influence the cancer survivor's quality of life. A study that evaluated survivors of breast cancer found that the current state of the medical condition, social support, and income level were positively associated with quality of life (Mols, Vingerhoets, Coebergh, & van de Poll-Franse, 2005).

Long-term survivorship is also very common among children who encounter cancers. Lund, Schmiegelow, Rechnitzer, and Johansen (2011) evaluated psychosocial late effects in childhood cancer and found that patients rated their health-related quality of life equal to or better than sibling or population controls. Certain factors were also predictors of increased psychosocial issues, including central nervous system tumors, cranial radiation therapy, female gender, and younger age at diagnosis (Lund et al., 2011).

A number of theories can be incorporated into the survivorship state, which in the best of circumstances will remain throughout a fully realized life trajectory. With the encouragement of healthcare providers, many adult survivors of cancer will have the incentive to live an overall healthier lifestyle than the one they may have lived prior to their cancer diagnosis. This may include better nutrition, exercise, reduction of alcohol consumption, and smoking cessation. The Transtheoretical Model can aid in the adaptation and adherence to such behavioral changes (Pinto & Floyd, 2008). In addition to behavioral changes, patients and their loved ones go through stages of change and ultimately adapt to living with the history of cancer and constant possibility of recurrence. Motivational interviewing as a technique and the social learning and social cognitive theories can aid in this process (Pinto & Floyd, 2008). The social cognitive theory also can aid in making behavior changes with emphasis placed on setting realistic goals and expectations to make the goals more obtainable with sustained success (Pinto & Floyd, 2008). Cognitive-behavioral theory (CBT) and the Roy Adaptation Model have also been used in survivorship with success (Pinto & Floyd, 2008). CBT assumes an interconnection among thoughts, feelings, and behaviors. CBT interventions can include components to enhance education about the behavior, establish goals, self-monitor, analyze behaviors, and enhance coping and social skills to alter underlying negative emotions that may be driving undesirable behaviors (Pinto & Floyd, 2008). The Roy Adaptation Model focuses on adapting to the altered environment through physiologic and psychological perspectives (Pinto & Floyd, 2008). Adding to this armament of theories guiding change, the social scientist Everett Rogers' Diffusion of Innovations Theoretical Model incorporates the domains of innovation, adoption, communication, and social relationships (Dooks, 2001; Rogers, 2004). Although this model has evolved since its inception in the early 1950s, the underlying premise of how innovation diffuses through communication channels into a social system has remained (Rogers, 2004). In the context of adapting to a lifestyle change in cancer survivorship, the innovation may be thought of as an individual's new desire to make the change required to lead a healthier lifestyle. Communication and social relationships in support of this change, in this example, would come from the healthcare team and family caregivers.

Nurses working with patients who have entered the survival state can apply these theories in encouraging and aiding patients to adapt to their new life (Ferrell, Virani, Smith, & Juarez, 2003). Because each patient's cancer experience can differ both physiologically and psychologically, consideration of individualized needs is essential. Much attention is now being focused on the survivorship phase of cancer. The growing number of guidelines and other evidence-based resources that address survivorship coupled with research that includes the patients and family members' report of symptoms, associated distress, and impact on the physical, psychological, social, spiritual, cultural, and financial aspects of care (ASCO, 2005–2011; NCCN, 2011; ONS, n.d.; SIO, 2009) will help to refine important research questions and hypotheses. Careful review and selection of the quality-of-life–associated guidelines that these organizations have published as well as the aforementioned theories and numerous others will guide this research and ensure that important concepts are considered.

Uncertainty in Illness

Mishel's Model of Uncertainty in Illness encompasses the art of mastery over uncertainty and an adverse situation as being either a danger or an opportunity (Mishel, Padilla, Grant, & Sorenson, 1991). Mastery, in this context, refers to the belief of being able to alleviate or transcend the impact of an adverse event and uncertainty within the context of it having the quality of vagueness. It is the vagueness within uncertainty that mastery can overcome in evaluating a situation and determining if it is a danger or opportunity (Mishel et al., 1991). Within the context of illness, uncertainty has a psychological impact that can influence outcomes (Wallace Kazer, Bailey, & Whittemore, 2010).

The Uncertainty in Illness model has been used in oncology nursing for patients of all ages with various malignancies and in various phases of the cancer experience. Stewart, Mishel, Lynn, and Terhorst (2010) applied this model to children and adolescents with cancer and found that uncertainty about the disease and long-term survival was associated with psychological distress, notably anxiety and depression. The Uncertainty model was also used in a study evaluating parental uncertainty in Taiwanese children with cancer. Personal growth through coping strategies was achieved; however, a negative influence was also seen within the context of family interactions (Lin, Yeh, & Mishel, 2010).

The Uncertainty model has also been adapted as an intervention for the management of patients with breast and prostate cancers by creating a cognitive schema about the uncertainty and then using it as a tool for finding ways to take control over areas that initially appear without control (Wallace Kazer et al., 2010). Mishel et al. (2009) applied this tool to men with prostate cancer during their treatment decision-making process. Uncertainty areas that showed improvement in both Caucasian and African American men included knowledge about the cancer, problem-solving ability, communication (both provider-patient communication and medical communication competence), informational resources, and decisional regret (Mishel et al., 2009). Similarly, a study in Caucasian and African American older women who were long-term survivors of breast cancer found this tool useful within the context of uncertainty management and also found improvements in the areas of knowledge and communication (Mishel et al., 2005). Additionally, this study revealed improvements in cognitive reframing and coping mechanisms when the uncertainty intervention was applied in this cohort of older adult long-term survivors of breast cancer (Mishel et al., 2005).

Oncology nurses can use the Uncertainty in Illness model as a point of understanding the psychological distress that uncertainty brings to patients with cancer. Furthermore, they can incorporate the instrument to help patients find areas of control, thus decreasing the level of distress the uncertainty causes. This model can be used throughout all phases of the cancer experience and can aid the family/caregiver as well.

Rogers' Science of Unitary Human Beings

Perhaps one of the more functional, yet often viewed as esoteric, theories underlying nursing practice is Martha Rogers' Science of Unitary Human Beings (SUHB). The SUHB can be used as an overarching theory in all aspects of the cancer experience. From the viewpoint of both humans and the environment existing as energy fields, each is both unitary and integrated with the other, thus creating the universe as a whole (Phillips, 2010). Furthermore, energy fields are defined by their patterns or characteristics that distinguish them. It is the fluid interaction of the human and environmental energy fields that can lead to a pattern alteration, and indeed, patterns change continuously (Barrett, 1988; Phillips, 2010), thus emphasizing the dynamic nature of life and the environment in which we live.

Applying the SUHB theory to patient care can be actualized in any number of ways. In patients with cancer, for example, the patients' values and beliefs about their disease manifests as their energy pattern (Wall, 2000). Additionally, the power of understanding contributes to the process of being able to change this pattern. Using Rogers' theory, Barrett (1988) created the Power as Knowing Participation in Change Tool to assist with this process. This tool is a questionnaire designed to help assess patients' states of being and understanding, which can further help guide them in their health-related decision-making processes (Barrett, 1988). Additionally, the SUHB theory promotes health and well-being at all stages of health and disease. Wall (2000) used Rogers' SUHB theory to evaluate hope and power changes in patients with lung cancer who exercised. Those who exercised increased their perception of power, although not their hope. The change in power through exercise is viewed as a pattern change (Wall, 2000). In another study, Rogers' SUHB theory was incorporated as part of the underlying mechanism for improving symptoms in patients with cancer through the use of massage therapy (Smith, Kemp, Hemphill, & Vojir, 2002). Pain, sleep quality, symptom distress, and anxiety improved in patients who received massage compared to the control group who received standard care without massage (Smith et al., 2002), thus supporting meaningful pattern changes. Understanding patients' inner power in relation to the environment is a strong tool for maximizing quality of life and overall well-being. Additionally, understanding how these energy fields are dynamic in nature can guide oncology nurses in helping patients to adapt to these changes over the course of the cancer experience as fluctuations occur throughout the health-illness continuum.

Phases of the Cancer Experience

The cancer experience includes the following phases: screening, diagnosis, treatment, immediate recovery, ongoing recovery and survivorship, and end-of-life care.

Treatment intention is conceptualized as curative, control, or palliation (NCCN, 2011). In this section and in Figure 4-2, we discuss each phase as an isolated occurrence; however, these phases overlap and blend into one another. In fact, some may occur concurrently, and the order in which they occur may vary from how we will discuss them. Concerns and needs continue to fluctuate based on the phase of the diagnosis and individualized patient and family priorities and needs.

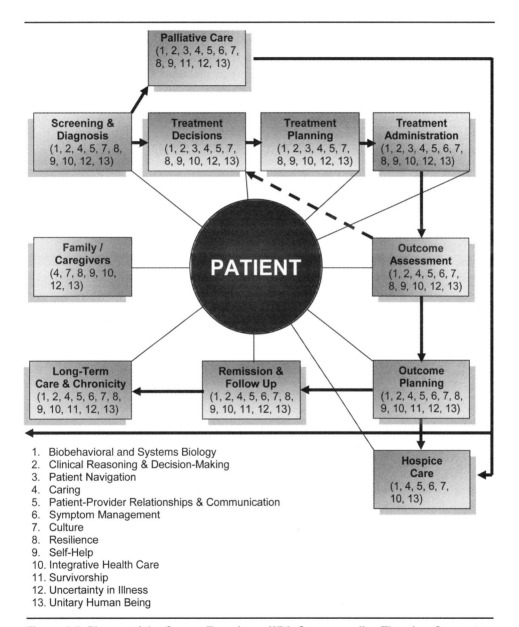

1. Biobehavioral and Systems Biology
2. Clinical Reasoning & Decision-Making
3. Patient Navigation
4. Caring
5. Patient-Provider Relationships & Communication
6. Symptom Management
7. Culture
8. Resilience
9. Self-Help
10. Integrative Health Care
11. Survivorship
12. Uncertainty in Illness
13. Unitary Human Being

Figure 4-2. Phases of the Cancer Experience With Corresponding Theories, Concepts, and Models Driving Nursing Practice

Note how palliative care surrounds all phases of the cancer experience.

Screening and Diagnosis

The moment of cancer diagnosis can often be met with extreme fear, anxiety, disbelief, anger, and myriad other emotions. Often symptoms precede the diagnosis, and the process of examinations, tests, and evaluations can be just as frightening. Uncertainty and anxiety can be tremendous and even higher during the diagnostic period than once a diagnosis of cancer is made (Liao, Chen, Chen, & Chen, 2008). In the prediagnosis phase, however, the patient has the underlying element of hope that the symptoms mean something other than cancer, that the resolution of the underlying problem is a simple one, and that this period is just a hiccup of uncertainty along life's path and that life will resume as "normal" in a relatively short time. In other cases, the patient experiences few or no symptoms, and the cancer is diagnosed through routine screening or as an incidental finding when dealing with another health issue. Whatever precedes it, the cancer diagnosis can replace hope with despair. More frequently, though, cancer can now be considered a chronic condition and one in which the individual can live out a full life. However, the life that will be lived will never be the same because a cancer diagnosis is life changing.

Throughout the diagnostic phase, many theories, models, and concepts can be applied to help the patient through this anxiety-inducing process. Rogers' SUHB can be applied at any phase and certainly merits application during this time. Biobehavioral and systems biology are driving forces for the actual physiologic underpinning. Clinical reasoning and decision making come into play in terms of directing diagnostic tests based on patient presentation. Similar to the SUHB, caring cannot be overemphasized or absent in any phase. This is also a key point at which patient-provider relationships can begin to be established with strong emphasis on communication. Culture, resilience, self-help, and mind-body are also important considerations. Overall, the diagnostic phase of the cancer diagnosis is the springboard to a life-changing event should the diagnosis be positive. Nurses who provide understanding and empathy can aid patients through this process tremendously.

Treatment Decisions, Planning, and Administration

Once the cancer diagnosis is confirmed, treatment decisions need to be made, followed by planning and treatment administration. Treatment decisions are not exclusively at the discretion of the oncologist. Ultimately, the patient makes treatment decisions based on weighing the factors of prognosis, survivability, treatment involvement, treatment-related symptoms, and quality of life with the guidance of the healthcare team. The degree of involvement can vary, and some patients prefer to leave all decision making to the healthcare provider. Hubbard, Kidd, and Donaghy (2008) found that a majority of patients prefer a collaborative role with their healthcare provider in treatment decision making with the minority preferring either a passive role in letting the provider make the full decisions or the patient making the decision in the absence of the provider recommendation. Some diagnoses do not have exact treatment guidelines; therefore, treatment recommendations cannot always be clearly defined. In patients with prostate cancer, for example, different therapies can have the same prognostic outcome, but the side effects vary and must be weighed by the patient. The oncologist can evaluate the tumor characteristics, state of patient health at the time of diagnosis, and prognosis and make recommendations based on those parameters; however, the patient's health-related quality of life needs to be considered before making the decision about the therapeutic approach to use (Singh, Trabulsi, & Gomella, 2010). This type of individualized care can support patient autonomy and give a sense of control. Individualized care is especially imperative when patients are in advanced stages of cancer (Peppercorn et al., 2011). Optimizing quality of life for the patient at whatever level can be achieved is paramount.

Once the decision on treatment has been established, the planning phase begins. The healthcare team will coordinate delivery of the therapy and related activities while the patient must start to plan life around the impending treatment schedule. Additionally, once treatment begins, life can further change when symptoms present. Even with the best planning, unanticipated events can occur. During these phases of treatment decisions, planning, and administration, as in other phases, many theories, concepts, and models can drive nursing practice as shown in Table 4-1 and Figure 4-2. Through each of these phases, the nurse is an essential support system and advocate who can also play a pivotal role in helping the patient reach an informed decision. The nurse is also the primary provider who delivers treatments and assesses the patient's tolerance to the treatment and side effects. Working with patients through this process requires a solid driving force of the theories for the most successful patient experience.

Outcome Planning

Treatment completion is a time for celebration concurrently with new fears and anxiety. Celebration is often accompanied by fear and anxiety about the treatment's success. Once a patient is in remission, discharge planning, including follow-up, continuation of or new post-treatment medication plans, and return to life, can be daunting. Often patients will be able to continue their lives with minimal disruptions. In other cases, hospitalization removes patients completely from their home life for periods of time. In both situations, separation anxiety from the healthcare team can ensue.

When post-treatment evaluation reveals that the cancer has not been fully eradicated, treatment decisions have to be made again. If the choice is made for active treatment, the cycle of treatment planning through outcome assessment begins again. If the prognosis is not good, discussions about palliative and hospice care may be warranted. In either situation, understanding and support from the healthcare team are essential. The theories, concepts, and models that underlie this support are shown in Table 4-1.

Remission, Follow-Up, Long-Term Care, and Chronicity

Entering remission is an exciting time in the life of someone who has been going through the cancer experience. Many new challenges can present themselves, however, as patients (and their loved ones) try to reenter a new form of "normalized" life. Physiologic and psychological challenges can persist long after the treatments end (Recklitis, Sanchez-Varela, & Bober, 2008; Royer, Phelan, & Heidrich, 2009). Additionally, reentering routines, such as returning to work, can be difficult and stressful and necessitates a supportive and understanding environment from employers—something that is not always in place (Tighe, Molassiotis, Morris, & Richardson, 2011).

Patients who survive five years or more are considered long-term survivors (Foster et al., 2009), and indeed, cancer can now be thought of as a chronic condition because patients with cancer are living longer, many fully living out their lives (Ber-linger & Gusmano, 2011; Lage & Crombet, 2011). Even in situations where can-cers cannot be cured, they can often be treated or managed over long periods of time (Berlinger & Gusmano, 2011). Furthermore, patients with advanced cancers can also live longer because of multiple, sequential treatment regimens through the advent of advanced therapies, including antibodies and cancer vaccines (Lage & Crombet, 2011).

Along with living longer with cancer or in remission from cancer are comorbidities that are common in aging (Lage & Crombet, 2011) and prolonged symptoms from the cancer and treatment experience. Symptoms can persist for many years into re-mission. Aside from ongoing worry and fear, chronic physical symptoms can be ex-tremely burdensome. Royer et al. (2009) reported on the perspective of symptoms among older women who survived breast cancer. The women in this sample report-ed that their symptoms were constant, unresolvable, and not easily managed (Royer et al., 2009). Patients also have an ongoing fear of cancer recurrence, and indeed, this is something evaluated for during their ongoing follow-up visits. Nursing care can provide tremendous support for the patient with a history of cancer. Among the many theories that can drive nursing practice at this stage, caring and symptom man-agement may be paramount for many patients.

Palliative Care and Hospice Care

When a patient reaches a terminal illness stage where aggressive treatment is no longer an option, hospice care can provide extensive comfort measures. Palliative care fits within this domain of comfort care but is not exclusive to end-of-life care. The pa-rameters of palliative care have shifted from an end-of-life focus to one that includes all time points (Ferris et al., 2009). Otis-Green et al. (2009) described the "transdisci-plinary model" in providing palliative care education that will address patient and fam-ily needs and concerns across the phases of the diagnosis and treatment. Ferrell and Virani (2008) provided a comprehensive overview of national guidelines for palliative care and the role of the nurse in incorporating them. Through this seminal work on palliative care at the City of Hope, many institutions have adopted the process of pro-viding this new paradigm in palliative care for their patients (Ferrell, Virani, Malloy, & Kelly, 2010). The Pain and Supportive Care Program, a palliative care program at the Joan Karnell Cancer Center at Pennsylvania Hospital, for example, enrolls some patients from the time of early diagnosis (Granda-Cameron, Viola, Lynch, & Poloma-no, 2008). Emphasizing the expansion of palliative care, ASCO defined palliative care as "the integration into cancer care of therapies that address the multiple issues that cause suffering for patients and their families and impact their life quality" (Ferris et al., 2009, p. 3052). The World Health Organization has an even broader view of palli-ative care that includes the "physical, psychosocial, and spiritual problems of patients with life-threatening illness and of their families" (Borasio, 2011, p. 1).

Hospice care is reserved for those who will not increase survival through fur-ther cancer treatments. The decision to transition into hospice care can be a difficult one, filled with new levels of fear and anxiety. The element of hope is redefined with end-of-life priorities identified and addressed including ex-istential concerns. At this stage, the focus shifts completely to comfort mea-sures. Quality of life also becomes redefined, although it certainly can be op-timized at a new level of meaning. To facilitate the need, understanding, and implementation of both palliative and hospice care in earlier stages than they are often initiated, ASCO, in collaboration with the National Cancer Institute, created the Education in Palliative and End-of-Life Care for Oncology (EPEC-Oncology) curriculum (Ferris et al., 2009).

Palliative care can encompass all theories and models discussed in this chapter. Underlying theories, concepts, and models that highly support the end-of-life component include SUHB, Biobehavioral and Systems Biology, Caring, Patient-Provider Relationships and Communication, Symptom Experience, Culture, and Mind-Body. In addition, Lazarus and Folkman's Theory of Stress and Coping can be applied for both patients and family caregivers when dealing with advanced cancer (Thomsen, Rydahl-Hansen, & Wagner, 2010). Thomsen et al. (2010) showed that at stages of advanced cancer the areas of meaning, support systems, minimizing the impact of cancer, physical and mental function, control, uncertainty, and emotions were of most importance to the patients. The stress and coping theory incorporating the processes of stress, appraisal, and coping ties together stressful factors (in this example, advanced cancer/poor prognosis), the environment, and coping mechanisms (Thomsen et al., 2010). Having an understanding of the processes that patients and family members go through and what their individualized needs are can guide oncology nurses in coordinating activities and services that will best meet these needs. In this context, patients can live out the remainder of the lives not only in comfort, but also with a sense of self, autonomy, and completion. Such an atmosphere will also support the family caregivers as they cope with the impending loss.

Family Caregiver Experiences

Although the focus of cancer is usually on the patient, the family caregivers of the patient undergo tremendous life alterations themselves. They can easily lose their own sense of self-care with focusing attention on and providing service to the patient. Family caregivers can even feel a sense of guilt if they do things for themselves while their loved ones are going through the cancer process. Added stress can be incurred from family financial burdens due to the illness in addition to overall life disruption. Dovetailing family stress from dealing with their loved one's illness is family members' own potential increased risk for cancer because of genetic predisposition (Mai et al., 2011). For example, individuals with a family history of breast or ovarian cancer who have *BRCA1* and *BRCA2* mutations are at high risk for the malignancies themselves (De Leeneer et al., 2011); therefore, it is imperative for family members to know of this familial predisposition, be proactive with regular screenings, and ensure their healthcare providers know of the history.

The healthcare community has recognized and acknowledged the role of family caregivers as a vital part of the experience for individuals with cancer in addition to the extreme stress placed on them compounded by their potential own increased risk of cancer. Rabow, Hauser, and Adams (2004) identified family caregiver burdens as time and logistics, physical tasks, financial costs, emotional burdens and mental health risks, and physical health risks. Healthcare provider support for family caregivers, particularly during end-of-life care, was noted to include promoting communication, advanced care planning and decision making, homecare support, empathy, and grief and bereavement (Ferris et al., 2009). Honea et al. (2008) conducted a review and synthesis of the literature that examines interventions to target caregiver strain and burden and concluded that supportive strategies to reduce caregiver strain and burden are scarce. Oncology nurses in particular can be a tremendous support system for family caregivers with an emphasis on establishing relationships with family caregivers and actively working with them to address issues (McLeod, Tapp, Moules, & Campbell, 2010). Underlying theories, models, and concepts supporting family caregiver care include SUHB, Caring, Culture, Resilience, Self-Help, Mind-Body, and Survivorship.

Conclusion

Concepts, theories, and models are essential components that drive oncology nursing practice. Through the many complex facets of care from a cancer diagnosis through long-term survival or imminent death, the oncology nurse is at the heart of patient care and family caregiver support. This chapter highlighted a number of selected concepts, theories, and models that can act as a foundation for oncology nursing practice. It is also prudent to note that as nursing has an autonomous quality, nurses may gravitate toward some theories more than others, and indeed many can be incorporated into various aspects of care beyond how they are outlined in this chapter.

As the platform on which nursing practice, health care, and research are based, these concepts, theories, and models serve to guide and direct our decisions from acute to long-term care. Particularly in oncology nursing practice with the many complexities that are threaded throughout the various stages and phases of care and where partnering with the patient and family is integral in all aspects of care, this platform cannot be overemphasized.

To recap, theories are built on concepts or the formation of ideas that developed from certain observations. Theories add meaning to scientific findings and are used to develop operational definitions that, in turn, are used for the development and refinement of research, education, and practice. Making this tangible, a model illustrates the related concepts that describe a specific theory, clarifying the symbolic representation. Hypotheses, in turn, can test and refine the theory or question that is based on the theory and concepts. For example, in oncology nursing practice, caring is an underlying theory based on the concept that patients and family caregivers have a need to be care for; this is illustrated through the caring model, which details the various components of the theory. In practice this would translate to the oncology nurse having an in-depth understanding and empathy with patients and their family caregivers throughout the cancer experience. Caring would include such attributes as listening to patients' needs and concerns, advocating for the best care while respecting patients' needs, and working toward optimizing quality of life, for example. Practice also guides the development of theory as we continually learn from our patients, creating new concepts that can turn into theories. We can create and test hypotheses about new theories and illustrate the process through visual models that then, in turn, can be used to drive practice. Through this process, key variables are tested that oncology nurses can be sensitive to in practice. This continuous and reciprocal process enhances patient care. Whether we are caught up in the moment of an acute event or planning long-term care for patients with cancer, concepts, theories, and models are essential to the process.

References

Adamsen, L., & Rasmussen, J.M. (2003). Exploring and encouraging through social interaction: A qualitative study of nurses' participation in self-help groups for cancer patients. *Cancer Nursing, 26,* 28–36. doi:10.1097/00002820-200302000-00004

Al-Majid, S., & Gray, D.P. (2009). A biobehavioral model for the study of exercise interventions in cancer-related fatigue. *Biological Research for Nursing, 10,* 381–391. doi:10.1177/1099800408324431

American Heart Association. (2012). Statistical fact sheet 2012 update: Smoking and cardiovascular disease. Retrieved from http://www.heart.org/idc/groups/heart-public/@wcm/@sop/@smd/documents/downloadable/ucm_319590.pdf

American Society of Clinical Oncology. (2005–2011). Clinical practice guidelines. Retrieved from http://www.asco.org/ascov2/Practice+&+Guidelines/Clincal+Practice+Guidelines

Andersen, B.L., Shapiro, C.L., Farrar, W.B., Crespin, T., & Wells-Digregorio, S. (2005). Psychological responses to cancer recurrence. *Cancer, 104,* 1540–1547. doi:10.1002/cncr.21309

Armstrong, T.S. (2003). Symptoms experience: A concept analysis. *Oncology Nursing Forum, 30,* 601–606. doi:10.1188/03.ONF.601-606

Barrett, E.A. (1988). Using Rogers' science of unitary human beings in nursing practice. *Nursing Science Quarterly, 1*(2), 50–51. doi:10.1177/089431848800100204

Bassett, C. (2002). Nurses' perceptions of care and caring. *International Journal of Nursing Practice, 8,* 8–15. doi:10.1046/j.1440-172x.2002.00325.x

Beckman, H.B., & Frankel, R.M. (2003). Training practitioners to communicate effectively in cancer care: It is the relationship that counts. *Patient Education and Counseling, 50,* 85–89. doi:10.1016/S0738-3991(03)00086-7

Bergner, S. (2011). Seductive symbolism: Psychoanalysis in the context of oncology. *Psychoanalytic Psychology, 28,* 267–292. doi:10.1037/a0021076

Berlinger, N., & Gusmano, M. (2011). Cancer chronicity: New research and policy challenges. *Journal of Health Services Research and Policy, 16,* 121–123. doi:10.1258/jhsrp.2010.010126

Berry, D.L., Wilkie, D.J., Thomas, C.R., Jr., & Fortner, P. (2003). Clinicians communicating with patients experiencing cancer pain. *Cancer Investigation, 21,* 374–381. doi:10.1081/CNV-120018228

Borasio, G.D. (2011). Translating the World Health Organization definition of palliative care into scientific practice. *Palliative and Supportive Care, 9,* 1–2. doi:10.1017/S1478951510000489

Brant, J.M., Beck, S., & Miaskowski, C. (2010). Building dynamic models and theories to advance the science of symptom management research. *Journal of Advanced Nursing, 66,* 228–240. doi:10.1111/j.1365-2648.2009.05179.x

Budin, W., Cartwright-Alcarese, F., & Hoskins, C. (2008). The breast cancer treatment response inventory: Development, psychometric testing, and refinement for use in clinical practice and research. *Oncology Nursing Forum, 35,* 209–215. doi:10.1188/08.ONF.209-215

Budin, W., Hoskins, C.N., Haber, J., Sherman, D.W., Maislin, G., Cater, J.R., ... Shukla, S. (2008). Breast cancer: Psycho-education, counseling, and adjustment among patients and partners—A randomized controlled trial. *Nursing Research, 57,* 199–213. doi:10.1097/01.NNR.0000319496.67369.37

Cassileth, B., & Gubili, J. (2008). The integrative medicine service at Memorial Sloan-Kettering Cancer Center. In L. Cohen & M. Markman (Eds.), *Integrative oncology: Incorporating complementary medicine into conventional cancer care.* Totowa, NJ: Humana Press.

Chin, P.L., & Jacobs, M.K. (1997). A model for theory development in nursing. In L.H. Nicoll (Ed.), *Perspectives on nursing theory* (3rd ed., pp. 452–460). Philadelphia, PA: Lippincott Williams & Wilkins.

Cohen, S., Janicki-Deverts, D., & Miller, G.E. (2007). Psychological stress and disease. *JAMA, 298,* 1685–1687. doi:10.1001/jama.298.14.1685

Consortium of Academic Health Centers for Integrative Medicine. (2009, November). About us. Retrieved from http://www.imconsortium.org/about/home.html

Coolbrandt, A., & Grypdonck, M.H. (2010). Keeping courage during stem cell transplantation: A qualitative research. *European Journal of Oncology Nursing, 14,* 218–223. doi:10.1016/j.ejon.2010.01.001

De Leeneer, K., Coene, I., Crombez, B., Simkens, J., Van den Broecke, R., Bols, A., ... Claes, K. (2011). Prevalence of BRCA1/2 mutations in sporadic breast/ovarian cancer patients and identification of a novel de novo BRCA1 mutation in a patient diagnosed with late onset breast and ovarian cancer: Implications for genetic testing. *Breast Cancer Research and Treatment, 7,* 7. doi:10.1007/s10549-011-1544-9

Deng, G.E., Frenkel, M., Cohen, L., Cassileth, B.R., Abrams, D.I., Capodice, J.L., … Sagar, S. (2009). Evidence-based clinical practice guidelines for integrative oncology: Complementary therapies and botanicals. *Journal of the Society for Integrative Oncology, 7,* 85–120. doi:10.2310/7200.2009 .0019

Devaraj, S., Venugopal, S.K., Singh, U., & Jialal, I. (2005). Hyperglycemia induces monocytic release of interleukin-6 via induction of protein kinase c-{alpha} and -{beta}. *Diabetes, 54,* 85–91. doi:10.2337/diabetes.54.1.85

Dodd, M.J., Miaskowski, C., & Lee, K.A. (2004). Occurrence of symptom clusters. *Journal of the National Cancer Institute Monographs, 2004*(32), 76–78. doi:10.1093/jncimonographs/lgh008

Dooks, P. (2001). Diffusion of pain management research into nursing practice. *Cancer Nursing, 24,* 99–103. doi:10.1097/00002820-200104000-00004

Dulock, H.L., & Holzemer, W.L. (1991). Substruction: Improving the linkage from theory to method. *Nursing Science Quarterly, 4*(2), 83–87. doi:10.1177/089431849100400209

Erickson, H.C., Tomlin, E.M., & Swain, M.A. (1983). *Modeling and role modeling: A theory and paradigm for nurses.* Upper Saddle River, NJ: Prentice-Hall.

Feldman-Stewart, D., & Brundage, M.D. (2009). A conceptual framework for patient-provider communication: A tool in the PRO research tool box. *Quality of Life Research, 18,* 109–114. doi:10.1007/s11136-008-9417-3

Ferrell, B.R., & Virani, R. (2008). National guidelines for palliative care: A roadmap for oncology nurses. *Oncology, 22*(2, Suppl. Nurse Ed.), 28–24.

Ferrell, B., Virani, R., Malloy, P., & Kelly, K. (2010). The preparation of oncology nurses in palliative care. *Seminars in Oncology Nursing, 26,* 259–265. doi:10.1016/j.soncn.2010.08.001

Ferrell, B.R., Virani, R., Smith, S., & Juarez, G. (2003). The role of oncology nursing to ensure quality care for cancer survivors: A report commissioned by the National Cancer Policy Board and Institute of Medicine [Online exclusive]. *Oncology Nursing Forum, 30,* E1–E11. doi:10.1188/03.ONF.E1-E11

Ferris, F.D., Bruera, E., Cherny, N., Cummings, C., Currow, D., Dudgeon, D., … Von Roenn, J.H. (2009). Palliative cancer care a decade later: Accomplishments, the need, next steps—From the American Society of Clinical Oncology. *Journal of Clinical Oncology, 27,* 3052–3058. doi:10.1200/ JCO.2008.20.1558

Foster, C., Wright, D., Hill, H., Hopkinson, J., & Roffe, L. (2009). Psychosocial implications of living 5 years or more following a cancer diagnosis: A systematic review of the research evidence. *European Journal of Cancer Care, 18,* 223–247. doi:10.1111/j.1365-2354.2008.01001.x

Founds, S.A. (2009). Introducing systems biology for nursing science. *Biological Research for Nursing, 11,* 73–80. doi:10.1177/1099800409331893

Gage, E.A., Pailler, M., Zevon, M.A., Ch'ng, J., Groman, A., Kelly, M., … Gruber, M. (2011). Structuring survivorship care: Discipline-specific clinician perspectives. *Journal of Cancer Survivorship: Research and Practice, 11,* 217–225. doi:10.1007/s11764-011-0174-x

Gallo, L.C., Penedo, F.J., Espinosa de los Monteros, K., & Arguelles, W. (2009). Resiliency in the face of disadvantage: Do Hispanic cultural characteristics protect health outcomes? *Journal of Personality, 77,* 1707–1746. doi:10.1111/j.1467-6494.2009.00598.x

Gaut, D.A. (1983). Development of a theoretically adequate description of caring. *Western Journal of Nursing Research, 5,* 313–324. doi:10.1177/019394598300500405

Godbout, J.P., & Glaser, R. (2006). Stress-induced immune dysregulation: Implications for wound healing, infectious disease and cancer. *Journal of Neuroimmune Pharmacology, 1,* 421–427. doi:10.1007/s11481-006-9036-0

Goodell, T.T., & Nail, L.M. (2005). Operationalizing symptom distress in adults with cancer: A literature synthesis [Online exclusive]. *Oncology Nursing Forum, 32,* E42–E47. doi:10.1188/05.ONF.E42-E47

Grafton, E., Gillespie, B., & Henderson, S. (2010). Resilience: The power within. *Oncology Nursing Forum, 37,* 698–705. doi:10.1188/10.ONF.698-705

Granda-Cameron, C., Viola, S.R., Lynch, M.P., & Polomano, R.C. (2008). Measuring patient-oriented outcomes in palliative care: Functionality and quality of life. *Clinical Journal of Oncology Nursing, 12,* 65–77. doi:10.1188/08.CJON.65-77

Gullatte, M. (2006). The influence of spirituality and religiosity on breast cancer screening delay in African American women: Application of the Theory of Reasoned Action and Planned Behavior (TRA/TPB). *ABNF Journal, 17,* 89–94.

Haase, J.E. (2004). The adolescent resilience model as a guide to interventions. *Journal of Pediatric Oncology Nursing, 21,* 289–299. doi:10.1177/1043454204267922

Hacker, E. (2009). Exercise and quality of life: Strengthening the connections. *Clinical Journal of Oncology Nursing, 13,* 31–39. doi:10.1188/09.CJON.31-39

Hammer, M.J., Casper, C., Gooley, T.A., O'Donnell, P.V., Boeckh, M., & Hirsch, I.B. (2009). The contribution of malglycemia to mortality among allogeneic hematopoietic cell transplant recipients. *Biology of Blood and Marrow Transplantation, 15,* 344–351. doi:10.1016/j.bbmt.2008.12.488

Hammer, M.J., Motzer, S.A., Voss, J.G., & Berry, D.L. (2010). Glycemic control among older adult hematopoietic cell transplant recipients. *Journal of Gerontological Nursing, 36,* 40–50. doi:10.3928/00989134-20091207-99

Haylock, P.J. (2010). Advanced cancer: A mind-body-spirit approach to life and living. *Seminars in Oncology Nursing, 26,* 183–194. doi:10.1016/j.soncn.2010.05.005

Hochedlinger, K., & Plath, K. (2009). Epigenetic reprogramming and induced pluripotency. *Development, 136,* 509–523. doi:10.1242/dev.020867

Honea, N.J., Brintnall, R., Given, B., Sherwood, P., Colao, D.B., Somers, S.C., & Northouse, L.L. (2008). Putting evidence into practice: Nursing assessment and interventions to reduce family caregiver strain and burden. *Clinical Journal of Oncology Nursing, 12,* 507–516. doi:10.1188/08.CJON.507-516

Hoskins, C.N. (1998). *Developing research in nursing and health: Quantitative and qualitative methods.* New York, NY: Springer.

Huang, Y.L., Yates, P., & Prior, D. (2009). Factors influencing oncology nurses' approaches to accommodating cultural needs in palliative care. *Journal of Clinical Nursing, 18,* 3421–3429. doi:10.1111/j.1365-2702.2009.02938.x

Hubbard, G., Kidd, L., & Donaghy, E. (2008). Preferences for involvement in treatment decision making of patients with cancer: A review of the literature. *European Journal of Oncology Nursing, 12,* 299–318. doi:10.1016/j.ejon.2008.03.004

Kemp, C. (2005). Cultural issues in palliative care. *Seminars in Oncology Nursing, 21,* 44–52. doi:10.1053/j.soncn.2004.10.007

Khalil, I.G., & Hill, C. (2005). Systems biology for cancer. *Current Opinion in Oncology, 17,* 44–48. doi:10.1097/01.cco.0000150951.38222.16

Kim, H.J., McGuire, D.B., Tulman, L., & Barsevick, A.M. (2005). Symptom clusters: Concept analysis and clinical implications for cancer nursing. *Cancer Nursing, 28,* 270–282.

King, C.R., Hinds, P., Dow, K.H., Schum, L., & Lee, C. (2002). The nurse's relationship-based perceptions of patient quality of life. *Oncology Nursing Forum, 29,* E118–E126. doi:10.1188/02.ONF.E118-E126.

Knobf, T., & Sun, Y. (2005). A longitudinal study of symptoms and self-care activities in women treated with primary radiotherapy for breast cancer. *Cancer Nursing, 28,* 210–218. doi:10.1097/00002820-200505000-00010

Koul, A., & Arora, N. (2010). Celecoxib mitigates cigarette smoke induced oxidative stress in mice. *Indian Journal of Biochemistry and Biophysics, 47,* 285–291.

Lage, A., & Crombet, T. (2011). Control of advanced cancer: The road to chronicity. *International Journal of Environmental Research and Public Health, 8,* 683–697. doi:10.3390/ijerph8030683

Lazarus, R.S., & Folkman, S. (1984). *Stress, appraisal and coping.* New York, NY: Springer.

Leininger, M. (2002). Culture care theory: A major contribution to advance transcultural nursing knowledge and practices. *Journal of Transcultural Nursing, 13,* 189–192. doi:10.1177/10459602013003005

Liao, M.N., Chen, M.F., Chen, S.C., & Chen, P.L. (2008). Uncertainty and anxiety during the diagnostic period for women with suspected breast cancer. *Cancer Nursing, 31,* 274–283. doi:10.1097/01.NCC.0000305744.64452.fe

Lin, L., Yeh, C.H., & Mishel, M.H. (2010). Evaluation of a conceptual model based on Mishel's theories of uncertainty in illness in a sample of Taiwanese parents of children with cancer: A cross-sectional questionnaire survey. *International Journal of Nursing Studies, 47,* 1510–1524. doi:10.1016/j.ijnurstu.2010.05.009

Liu, J.E., Mok, E., & Wong, T. (2006). Caring in nursing: Investigating the meaning of caring from the perspective of cancer patients in Beijing, China. *Journal of Clinical Nursing, 15,* 188–196. doi:10.1111/j.1365-2702.2006.01291.x

Lu, H.Y., Shaw, B.R., & Gustafson, D.H. (2011). Online health consultation: Examining uses of an interactive cancer communication tool by low-income women with breast cancer. *International Journal of Medical Informatics, 27,* 518–528. doi:10.1016/j.ijmedinf.2011.03.011

Lund, L.W., Schmiegelow, K., Rechnitzer, C., & Johansen, C. (2011). A systematic review of studies on psychosocial late effects of childhood cancer: Structures of society and methodological pitfalls may challenge the conclusions. *Pediatric Blood and Cancer, 56,* 532–543. doi:10.1002/pbc.22883

Mai, P.L., Garceau, A.O., Graubard, B.I., Dunn, M., McNeel, T.S., Gonsalves, L., … Wideroff, L. (2011). Confirmation of family cancer history reported in a population-based survey. *Journal of the National Cancer Institute, 103,* 788–797. doi:10.1093/jnci/djr114

Maier-Lorentz, M.M. (2008). Transcultural nursing: Its importance in nursing practice. *Journal of Cultural Diversity, 15,* 37–43.

Mantovani, A., Allavena, P., Sica, A., & Balkwill, F. (2008). Cancer-related inflammation. *Nature, 454,* 436–444. doi:10.1038/nature07205

Mason, T.A., Thompson, W.W., Allen, D., Rogers, D., Gabram-Mendola, S., & Jacob Arriola, K.R. (2011). Evaluation of the Avon Foundation Community Education and Outreach Initiative Community Patient Navigation Program. *Health Promotion Practice, 8.* Advance online publication. doi:10.1177/1524839911404229

McLeod, D.L., Tapp, D.M., Moules, N.J., & Campbell, M.E. (2010). Knowing the family: Interpretations of family nursing in oncology and palliative care. *European Journal of Oncology Nursing, 14,* 93–100. doi:10.1016/j.ejon.2009.09.006

Meleis, A.I. (Ed.). (2007). *Theoretical nursing: Development and progress* (4th ed.). Philadelphia, PA: Lippincott Williams & Wilkins.

Miaskowski, C., Aouizerat, B.E., Dodd, M., & Cooper, B. (2007). Conceptual issues in symptom clusters research and their implications for quality-of-life assessment in patients with cancer. *Journal of the National Cancer Institute Monographs, 2007*(37), 39–46. doi:10.1093/jncimonographs/lgm003

Mishel, M.H., Germino, B.B., Gil, K.M., Belyea, M., Laney, I.C., Stewart, J., ... Clayton, M. (2005). Benefits from an uncertainty management intervention for African-American and Caucasian older long-term breast cancer survivors. *Psycho-Oncology, 14,* 962–978. doi:10.1002/pon.909

Mishel, M.H., Germino, B.B., Lin, L., Pruthi, R.S., Wallen, E.M., Crandell, J., & Blyler, D. (2009). Managing uncertainty about treatment decision making in early stage prostate cancer: A randomized clinical trial. *Patient Education and Counseling, 77,* 349–359. doi:10.1016/j.pec.2009.09.009

Mishel, M.H., Padilla, G., Grant, M., & Sorenson, D.S. (1991). Uncertainty in illness theory: A replication of the mediating effects of mastery and coping. *Nursing Research, 40,* 236–240. doi:10.1097/00006199-199107000-00013

Mols, F., Vingerhoets, A.J., Coebergh, J.W., & van de Poll-Franse, L.V. (2005). Quality of life among long-term breast cancer survivors: A systematic review. *European Journal of Cancer Care, 41,* 2613–2619. doi:10.1016/j.ejca.2005.05.017

Muir, N. (2004). Clinical decision making: Theory and practice. *Nursing Standard, 18*(36), 47–52.

National Cancer Institute. (2011). Tobacco facts. Retrieved from http://www.cancer.gov/cancertopics/tobacco/smoking

National Coalition for Cancer Survivorship. (n.d.). About us: Who we are. Retrieved from http://www.canceradvocacy.org/about-us/who-we-are

National Comprehensive Cancer Network. (2011). *NCCN Clinical Practice Guidelines in Oncology.* Retrieved from http://www.nccn.org

National Marrow Donor Program. (2011). You and survivorship. Retrived from http://marrow.org/Patient/You_and_Survivorship/You_and_Survivorship.aspx

Oncology Nursing Society. (n.d.). ONS PEP—Putting evidence into practice. Retrieved from http://ons.org/Research/PEP

Orgel, E., McCarter, R., & Jacobs, S. (2010). A failing medical educational model: A self-assessment by physicians at all levels of training of ability and comfort to deliver bad news. *Journal of Palliative Medicine, 13,* 677–683. doi:10.1089/jpm.2009.0338

Otis-Green, S., Ferrel, B.R., Spolum, M., Uman, G., Mullan, P., & Grant, M. (2009). An overview of the ACE project—Advocating for clinical excellence: Transdisciplinary palliative care education. *Journal of Cancer Education, 24,* 120–126. doi:10.1080/08858190902854616

Pedersen, A.E., & Hack, T.F. (2011). The British Columbia Patient Navigation Model: A critical analysis. *Oncology Nursing Forum, 38,* 200–206. doi:10.1188/11.ONF.200-206

Peppercorn, J.M., Smith, T.J., Helft, P.R., Debono, D.J., Berry, S.R., Wollins, D.S., ... Schnipper, L.E. (2011). American Society of Clinical Oncology statement: Toward individualized care for patients with advanced cancer. *Journal of Clinical Oncology, 29,* 755–760. doi:10.1200/JCO.2010.33.1744

Phillips, J.R. (2010). The universality of Rogers' Science of Unitary Human Beings. *Nursing Science Quarterly, 23*(1), 55–59. doi:10.1177/0894318409353795

Pinto, B.M., & Floyd, A. (2008). Theories underlying health promotion interventions among cancer survivors. *Seminars in Oncology Nursing, 24,* 153–163. doi:10.1016/j.soncn.2008.05.003

Rabow, M.W., Hauser, J.M., & Adams, J. (2004). Supporting family caregivers at the end of life: "They don't know what they don't know." *JAMA, 291,* 483–491. doi:10.1001/jama.291.4.483

Raleigh, Z.T. (2010). A biopsychosocial perspective on the experience of lung cancer. *Journal of Psychosocial Oncology, 28,* 116–125. doi:10.1080/07347330903438990

Recklitis, C.J., Sanchez-Varela, V., & Bober, S. (2008). Addressing psychological challenges after cancer: A guide for clinical practice. *Oncology, 22*(11, Suppl. Nurse Ed.), 11–20.

Robie, L., Alexandru, D., & Bota, D.A. (2011). The use of patient navigators to improve cancer care for Hispanic patients. *Clinical Medicine Insights: Oncology, 5*, 1–7. doi:10.4137/CMO.S6074

Rogers, E.M. (2004). A prospective and retrospective look at the diffusion model. *Journal of Health Communication, 9*(Suppl. 1), 13–19. doi:10.1080/10810730490271449

Royer, H.R., Phelan, C.H., & Heidrich, S.M. (2009). Older breast cancer survivors' symptom beliefs. *Oncology Nursing Forum, 36*, 463–470. doi:10.1188/09.ONF.463-470

Saintsing, D., Gibson, L.M., & Pennington, A.W. (2011). The novice nurse and clinical decision making: How to avoid errors. *Journal of Nursing Management, 19*, 354–359. doi:310.1111/j.1365-2834.2011.01248.x

Salander, P. (2010). Facilitating interventions and/or relationships in malignant brain tumors. *Advances in Therapy, 27*, 17–27. doi:10.1007/s12325-010-0003-z

Schallom, L., Thimmesch, A.R., & Pierce, J.D. (2011). Systems biology in critical-care nursing. *Dimensions of Critical Care Nursing, 30*, 1–7. doi:10.1097/DCC.0b013e3181fd0169

Schim, S.M., Doorenbos, A., Benkert, R., & Miller, J. (2007). Culturally congruent care: Putting the puzzle together. *Journal of Transcultural Nursing, 18*, 103–110. doi:10.1177/1043659606298613

Simmons, B. (2010). Clinical reasoning: Concept analysis. *Journal of Advanced Nursing, 66*, 1151–1158. doi:10.1111/j.1365-2648.2010.05262.x

Singh, J., Trabulsi, E.J., & Gomella, L.G. (2010). The quality-of-life impact of prostate cancer treatments. *Current Urology Reports, 11*, 139–146. doi:10.1007/s11934010-0103-y

Skrutkowski, M., Saucier, A., & Meterissian, S. (2011). The Breast Cancer Patient Navigation Kit: Development and user feedback. *Journal of Cancer Education, 26*, 782–792. doi:10.1007/s13187-011-0216-0

Smith, M.C., Kemp, J., Hemphill, L., & Vojir, C.P. (2002). Outcomes of therapeutic massage for hospitalized cancer patients. *Journal of Nursing Scholarship, 34*, 257–262. doi:10.1111/j.1547-5069.2002.00257.x

Society for Integratvie Oncology. (2009). SIO practice guidelines 2009. Retrieved from http://www.integrativeonc.org/index.php/Search?ordering=&searchphrase=all&searchword=guidelines

St. Clair, A., & McKenry, L. (1999). Preparing culturally competent practitioners. *Journal of Nursing Education, 38*, 228–234.

Stewart, J.L., Mishel, M.H., Lynn, M.R., & Terhorst, L. (2010). Test of a conceptual model of uncertainty in children and adolescents with cancer. *Research in Nursing and Health, 33*, 179–191. doi:10.1002/nur.20374

Thomsen, T.G., Rydahl-Hansen, S., & Wagner, L. (2010). A review of potential factors relevant to coping in patients with advanced cancer. *Journal of Clinical Nursing, 19*, 3410–3426. doi:10.1111/j.1365-2702.2009.03154.x

Tighe, M., Molassiotis, A., Morris, J., & Richardson, J. (2011). Coping, meaning and symptom experience: A narrative approach to the overwhelming impacts of breast cancer in the first year following diagnosis. *European Journal of Oncology Nursing, 15*, 226–232. doi:10.1016/j.ejon.2011.03.004

Wall, L.M. (2000). Changes in hope and power in lung cancer patients who exercise. *Nursing Science Quarterly, 13*, 234–242. doi:10.1177/08943180022107627

Wallace Kazer, M.W., Bailey, D.E., Jr., & Whittemore, R. (2010). Out of the black box: Expansion of a theory-based intervention to self-manage the uncertainty associated with active surveillance (AS) for prostate cancer. *Research and Theory for Nursing Practice, 24*, 101–112. doi:10.1891/1541-6577.24.2.101

Wang, E. (2010). Cancer systems biology and personalized medicine. In E. Wang (Ed.), *A roadmap of cancer systems biology*. Boca Raton, FL: CRC Press. Retrieved from http://precedings.nature.com/documents/4322/version/2

Webb, M.S., de Ybarra, D.R., Baker, E.A., Reis, I.M., & Carey, M.P. (2010). Cognitive-behavioral therapy to promote smoking cessation among African American smokers: A randomized clinical trial. *Journal of Consulting and Clinical Psychology, 78*, 24–33. doi:10.1037/a0017669

Wilson, A.G. (2008). Epigenetic regulation of gene expression in the inflammatory response and relevance to common diseases. *Journal of Periodontology, 79*(8, Suppl.), 1514–1519. doi:10.1902/jop.2008.080172

CHAPTER 5

Oncology Nursing Leadership and Healthcare Policy

Carlton G. Brown, PhD, RN, AOCN®

Making your mark on the world is hard. If it were easy, everybody would do it. But it's not. It takes patience, it takes commitment, and it comes with plenty of failure along the way. The real test is not whether you avoid this failure, because you won't. It's whether you let it harden or shame you into inaction, or whether you learn from it; whether you choose to persevere.
—Barack Obama, July 12, 2006

Introduction

Nurses are tremendously vital to the future transformation of health care in the United States. What we do today will influence how our healthcare system will look in 10 years. Again and again in Gallup polls over the past several years, the American public has ranked nursing as the most trusted profession in the country (Jones, 2010). The healthcare community, legislators, patients, and families are calling on nurse leaders to contribute to the current discussions of how best to meet the needs of all patients for quality health care. Nurses are being asked to take the proverbial seat at the table of change—and we must accept that invitation or others less qualified will take that seat and attempt to speak on our behalf. The stakes are very high for nurse leaders to design a healthcare system today that will serve all Americans in coming years.

To take it a step further, oncology nurses are positioned perfectly to focus their leadership on promoting excellence in oncology nursing and to work diligently for high-quality care of patients with cancer and their families. No one knows the patient and family with cancer better than the oncology nurse. We spend numerous hours with them beginning at diagnosis and remain with them through survivorship and even to the end of life if that is where their journey leads them. Yet, nurses unfortunately cannot transform the future of health care alone; if they could, that transformation would have already occurred successfully. Instead, this successful transformation will need to include federal and state governments, healthcare institutions, professional organizations, other health professionals, and the insurance industry. Still, oncology nurses are important leaders in the creation of future healthcare models for patients with cancer. Yet, nurses often do not realize their own power and prestige in the current healthcare arena and sometimes give their authority away to others who are less qualified to speak on issues related to oncology nursing and the patients in our care.

This chapter will focus on specific recent health policy initiatives and how they will affect the overall landscape of health care and nursing in the United States. Specifically, this chapter will focus on outcomes from the Patient Protection and Affordable Care Act (PPACA), the Institute of Medicine report on the future of nursing, and the Consensus Model for APRN Regulation: Licensure, Accreditation, Certification, and Education (LACE) (National Council of State Boards of Nursing [NCSBN], 2008), and how these initiatives will ultimately affect patients with cancer, their families, and the nurses who care for them. This chapter will also focus briefly on how these initiatives will potentially affect advanced practice registered nurses (APRNs). The chapter will conclude with some areas where oncology nurse leaders can advocate for other nurses and patients with cancer.

Patient Protection and Affordable Care Act

On March 23, 2010, President Barack Obama signed the PPACA into law. This law will undoubtedly change health care in innumerable ways and perhaps will become one the most important pieces of social legislation passed in the last half-century (Chaffee, Mason, & Leavitt, 2011). In 2009, approximately 50 million Americans (42 million adults and 8 million children) were without health insurance; thus, the effect of this legislation is monumental for many patients for years to come (Henry J. Kaiser Family Foundation, 2010). Of course, the legislation has great healthcare potential for all Americans, especially those uninsured, but specifically patients who will or have been diagnosed with cancer.

Benefits for Patients From the Patient Protection and Affordable Care Act

For patients with cancer, the PPACA has numerous impact outcomes. These include
- Immediate creation of high-risk pools for those with preexisting conditions who are uninsured
- More affordable coverage because of elimination of annual and lifetime caps on benefits and prohibition of gender rating
- Portability and continuity of coverage for people with cancer or history of cancer by eliminating preexisting condition limitations
- Guaranteed coverage, even if a patient becomes sick or has a recurrence of cancer
- Prohibition of eligibility based on health status
- Increased access to early detection, prevention, treatment, and follow-up care for those previously without coverage
- Improved access to and coverage of prescription drugs for Medicare beneficiaries
- Provision of evidence-based preventive and early detection measures without co-payments (private insurance/plans)
- Assured coverage of participation in clinical trials

• More education and focus on effective pain management strategies (PPACA, 2010).

Perhaps most importantly, in 2014 the PPACA makes it illegal for a patient to be denied medical coverage by being diagnosed with cancer. There have been recent reports of insurance companies canceling policies once the patient has been diagnosed with breast cancer, for example. In fact, this cancellation has continued to occur even after the PPACA was signed into law. For years, we have witnessed patients who have needed a stem cell transplant as treatment for cancer, yet insurance companies have refused to pay for that treatment. However, in 2014, it will be illegal to cancel any patient's insurance coverage because of a cancer diagnosis or recurrence.

Benefits for Nurses From the Patient Protection and Affordable Care Act

Many educational opportunities for nurses derive from the PPACA, ranging from grants, loans, fellowships, and more (Stokowski, 2010). It is clear that as more patients become eligible and seek health care in the United States, there will be a dire need for more nurses to provide nursing care. The bill seeks to address the projected shortage of nurses and retention of nurses through (PPACA, 2010)

• Nurse education, practice, and retention grants
• Education loan repayment and scholarship programs
• Nursing faculty loan programs
• Loan repayment for master's/doctoral graduates who serve as nursing faculty for four years
• Advanced nursing education grants
• Workforce diversity grants
• Nursing education, practice, and retention grants
• Grant program to support nurse-managed health clinics that provide primary care.

This is a great time for nurses to return to school for further education for not only bachelor's, master's, or doctoral degrees, but also APRN degrees, such as a clinical nurse specialist (CNS), nurse practitioner (NP), or certified nurse midwife. For example, under the PPACA, the Nursing Student Loan Program will witness increases in loans for a nursing education from $13,000 to $17,000 with a set 5% interest rate (Stokowski, 2010). Furthermore, a loan repayment plan will be available for master's and doctoral graduates who serve as nursing faculty for four years in accredited schools (loan repayment up to $40,000 for master's student and $80,000 for doctoral) (Stokowski, 2010). Thus, numerous opportunities are available for nurses to more effectively prepare themselves for higher levels of nursing practice. Questions arise as to whether students will be attracted to the profession of nursing and if current nurses will seek these opportunities within the PPACA to seek more education in nursing practice.

The Role of the Advanced Practice Registered Nurse and the Patient Protection and Affordable Care Act

APRN is an umbrella term referring to the four advanced practice roles: the certified NP, certified CNS, certified nurse midwife, and certified registered nurse anesthetist (NCSBN, 2008). APRNs potentially have the greatest future opportunities within healthcare reform. In fact, the PPACA provided "a number of astounding opportunities for APRNs" (O'Grady & Ford, 2011, p. 397). Specifically, there will be instances where APRNs will have independent practices in cancer survivorship clinics, nurse-managed health centers, private practice, and school-based health centers. The PPACA provides a funded demonstration where Medicare will appropriate $50 million (2012–2015) to fund APRN graduate programs that will teach the needed skills so that these specially trained nurses can work in numerous areas to include primary care, chronic case management, preventive care, and numerous other options (O'Grady & Ford, 2011). In a recent interview, Susan Hassmiller, PhD, RN, stated, "This could be the day of the nurse practitioner" (Stokowski, 2011).

Many researchers have shown the effectiveness of the APRN. A Cochrane Collaboration article suggested that in many healthcare settings, care is comparable between NPs and physicians, and NPs often score better on subjective measures such as patient satisfaction (Laurant et al., 2005). Just as new opportunities for APRNs become reality, there also has been an increased debate and opposition to APRNs practicing independently. In reality, it is a turf war where certain physicians are trying to protect their own practice and their livelihood, but there will be a tremendous need for all healthcare professionals to provide care to millions of Americans who do or will have need. Still, some physician groups continue to attempt to limit the practice of APRNs (O'Grady & Ford, 2011). According to O'Grady and Ford (2011, p. 394), "This relationship deteriorated into turf battles as medical organizations sought to control the NP's expanding scope of practice. The belief that physicians were 'Captains of the Ship' fueled a growing animosity between nursing and medical organizations."

Perhaps the tides are changing in relation to utilizing NPs in oncology practices and patients are verbalizing high satisfaction when cared for by nonphysician providers (NPPs) (both NPs and physician assistants [PAs]). In a recent study, Towle and Barr (2011) found that more than 92.5% of patients were extremely satisfied with the care they received from an NPP and that 98.3% of patients were aware when a NPP was caring for them. Yet it is not just the patients who were satisfied when an NP or PA was caring for them; the members of the healthcare team also were satisfied. Towle and Barr (2011) noted that in practices in which NPPs worked with all physicians and saw a wide variety of patients, a 19% increase in overall productivity was demonstrated. Although some variability existed, the overall satisfaction of physicians working with NPPs in the study group was 7.98 of 10 (79.8%). Similarly, the overall NPP satisfaction score was 7.82 (78.2%) of NPPs. These findings suggest that NPPs are productive and helpful to the practice. These findings also suggest that both physicians and NPPs are satisfied with a collaborative practice. With an increase in the number of patients with cancer, using NPPs effectively could lessen physicians' workloads, improve patient outcomes, and result in positive professional experiences for all healthcare providers. This study is just one example of the much-needed research to support the use of NPs in the care of patients with cancer and other diseases. Obviously, much more research is needed that shows the value in using NPs.

Until recently, the licensure of APRNs was confusing because each of the individual state boards of nursing decided the practice level of these nurses. There was a high degree of variability in APRN practice depending on where the nurse practiced. For instance, an NP practicing in Maryland might have different responsibilities and privileges when compared to an NP in Iowa. In some states, APRNs were required to hold a certification in order to practice while other states required no certification. This variability created barriers to practice for APRNs and allowed for vulnerable criticism from those who opposed more individualized practice, such as certain physician groups (O'Grady & Ford, 2011).

The LACE Model

In 2008, NCSBN and 72 participating organizations created the Consensus Model for APRN Regulation: Licensure, Accreditation, Certification, and Education, also known as the LACE Model (NCSBN, 2008). The LACE document set forth a clear model of licensure, certification, accreditation, and education for APRNs that was endorsed by numerous professional nursing organizations including the American Nurses Association (ANA), the Oncology Nursing Society (ONS), and the Oncology Nursing Certification Corporation. Although individual state boards of nursing still determine APRN practice, the LACE model framework provides clear definitions of how APRNs are educated, licensed, certified, and accredited and in essence ascertains that APRNs meet the same consistent qualifications in all 50 states. Furthermore, the LACE model provides a foundation for all APRNs and should help to confront those who are resistant to the individual practice of APRNs.

Healthcare reform, specifically the PPACA, has begun to convert a once rocky road with limited opportunity for APRNs into a street of possible golden opportunity. However, other variables and events are also creating new opportunities for APRNs, especially in oncology nursing. By 2020, according to the American Society of Clinical Oncology (ASCO), a significant shortage of medical and gynecologic oncologists will result in a deficit of 2,550–4,080 oncologists. As the general population lives longer, people are more likely to be diagnosed with a cancer. Millions of Americans in coming years will have better access to care thanks to PPACA. The bottom line is that this increased number of patients who will likely be diagnosed with cancer coupled with a shortage of oncology healthcare providers will mean that an interdisciplinary team will become more important and relevant. An article in a 2011 issue of *ASCO Post* noted the relationship to a team approach to cancer care:

> There is room for excellent cancer care provided by numerous healthcare providers including physicians, nurse practitioners, and physician assistants. Many of us have worked in successful teams while caring for patients with cancer. That teamwork will become more important than ever if we are to provide quality cancer care, while eliminating errors, and surviving likely burnout. None of us can do it alone—but together we can provide cancer care more successfully and safely. (Brown, 2011, p. 2)

While APRNs try to make arguments for the strength and reputation of quality in the care they provide, and while some physicians try to protect the practice that historically belonged to them, patients are still diagnosed with many chronic illnesses such as cancer. The real reason for this move toward a multidisciplinary team approach to cancer care is to benefit the thousands of patients and families.

The Institute of Medicine Report on the Future of Nursing

Recently, the Robert Wood Johnson Foundation (RWJF) in conjunction with the Institute of Medicine (IOM) completed a study on the future of nursing titled *The Fu-*

ture of Nursing: Leading Change, Advancing Health (IOM, 2010). This was a landmark study conducted over two years that made specific recommendations for the future of nursing. The four major recommendations derived from the study are as follows.

- Nurses should practice to the full extent of their education and training.
- Nurses should achieve higher levels of education and training through an improved education system that promotes seamless academic progression.
- Nurses should be full partners with physicians and other healthcare professionals in redesigning health care in the United States.
- Effective workforce planning and policy making require better data collection and information infrastructure.

   These key messages are intended to transform nursing for the future. IOM (2010) also created recommendations for how these four key messages will be accomplished. Not all of those will be discussed, but a few will be mentioned in relationship to the immediate importance to nursing.

- Remove scope-of-practice barriers. This recommendation notes the importance of all nurses, including APRNs, to be allowed to practice to the fullest extent that their license state allows. For example, all state boards of nursing should band together to have the same practice for NPs instead of fractionating the NP practice rights from state to state. Another tactic in this recommendation is to allow Medicare to pay for NP coverage of similar skills provided to patients (such as admission assessments) that physicians are currently providing and receiving reimbursement.
- Increase the proportion of nurses with a baccalaureate degree to 80% by 2020. Considering that only 50% of RNs practicing nursing today possess a baccalaureate degree, this will be a very difficult recommendation to accomplish. Perhaps the largest barrier to this recommendation is the ongoing nursing faculty shortage. Faculty shortages will play an important role in the preparedness of all nurses in the very near future. Without attention to the faculty shortage, this recommendation of increasing the number of bachelor's-prepared nurses by 30% in the next eight or so years will not be accomplished.
- Double the number of nurses with a doctorate by 2020. This recommendation focuses interest on the faculty shortage discussed in the second item. IOM (2010) encouraged university trustees and academic administrators to create salary and benefit packages that recruit and retain highly qualified academic and clinical nurse faculty.
- Prepare and enable nurses to lead change to advance health. This is perhaps one of IOM's most important recommendations because it challenges nurses to take a more specific and prominent role in leading healthcare change in America. On numerous fronts, nurses have been invited to "seats at the table" in relation to the important transformation of the future of health care. If nurse leaders do not actively speak on behalf of the three million nurses in the United States, someone else will speak for them, thereby allowing the future of nursing to be decided by non-nurses. According to the IOM (2010) report, "Nurses should take responsibility for their personal and professional growth by continuing their education and seeking opportunities to develop and exercise their leadership skills" (p. 14). Furthermore, nursing associations, such as ONS and ANA, should provide their members with leadership opportunities and mentorship that will provide them the training and experience necessary to lead at the local, state, national, and international levels within nursing and health care.

Advocacy and the Oncology Nurse Leader

Every oncology nurse is a leader, whether working in inpatient or outpatient settings, hospices, schools of nursing, or industry or actively participating in an organization such as ONS. Some will say that the presence of oncology nursing is still somewhat or largely invisible at decision-making meetings in some healthcare organizations and in the U.S. federal government. Nurses have a strong history of advocating for patients, families, and communities for the promotion and equality of health care for all (Priest, 2011). Famous nurses such as Florence Nightingale, Dorothea Dix, and more recently, Dr. Mary Wakefield, a nurse and administrator of the Health Resources and Services Administration (HRSA), advocated and continued to work tirelessly on behalf of nurses and patients. Oncology nurses now more than ever are answering the call to be involved in more decisions surrounding the future of health care. Although our initial training as nurses prepared us to serve as advocates for patients and families, it did not truly prepare us for the types of advocacy needed today. Nurse leaders today must be prepared to speak about the needs of patients, present data and evidence to support their thoughts and ideals, use financial facts and figures to justify the patients' needs, and be comfortable in a boardroom or on Capitol Hill making the case for the needs of those in their care. Historically, nurses have not been prepared to take on these roles; thus, it is easy to understand why they sometimes have difficulty taking on these new responsibilities. Make no mistake, nurses across history have always learned the skills that were needed in order to advocate for patients and their own profession. As a case in point, look to comments from President Obama on the importance of nurses in the passing of healthcare reform in spring 2010:

> Nurses aren't in health care to get rich. Last I checked, they're in it to care for all of us, from the time they bring a new life into this world to the moment they ease the pain of those who pass from it. If it weren't for nurses, many Americans in underserved and rural areas would have no access to health care at all. (Wakefield, 2010, para. 6)

Yet the question always arises about where nurses can best fit in the area of advocacy, especially in policy and politics. According to Chaffee et al. (2011), there is a framework for action, also considered the spheres of influence where nurses shape policy. The spheres of influence consist of four important areas: (a) the workplace and workforce, (b) the government, (c) associations and interest groups, and (d) the community. Oncology nurse leaders can use these four spheres to focus specific energies for the advocacy of patients with cancer, their families, and the nurses who care for them.

The Workplace

As previously mentioned, nurses work in numerous settings from chairside or bedside to schools of nursing, industry, and government settings, just to mention a few. In each of these settings, nurses have tremendous authority and stature when it comes to issues specific to oncology nursing and caring for patients with cancer. All of these workplaces are political in that nurses must work diligently to influence the allocation of finite resources (Chaffee et al., 2011). The workplace is where oncology nurse leaders can negotiate and advocate for patients with cancer and their care providers. Examples of negotiation might include nurse-to-patient ratios, resources needed to provide safe and adequate care, proper space to provide care, and initial and continued education for nurses so that they may remain competent in the care they provide.

The Government

While much of health care is funded and provided by the private sector, the U.S. government does fund and control a portion of that health care (Chaffee et al., 2011). The government plays an important role in influencing nursing and nursing practice as is evident by legislation, including the PPACA. Because the government makes many decisions about nursing practice and care for patients with cancer, obviously nurses would want to be interactive with the government. Chaffee et al. (2011) noted numerous ways that nurses can influence all levels of local, state, and federal government, including
- Serving as an elected official (e.g., Congresswomen Lois Capps (D-CA), Delaware State Senator Bethany Hall Long)
- Serving in federal, state, and local agencies (e.g., Mary Wakefield, RN, PhD, administrator of HRSA)
- Providing testimony at government hearings (I myself serve as an example because as president of ONS, I gave testimony to the U.S. Food and Drug Administration in July 2010.)
- Communicating to policy makers about their support or opposition for respective legislation.

Oncology nurse leaders should establish relationships with their local, state, and federal leaders well in advance of approaching these leaders for an "ask." If nurse leaders do not know who their congressperson or senator is, they can go to www.senate.gov/general/contact_information/senators_cfm.cfm or www.house.gov/leadership and simply put in a zip code to find out who represents them on a federal level. ONS also provides information on legislative issues at the Legislative Action Center at www.ons.org/LAC. Although many oncology nurses may not have an opportunity to influence policy at the highest levels, there are numerous ways to get involved. Nurses know the stories of patients and families with cancer firsthand, and this knowledge of the patient experience often sells our government leaders on legislation for these respective patients. Nurses are paramount to this legislative process and should never overlook an opportunity to advocate at the governmental level.

Associations and Interest Groups

Perhaps one of the easiest ways to advocate for oncology nursing and patients with cancer is through membership with professional nursing associations. ONS (www.ons.org), ANA (www.nursingworld.org), and the Hospice and Palliative Nurses Association (www.hpna.org) are three examples. These nursing organizations have extensive legislative and policy initiatives as part of their overall strategic plan. ONS has developed legislation (Improving Cancer Treatment Education Act of 2011) focused on funding one hour of nursing education for patients before beginning treatment such as chemotherapy or radiation. Nurse leaders who want to learn more about the legislative process and also learn techniques on how to approach and talk with government leaders can attend programs such as the Nurse in Washington Internship (NIWI) (www.nursing-alliance.org/content.cfm/id/niwi). NIWI is open to any RN or nursing student (all levels of education) who is interested in an orientation to the legislative process.

The Community

The final sphere of influence is the community, which is a group of people who share a common goal and are focused on accomplishing that goal together. Oncology nurse leaders can participate in many community events to advocate for patients with cancer, their families, and their caregivers. The communities can be a neighborhood, city, state, or even an online group that has a common interest such as Susan G. Komen for the Cure (ww5.komen.org) or the Leukemia and Lymphoma Society (www.lls.org).

Given all these opportunities within the sphere of influence, there are numerous ways that oncology nurse leaders can become involved in health policy and advocacy for patients and families with cancer. As mentioned previously, if oncology nurses do not become involved, do not use their voice and their authority, do not accept a seat at the proverbial table of quality health care for patients with cancer, someone else will. And it is likely that the person who takes the place of the nurse in that seat will not represent nurses and patients with cancer appropriately.

Conclusion

This chapter has provided an overview of specific recent health policy initiatives and how they will affect the overall landscape of health care and nursing in the United States. This chapter also focused on how these initiatives will potentially affect APRNs. Finally, the chapter concluded with a discussion of areas where oncology nurse leaders can advocate for other nurses and patients with cancer. The opportunities are immense and the climate is ripe for oncology nurse leaders to help shape the healthcare system for the coming decade and beyond. What will you do to advocate for patients and families with cancer and those oncology nurses who care for them?

References

Brown, C.G. (2011). Teamwork in cancer care: More important than ever. *ASCO Post, 2*(6), 1–2. Retrieved from http://www.ascopost.com/articles/april-15-2011/teamwork-in-cancer-care-more-important-than-ever/

Chaffee, M.W., Mason, D.J., & Leavitt, J.K. (2012). A framework for action in policy and politics. In D.J. Mason, J.K. Leavitt, & M.W. Chaffee (Eds.), *Policy and politics in nursing and health care* (6th ed., pp. 1–11). St. Louis, MO: Elsevier Saunders.

Henry J. Kaiser Family Foundation. (2009). The Kaiser Commission on Medicaid and the Uninsured key facts: Five facts about the uninsured. Retrieved from http://www.kff.org/uninsured/upload/7806-03.pdf

Institute of Medicine. (2010). *The future of nursing: Leading change, advancing health.* Retrieved from http://www.iom.edu/Reports/2010/The-Future-of-Nursing-Leading-Change-Advancing-Health.aspx

Jones, J.M. (2010, December 3). Nurses top honesty and ethics list for 11th year. Retrieved from http://www.gallup.com/poll/145043/nurses-top-honesty-ethics-list-11-year.aspx

Laurant, M., Reeves, D., Hermens, R., Braspenning, J., Grol, R., & Sibbald, B. (2005). Substitution of doctors by nurses in primary care. Retrieved from http://www.mrw.interscience.wiley.com/cochrane/clsysrev/articles/CD001271/frame.html

National Council of State Boards of Nursing. (2008, July 7). Consensus model for APRN regulation: Licensure, accreditation, certification and education. Retrieved from https://www.ncsbn.org/Consensus_Model_for_APRN_Regulation_July_2008.pdf

O'Grady, E.T., & Ford, L.C. (2011). The politics of advanced practice nursing. In D.J. Mason, J.K. Leavitt, & M.W. Chaffee (Eds.), *Policy and politics in nursing and health care* (6th ed., pp. 393–400). St. Louis, MO: Elsevier Saunders.

Patient Protection and Affordable Care Act. (2010). Retrieved from http://docs.house.gov/energycommerce/ppacacon.pdf

Priest, C. (2011). Advocacy in nursing and health care. In D.J. Mason, J.K. Leavitt, & M.W. Chaffee (Eds.), *Policy and politics in nursing and health care* (6th ed., pp. 39–48). St. Louis, MO: Elsevier Saunders.

Stokowski, L.A. (2010). Healthcare reform and nurses: Challenges and opportunities. Retrieved from http://www.medscape.com/viewarticle/721049

Towle, E.L., & Barr, T.R. (2011). Results of the ASCO study of collaborative practice arrangements. *Journal of Oncology Practice, 7,* 286–290. doi:10.1200/JOP.2011.000385

Wakefield, M.K. (2010, May 7). Remarks to a 2010 Nursing Recognition Day ceremony. Retrieved from http://www.hrsa.gov/about/news/speeches/2010/050710nursing.html

CHAPTER 6

Basic Science of Genetics

Kristi L. Wiggins, MSN, RN, ANP-BC, AOCNP®, CCRC
Judith K. Payne, PhD, RN, AOCN®

Introduction

Is all cancer genetic? Simply put, yes, all cancer is genetic. This does not necessarily mean all cancer is inherited. Inherited gene mutations only account for approximately 10% of all cancers. This type of mutation is also called a *somatic* or *germline mutation*, something that is present in a person's genes at the time of birth. Most cancers arise from normal cells that undergo some type of transformation that alters the intended function of the cell. This happens because of damage to the genes of the cells, most commonly from environmental factors. These are acquired, sporadic cancers (American Cancer Society, 2011). So why do 90% of most cancers occur? Because we are made of DNA, and by a variety of factors, the DNA product becomes defective and no longer functions correctly.

Most laypeople are very familiar with the term *DNA* but do not fully comprehend the implications for health care. Genetics is on the forefront of medicine—the genomic age is now. Chapman (2007) noted that with the advances in molecular knowledge, the field of genetics will impact every facet of clinical care. Nurses are always on the front line of health care, establishing relationships, assessing, screening, teaching, treating, and monitoring. In the new era of genetics, nurses should have a basic understanding of the principles of genetics and how to educate patients. The application of genomic knowledge will allow nurses to be proactive instead of reactive. Nurses can no longer sit back and wait for someone else to address patients' and families' needs for genetic screening, education, and referrals. It is time for nurses to embrace this new frontier in which we are already a part.

Structures of Life

The majority of people tend to use the terms *genes*, *DNA*, and *chromosomes* interchangeably. These are the same, but different. To clarify, we must break down these concepts into the basic structures of life. Our very physical existence is dependent on four nitrogenous bases: adenine (A), thymine (T), cytosine (C), and guanine (G). Imagine that these four bases, much like our 26-letter English alphabet, create a language—the language of life. These four bases create the DNA double helix. Attached to each base is a sugar molecule. The sugar molecule is united by a phosphate molecule, which makes the sides of the helix strand. Two strands of bases create the two linear sides of the DNA strand, much like railroad tracks (see Figure 6-1). A always bonds with T, and C always bonds with G. These paired unions are considered "faithful" because they only bond in this fashion, creating the railroad ties for the tracks (Richards & Hawley, 2011).

Chromosomes

Imagine twisting the double helix over and over until it twists upon itself. Keep twisting the strand until the string of bases becomes a tightly wound piece of rope. This tightly wound piece of DNA is a chromosome. Humans have 23 pairs of chromosomes, 46 separate pieces of tightly wound DNA. Within each of these tightly wound pieces of material resides the different genes that compose all the information for the human body. The genes are sections along the double helix strand, defined by the differing sequences of bases (A, T, C, and G). The U.S. Department of Energy Genome Program (2008), through its work with the Human Genome Project, determined that the human body contains less than 30,000 genes. But imagine the different sequences of bases that it takes to create all of these genes! The sum of our genetic information in all these genes is referred to as our *genome*.

Chromosomes are best visualized when the cell cycle is in the metaphase of the cycle. This is the time in cell mitosis when the genetic material is most tightly compacted. To do a chromosomal analysis, the DNA in the nucleus of a cell in metaphase is examined. The 46 chromosomes located in the nucleus are arranged according to size, centromere location, and banding pattern. This chromosome arrangement is called a *karyotype*. The centromere is the bound area near the center of the chromosome. Centromeres can occur centrally, superior, or inferior to the middle section of a particular chromosome. Chromosomes are ordered 1 through 22, arranged by size, longest to shortest. After a karyotype sample is stained, the dark bands (G-bands, named for the Giemsa stain) that appear are unique to each

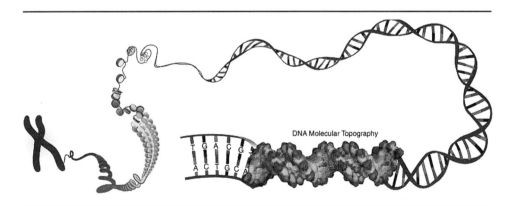

Figure 6-1. DNA Packaging and Topography

Note. Illustration by Darryl Leja, courtesy of the National Human Genome Research Institute. Retrieved from http://www.genome.gov/pressDisplay.cfm?photoID=20150.

pair of chromosomes. The arms of a chromosome above and below the centromere are also specifically characterized. These are described as the p arm, for the petite or shorter arms, and the longer q arms (named *q* because this letter follows *p* in the alphabet). Karyotypes are useful in detecting large chromosomal abnormalities (Richards & Hawley, 2011). For example, the *BRCA1* gene implicated in breast cancer is found on the long arm of chromosome 17 at gene location 21, written as 17q21 (Eggert & Kasse, 2010).

More than 99% of human DNA lives inside the cell's nucleus. It has two basic functions: (a) to replicate itself, make more of the same cell, and perform the same function, renewing itself, and (b) to code for proteins, products that the body needs to maintain homeostasis, such as mucus, enzymes, sweat, insulin, and hormones. To manufacture proteins, a section of a single strand of DNA has to be copied. A complementary, or mirror image, of the DNA is made. This copying process is called *transcription*, which is carried out by RNA. The messenger RNA (mRNA) regulates how and what genes are to be expressed. The transcribed information is taken out of the cell nucleus into the cytoplasm to be read, or translated by, RNA. For the transcribed information to travel outside the nucleus, the T must become uracil (U). Why? The T molecule contains a methyl group (written as CH3) as part of its structure. This methyl group does not allow T to cross the nuclear boundary. Think of T being the protector of your DNA, much like the sensor tags on clothing in the department store. You cannot leave the store with the item unless the tag is removed. Similarly, T drops the methyl group and the molecule becomes U, a nucleotide that replaces T that is found almost exclusively in RNA (National Institutes of Health [NIH] National Human Genome Research Institute [NHGRI], 2010). Once in the cytoplasm, ribosomes translate the information. In the copied strand of RNA, each set of three bases is called a *codon*. Each codon "codes" for a specific amino acid (see Figure 6-2). There are 64 possible codons for human genes. These codons manufacture the human body's 20 amino acids. One codon is the "start" codon (methionine), and three others are "stop" codons. The mRNA starts translating its copy messages at a "start" codon. It is the varied sequences of these amino acids that account for the multitude of different proteins our bodies make. During translation, transfer RNA (expressed as tRNA) carries the amino acids around awaiting ribosomal RNA (expressed as rRNA) to place the amino acids together into chains based on the codon sequence. As the amino acids are connected together in the prescribed order, they build and fold to create the appropriate protein. Each respective protein in the human body requires the exact same order of amino acids every time it is produced for it to become the correct protein and function the same way.

The code for our entire genome lives in every nucleus of every cell of the human body. Therefore, all DNA that codes for some type of protein must be replicated completely with each cell division. Replication is so specific that a mistake in copying only happens about once in every 10 billion copies. If the amino acids are not in the same sequence as the original DNA intended, it may be caused by a change in the DNA, a problem with transcription, or an error in translation. Changes in the DNA are called *gene mutations*. When a mutation occurs, a different product may be made, or the protein may not be made at all. When a different protein is made, this may or may not affect function. A variety of mutations can occur in human DNA. Mutations are defined by the change in the sequence of bases that change to the type of amino acid being provided in the production of a specific protein, thus changing the end product (Richards & Hawley, 2011).

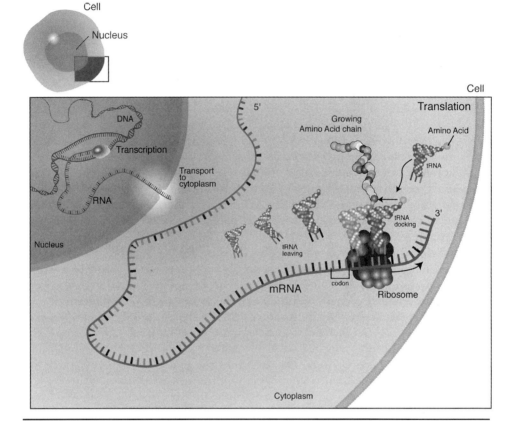

Figure 6-2. Translation

Note. Illustration by Darryl Leja, courtesy of the National Human Genome Research Institute. Retrieved from http://www.genome.gov/Glossary/resources/translation.pdf.

Mutations

Eggert and Kasse (2010) described different types of mutations known to occur in DNA. Point mutations are the change in a single point, or base. The base is not deleted or added, just changed, so the triad codon sequence remains intact, but the amino acid produced may be changed. If this type of change codes for the same amino acid, nothing happens; this is known as a *silent mutation.* If it changes the amino acid, the changes could be minimal, causing little noticeable change. Changes in protein production can range from decreased efficiency all the way to no protein function at all. A missense mutation is when a base change results in a stop codon. In other words, the amino acid the base change creates causes the protein to stop abruptly at a locale that was not intended, usually rendering the protein product useless. Some mutations involve the loss or addition of a base or bases. This causes a frameshift mutation. The codon triplet reading-frame for amino acids is either shifted forward with the addition of a base, or moved backward with the deletion. This causes an error in the entire reading frame, usually causing a deleterious change in the gene function (Eggert & Kasse, 2010).

Understanding mutations helps nurses conceptualize the types of errors that can occur in tumor suppressor genes or oncogenes. When these genes encounter errors in the DNA, which in turn create errors in the amino acids and/or reading frames, cancer is more likely to occur. Tumor suppressor genes and oncogenes are the "brakes" and the "gas pedal" for cell growth and replication, respectively. If the brakes are broken, the cell will continue to enter the cell cycle indefinitely. If the gas pedal is broken and stuck to the floor, the cell may turn on and never be able to turn off, therefore also continuing to enter the cell cycle.

Gene Alleles

Alleles refers to a version of a gene. There can be one or multiple versions. Humans have two copies of each chromosome, one copy provided by each biologic parent at the time of conception. Explaining this concept is important when discussing genetic defects with patients. When a gene mutation is present, typically one allele is healthy and one allele is affected by the mutation.

A genotype is the combination of alleles of all the various genes of one individual. Think of genotype as your gene type. The phenotype is the expression of the genotype. Common examples are hair and eye color, or having a widow's peak. It is important to remember that internal and external environmental factors play a role in phenotypic expression, whether it is a physically apparent trait or a disease process (NIH NHGRI, 2010).

Single nucleotide polymorphisms (SNPs) are benign mutations and normal variants found in the DNA of our alleles. In other words, there is a sequence variation of A, T, C, and G that is different than the majority of the population. These variations are present in approximately 1% of the general population. For example, after eating asparagus, some individuals notice a distinctive aroma in their urine. This odor is caused by chemicals called *methyl mercaptan* and *asparagine*. Asparagus contains both of these odiferous chemicals. There has been debate over whether the odor is present in the urine of individuals that lack an enzyme to break down these chemicals or if only certain individuals possess the olfactory capacity to smell this unusual odor. Pelchat, Bykowski, Duke, and Reed (2010) conducted genetic research that confirms the varying degrees to which humans metabolize the chemicals found in asparagus and varying degrees of one's ability to smell the odor in urine. This variation is due to a wide variety of polymorphisms—mutations that are not harmful, just different from person to person. Individuals experiencing the asparagus urine phenomenon can identify with this polymorphism. This is a simple, known example of how a gene mutation or variation is different, but not harmful to one's health.

Genetics, Genomics, and Proteomics

Genetics, genomics, and proteomics—so what's the difference? *Genetics* is the study of genes, how genetic traits are passed on to offspring, and how some traits occur as a result of mutations. *Genomics* goes a step further. Think what you have learned about genes. Now apply this information to how genes function, relating to their environments inside and outside the human body. Genomics is about the relationships genes have and how these relationships affect the growth and development of a living organism (NIH NHGRI, 2010).

Proteomics is the study of proteins, the product of genes. It evaluates the sum of an organism's proteins. The goal is to predict how proteins function, how they are expressed, how they relate to one another, and how they affect metabolic and cellular communication pathways (Beery & Hern, 2004). Each day more is understood about how proteins affect health and disease by examining biologic and chemical changes in the body. Protein biomarkers can aid in identifying particular physiologic conditions or processes.

Epigenetics and Biomarkers

Genetics alone cannot explain the diversity of phenotypes within a population or explain how, despite their identical DNA sequences, monozygotic twins can have different phenotypes and different susceptibilities to a disease (Esteller, 2008). Epigenetics is a promising field in the current biomedical and biobehavioral research landscape (Rodriguez-Paredes & Esteller, 2011). Today, the term *epigenetics* refers specifically to the study of mitotically and meiotically heritable changes in gene expression that occur without changes in the DNA sequence (Berger, Kouzarides, Shiekhattar, & Shilatifard, 2009). Others have defined *epigenetics* as the study of heritable changes in gene function that occur without a change in the sequence of the DNA (Silviera, Smith, Powell, & Sapienza, 2012). The field of epigenetics has exploded in large part because of advances in our understanding of how epigenetic changes are involved in modulating functional pathways that are key to the neoplastic phenotype and by showing the clinical usefulness of targeting epigenetics for the treatment of cancer. Finally, the fields of cancer and epigenetics have matured to a point where the intersection of the two fields is ready for sustained research (Issa, 2008). Strong evidence exists for an epigenetic component of early neoplasia, and data on the cancer preventive properties of epigenetic modulation are emerging (Issa, 2008). Silviera et al. (2012) have identified three main reasons that ascertain the value of epigenetic information. The first is that systemic epigenetic differences between individuals, such as differences that result from environmental and genetic factors that act very early in development, can help explain differences in gene expression between individuals of identical genotype. Second, these differences may serve as surrogate markers of gene activity in tissues that are inaccessible to analysis, and third, tissue-specific epigenetic differences between individuals may provide a mechanistic link between the genetic and environmental factors that contribute to disease risk. The challenge for oncology nurses experienced in biobehavioral research is to translate these epigenetic findings into clinical and testable hypotheses.

Biomarkers, or *biologic markers*, can be defined as a biochemical feature or characteristic that can be used to measure the progress of a disease or the effects of treatment (Payne, 2006). The NIH Biomarkers Definition Group (2001) defined a *biomarker* to be a characteristic that can be objectively measured and evaluated as an indicator of normal biologic processes, pathogenic processes, or pharmacologic responses to a therapeutic intervention. Other definitions provided by various organizations are tailored to be more relevant for their purpose. Therefore, the definition is generally expansive, and therapeutic interventions described in the definition may include psychosocial and behavioral interventions beyond pharmacologic interventions (Kang, Rice, Park, Turner-Henson, & Downs, 2010). These investigators suggest that "in these cases, biomarkers are used as prognostic indicators to assess a person's response to any treatment or intervention or to elucidate potential mechanisms underlying the relationship between the factors of interest" (Kang et al., 2010, p. 732).

The study of biomarkers and how they may be used to guide practice is an evolving area of exploration in genomic science. The use of biomarkers to define and guide clinical practice is not new to clinicians in other disciplines, such as physicians who have increasingly used various biomarkers to diagnose disease and measure response rates. The use of biomarkers offers significant opportunities for us to understand the biologic impact of cancer and various treatment modalities on individuals with cancer. Understanding the concept of biomarkers and how they relate to the science of symptom management will provide evidence that nursing professionals can use to design and test nursing interventions targeted at specific mechanisms (Payne, 2006).

Cancer and accompanying tumor load (burden) as well as many types of treatment regimens, such as surgery, radiation, chemotherapy, targeted biotherapies, and hormonal therapy, can cause a multitude of symptoms. However, the science of how symptom management interventions work is lacking. Today, at best, interventions are selected with little thought as to how the respective intervention works and whether it is the best intervention for an individual. Symptom management is a major focus of oncology nursing practice. Nursing research must move forward to continue the science of identifying and testing selected biomarkers to enhance symptom management for patients.

Pharmacogenomics

Since the completion of the Human Genome Project in 2003, scientists have attempted to fashion less-toxic gene-targeted therapies by tailoring molecular medicines for patients. This resulted in a huge paradigm shift of drug development. In the past, research largely focused on creating drugs for a particular symptom or disease. The drug was then tested for efficacy, basic trial and error. In the genomic era, research has shifted to targeting specific genes and proteins that play a role in particular diseases. This will continue to create a remarkable transformation in the way scientists search for cures (U.S. Department of Energy Genome Program, 2011).

Pharmacogenomics is the study of how an individual's genetic makeup affects the way he or she metabolizes drugs. With genetic knowledge, scientists will examine not only genes, but also proteins and SNPs to work toward tailor-made medicine. Investigating deeper into drug metabolism, scientists are discovering how to predict drug absorption and effect. One useful method of monitoring certain drugs is through pharmacokinetics. However, serial blood levels are obtained to adjust drug doses after a patient has been administered the drug. Beery and Hern (2004) noted what is currently known about the CYP450 family of enzymes in the liver supplies healthcare providers with critical information used in prescribing drugs prior to implementing treatment. We know that SNPs are specific to the individual and will provide even greater insight to an individual's response to pharmacologic therapeutics. SNPs will be especially important in predicting indirect responses to drugs. Adverse drug reactions are the leading cause of hospitalizations. Therefore, preemptive SNP analysis would eliminate most of the trial-and-error method we use now, as well as the dangers associated with this method.

Evans and McLeod (2003) performed a pharmacogenomic analysis that confirmed evidence of SNPs and multi-gene (polygenic) involvement in drug metabolism. They studied multiple substrates in CYP-450, noting differences in metabolism in the individual and also variations based on alleles commonly found in certain ethnic groups. However, clinicians must remain aware that the allele determines metabolism, not the assumed ethnicity of the individual receiving the drug. The genome of an individual never changes (how genes may express themselves can change), but technology will continue to move forward. Clinical trials are already being conducted to evaluate the metabolic rate of patients so that medication doses can be tailored (Evans & McLeod, 2003). The goal of pharmacogenomics is to provide clinicians with useful tools to assist in deciding the optimal therapies for treating an individual's illness with the least toxicity and with the best possible outcome.

Personalized Medicine: Changing the Meaning of Health, Illness, and Clinical Intervention

Clinical care is based largely on how the intervention for conditions will benefit the greatest number of individuals. Evidence-based research supports this method of care. Treatments are given to patients that are proven to work for the majority of patients with a specific illness. Although this approach is both ethical and logical, what are we doing about those individuals for whom these treatments do not work? We now enter the era of personalized medicine in hopes of answering this question. With completion of the Human Genome Project, the medical community assumed a vast majority of our genetic questions would be answered. They were wrong. This accomplishment provided us with a window into the amazing complexity of the human body. We are all 99.9% alike in our genetic makeup. The remaining 0.1% makes us unique and more complex, especially when considering treatment for illness. This 0.1% is the SNPs in the human genome. To date, more than two million known SNPs occur in human DNA (Beery & Hern, 2004). It seems that the very fine distinctions in our DNA are what may hold the key to the optimal treatment for diseases. Our knowledge of genetics and how to target treatments is in its infancy.

The Human Genome Project has provided a new way for scientists to go about developing new drugs, targeting errors in the human genome and the cancer genome, to build novel targeted agents. Generalizations regarding the best treatment for diseases will continue despite the current knowledge of genes and gene therapy. We must educate ourselves to the science of gene therapy in hopes of moving closer to personalized medicine.

Genomic medicine is clearly not a core part of standard nursing practice. Most nurses think that personalized care has been a long time coming, but some think that the genetic revolution has been exaggerated. This information was gleaned from Kirk, Lea, and Skirton's (2008) survey of nurse specialists in genetics. Many of these specialists noted that the completion of the Human Genome Project did not meet their expectations. However, they emphasized the impact that genetic information in the hands of nurses could have in improving patient health care. It is clearly nurses' role to be the agents for change in this rapidly changing field to improve patient outcomes through earlier and more accurate diagnoses and better targeted treatment and to overcome barriers. The primary barrier noted by the nurse specialists was lack of awareness and knowledge of genetics (Kirk et al., 2008).

Genetic knowledge is critical in providing insight to underlying causes of disease, rationale for cellular dysfunction that causes malignancy, and the amazing molecular targets and treatments for potential cures. This technical information is important to the future role of oncology nursing and personalized care. Nurses must enhance their genetic knowledge to accurately identify individuals who would benefit from genetic testing and potentially make a diagnosis earlier and more accurately. It is nurses' role to identify at-risk patients and families, perform a thorough family history, identify needed lifestyle changes, and refer for genetics counseling if increased risk for a genetic abnormality is suspected. Nurses are key in motivating patients and families to act on behalf of their health and have a responsibility to navigate them through the process.

Genetic Testing

Genetic testing is becoming ever more prevalent in clinical practice. The first gene was mapped in 1999, and a rough draft of the human genome map was published in June 2000. The Human Genome Project posted a near-complete map of the human genome in 2003. Since that time, more than 1,000 genetic tests have become available. Care providers are using these tests to improve prediction of occurrence, diagnose, determine prognosis, and treat both complex and common diseases. Close attention must be paid to the clinical validity of genetic tests as well as determining if they are clinically useful. Vast amounts of genetic information are publicly available, but most has no clinical utility (Burke, 2002). Once a clinician obtains genetic testing information, he or she must know how to apply the information to the patient and the specific clinical situation. Genetic information should always be viewed within the context of clinical information. As nurses, we must use genetic information as part of an individualized plan of care—that is truly individualized medicine.

Three basic types of genetic testing are biochemical, molecular, and cytogenetic. Biochemical genetic testing examines enzyme activity and metabolites, such as newborn screening for amino acid disorders. Molecular testing looks at DNA and RNA to examine specific genes, such as HFE for hemochromatosis, amino acid mutations that cause sickle-cell anemia, or HER2/neu through fluorescent in situ hybridization (known as FISH) analysis. Cytogenetic testing refers to chromosome analysis, such as looking for trisomy 21 (Down syndrome). Gaining a better understanding of these genetic abnormalities can lead to better preventive care. Nurses play a key role in managing care to prevent complications, provide longitudinal surveillance, and continue patient education (Burke, 2002).

Interestingly, patients take into consideration the level of competency of their care providers when deciding whether to undergo genetic testing. Historically, physicians performed most genetic counseling and testing. With nurses taking more of a lead role, we must consider how patients view the shift in the genetics paradigm. Basically, it comes down to whether the care provider is seen as an expert. The actual title means less if competence of the provider is determined and proven to the patient. Interestingly, a recommendation by a novice physician is seen as valid as an expert physician, but not so in nursing. An expert nurse is more influential in having a patient follow through with recommendations for genetic testing than a novice nurse, as noted by Barnoy, Levy, and Bar-Tal (2010). Nurses have a responsibility to competently explain genetic information to patients and families in such a way that they can make informed decisions about genetic testing. The way information is presented strongly influences an individual's decision whether to proceed with genetic testing (Beery & Hern, 2004).

Germ-Line Mutations

A common genetic test, BRACAnalysis® by Myriad Genetics Laboratories (2012), is used in the detection of a mutation in the *BRCA1* and *BRCA2* genes, which are implicated in an increased risk for breast and ovarian cancers. The *BRCA1* and *BRCA2* genes are tumor suppressor genes. Each person is born with two copies of normal *BRCA1* and *BRCA2* genes, one copy from each parent. If an individual inherits a copy of a mutated gene from either parent, he or she has one normal copy. This puts the individual one step into the process for cancer development but does not mean that the individual will certainly develop cancer. Unless the healthy copy also becomes mutated during that individual's life, cancer attributed to the genetic mutation will not occur. Having a mutation does not determine who will develop cancer or when, it only determines risk in the population of those having the mutation. Being born with *BRCA1* or *BRCA2* mutations increases the risk of developing breast cancer to 60% during one's lifetime, compared to 12% in the general population. The risk of developing ovarian cancer is 15%–40%, compared to 1.4% in the general population (National Cancer Institute, 2008, 2012).

Transitioning Our Knowledge of Genetic Testing to the Age of Genomics

One cancer diagnosis that illustrates the effect of genetic mutations in multiple ways is lymphoma. Non-Hodgkin lymphoma (NHL) is a very complicated hematologic malignancy. Although a single germ-line mutation is not known to be a direct cause of NHL, multiple mutations and environmental influences increase the risk of developing the disease. A family history of a lymphoid malignancy such as NHL, Hodgkin disease, or chronic lymphocytic leukemia has been associated with an increased risk of NHL in other family members (Chang et al., 2005). One of several genes implicated in the development of NHL is the *BCL6* gene, a proto-oncogene. Researchers have hypothesized that SNPs in the lymphogenesis pathways affecting the activity of *BCL6* are what lead to malignant transformation. These polymorphisms may be present at birth, increasing individuals' predisposition to developing cancer in their lifetime. This could be due to mutation in *BCL6* alone, but is more likely a result of the effect the mutated *BCL6* has on other genes with which it interacts. There are likely other promoting factors that are unknown at this time (Zhang et al., 2005). As care providers in this confusing environment, nurses have the responsibility to be able to explain these concepts and assist in navigating patients through this new world of genomics (Calzone, Lea, & Masney, 2006).

Tumor Mutation and Genomic Testing

Genetic fingerprinting, or tumor genetic profiling, is an advancing technology that is rapidly changing clinical practice. Scientists are analyzing the genome of tumors to determine how a specific tumor develops, survives, and develops resistance to treatment. One major breakthrough is the development of tests that predict outcomes for patients and provide vital information to clinicians regarding appropriate treatment strategies. One such test is the Oncotype DX® for Breast Cancer developed by Genomic Health, Inc. (n.d.). This test is used in women with a diagnosis of estrogen receptor–positive breast cancer that is diagnosed as stage I or II, without lymph node involvement. The 21-gene assay helps predict recurrence risk and provides information helpful in deciding whether an individual requires chemotherapy or if hormonal manipulation alone is adequate (Genomic Health, Inc., n.d.).

To develop the assay, researchers studied commonly occurring gene mutations in breast cancer. What they discovered is that the expression of certain genes provides a good prognosis, whereas others provide high-risk or poorer prognosis. A breast tumor sample is tested for the 21 genes. Depending on the propensity to overexpress particular genes, a risk score is calculated. A low score infers low risk; therefore, these women will benefit from hormone therapy alone. If the score is high, even if the tumor is small, a higher risk of recurrence is inferred, and that individual requires chemotherapy in addition to hormonal manipulation. This test has been proven as clinically valid and continues to help close the gap on recurrence rates for those women who would not have been treated with chemotherapy due to the small tumor size. Conversely, it eliminates unnecessary chemotherapy (and long-term risks from chemotherapy) for those women who are at reduced risk of recurrence. Habel et al. (2006) reevaluated the validity of Oncotype DX and noted that the outcomes for patients were best when the recurrence score provided by Oncotype DX was combined with risk associated with tumor size and grade. This consideration provided the best tool for determining treatment, rather than using one characteristic exclusively.

Genomic Health has also developed a 12-gene assay, Oncotype DX® for Colon Cancer. The design of this assay was somewhat different from the assay for breast cancer, but it is used in a similar fashion to determine if patients with stage II colon cancer require chemotherapy (Genomic Health, Inc., n.d.). Another evolving use for tumor profiling is to predict the chemosensitivity of certain tumors. One such test is Caris Target Now™ Molecular Profiling. This test measures proteins in cancer cells and predicts how the particular proteins will respond to a particular chemotherapy or combined therapy. Target Now is commonly used in patients who may have exhausted all conventional treatments for their cancer or have resistant disease (Caris Life Sciences, 2012). This and other molecular profiling tests are being increasingly used to determine chemosensitivity in cancers of unknown origin.

Genetic Counseling

Taking a thorough family history is still the foundational tool for genetic assessment. Nurses are well prepared to take excellent histories. We connect, query, and form working professional relationships with patients and families with ease. Remember that people are generally poor historians. Knowing the general ethnicity of parents and grandparents is common in most families, but little typically is known about the pedigree beyond the third generation (Ashcraft, Coleman, Lange, Enderlin, & Stewart, 2007). Most people identify themselves as how they are perceived through visual appearance. This is widely how we describe our current concept of race. Beware that looks can be deceiving. Race, as beauty, is only skin deep!

To identify individuals who may be eligible for genetic counseling, nurses can perform a general risk assessment (see Figure 6-3) and use or develop a family history questionnaire. To assist in creating a family history report, a variety of genealogy tools are available on the Internet. One common tool for collecting a family history is through the U.S. Department of Health and Human Services (http://familyhistory.hhs.gov). Inquire about the patient's interest in genetic testing and determine the patient's perceived risk.

- Early age at onset (e.g., premenopausal breast cancer)
- Multiple cancers in the same individual
- Clustering of the same cancer in close relatives
- Cancers occurring in two or more individuals in the same generation on the same side of the family
- Bilateral cancers in paired organs
- Unusual cancer presentations (e.g., male breast cancer)
- Rare cancers associated with birth defects (e.g., Wilms tumor)
- Uncommon tumor histology (e.g., medullary thyroid cancer)
- Occurrence of rare tumors
- Ethnic or geographic populations at high risk (e.g., Ashkenazi heritage and *BRCA1/BRCA2* mutations)
- Any known family member with a documented genetic mutation

Figure 6-3. Risk Assessment for Hereditary Cancer

Note. From "Cancer Genetics Risk Assessment and Counseling (PDQ®)" [Health professional version], by the National Cancer Institute, September 27, 2011. Retrieved from http://www.cancer.gov/cancertopics/pdq/genetics/risk-assessment-and-counseling/HealthProfessional.

Genograms

Learning how to draw a genogram will help nurses to provide patients with a visual representation of the patient's family history. Seeing the family history provides the opportunity to discuss patterns of inheritance and the likelihood, or not, of having a genetic-related diagnosis. In many cases, nurses first begin this process by doing their own family pedigree. This brings a certain sense of ownership and curiosity for discovery to the process when doing it for others (Tavernier, 2009). The usual practice of drawing a pedigree is to obtain information on three generations.

To begin, the nurse chooses the appropriate gender symbol (see Figure 6-4). The pedigree begins with the individual about whom the nurse is obtaining the family history information. Most people prefer to start at the bottom of the page and draw their first-degree relatives and other predecessors as they work their way upward through the generations. To determine relationships, the nurse will need to inquire about marriages, divorces, remarriage, consanguinity (intermarrying), offspring outside marriage, siblings (same parents or different parents), and deaths, including miscarriages and stillbirths. Lines connect the gender symbols to establish relationships between family members (see Figure 6-5). For each family member, the nurse should collect information on date of birth and current age, diagnoses, age at each diagnosis, age at death, and cause of death. Depending on the suspected disease, one might also collect information on congenital anomalies, occupational and environmental exposures, and medications (Skirton & Patch, 2002). Drawing a pedigree is extremely useful in determining patterns of inheritance of a suspected genetic disorder.

Once the pedigree is drawn, the nurse can discuss the family background with the individual and any other family members present to fill in any gaps in information. The nurse can then conduct a brief assessment of the individual's risk based on family history and any general recommendations for screening. This provides an opportunity for both recommending further genetics counseling as well as opening a discussion about health habits, disease prevention, and early disease detection. For a more specific calculation of risk, the clinician may use a risk model specific to

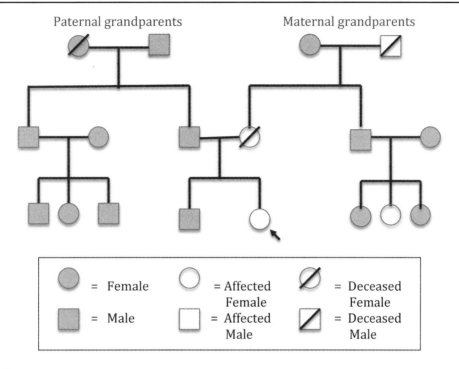

History:

Paternal GM deceased age 74 from MI. Maternal GF deceased age 50 from metastatic prostate cancer, diagnosed age 48. Mother deceased age 55 from ovarian cancer, diagnosed age 53. Maternal first cousin diagnosed with breast cancer age 42.
Proband/Patient (marked with arrow) diagnosed with breast cancer age 40, seeking genetic counseling for *BRCA1/2* testing.

Figure 6-4. Basic Pedigree

Note. Based on information from Bennett et al., 2008.

a particular diagnosis, based on statistics to predict chances of a gene mutation being present in the individual, such as the Claus Model for calculating breast cancer risk. In most cases, if the risk of possessing a gene mutation is calculated at greater than 10%, the individual is sent for genetic counseling and testing. Be aware that the decision to undergo genetic testing can precipitate both emotional and social angst for the patient and his or her family (Crockett-Maillet, 2010). Even if models show a low risk of genetic mutation, patterns of inheritance that are suspicious for a genetic mutation or familial cancer may be noted on the genogram. Some models are limited to certain variables for risk, not taking into account all of an individual's known risk factors. It is wise to refer these individuals despite the calculation of low risk. Also, some individuals have a low probability of genetic mutation and seem to have no patterns of inheritance on their genogram. However, individuals who are highly anxious would benefit from the additional education that genetic counseling provides (Hampel, Sweet, Westman, Offit, & Eng, 2004).

	Male	**Female**
Type of individual	☐	◯
Affected individual	☐	◯
Deceased individuals	◺	⊘
Proband	↗ ☐	↗ ◯
Relationship no longer exists	☐—//—◯	
Twins	☐ ☐	
Consanguinity	☐══◯	

Figure 6-5. Basic Pedigree Key

Note. Based on information from Bennett et al., 2008.

Most larger medical centers have access to genetics counselors to whom patients are referred for further counseling, testing, and post-test counseling. Smaller centers either refer patients to a larger center for this process or perform the tests from their private offices. In either case, the patient needs to be apprised of the possible results of testing and the implications for these. Most genetic tests will be reported with a negative result, a positive result, or a variant of uncertain significance (VUS), sometimes called an unclassified variant. The pretest counseling should include the possibility of each of these three results. If a VUS is found, most providers will recommend having other family members tested to confirm the finding and determine if there are any correlations in disease occurrence with the family history. Currently, there are no standard guidelines on how to make recommendations based on this type of result from genetic testing. Petrucelli, Lazebnik, Huelsman, and Lazebnik (2002) performed a qualitative study evaluating feedback from genetic testing participants. They discovered that the response to a VUS genetic test result was mainly affected by tested individuals' preconceived ideas of whether they thought their test results would be positive or negative. Negative results may impart a sense of false security, whereas positive results can create a sense of fatalism in the person being tested. However, many of the tested individuals continued to be confused by the result. Counseling was directed at explaining that the VUS could be a normal variant (like an SNP), or it could be a deleterious mutation not yet confirmed. What is most important to incorporate into the counseling sessions is the overall risk of the patient of developing cancer based on his or her personal and family history. With appropriate genetics counseling, patients can gain insight to what their results mean when applied to their unique situation. The goal of genetic testing is to glean answers that will help inform individualized healthcare decisions (Petrucelli et al., 2002).

Conclusion

The future of nursing in the field of genetics and genomics is exciting and challenging. Nurses are adept at considering the psychosocial, ethical, and cultural implications when providing clinical care. The nursing profession has grown in its advocacy of patient rights, access to care, and protection of privacy (Hamilton, 2009). In this genomic era, nurses must engage their skill to pursue genetic knowledge and engage in deeper clinical reasoning to manage the rapid pace of science for the better health of our patients and for future generations.

References

American Cancer Society. (2011, December 27). Heredity and cancer. Retrieved from http://www.cancer.org/Cancer/CancerCauses/GeneticsandCancer/heredity-and-cancer

Ashcraft, P.F., Coleman, E.A., Lange, U., Enderlin, C., & Stewart, C.B. (2007). Obtaining family histories from patients with cancer. *Clinical Journal of Oncology Nursing, 11,* 119–124. doi:10.1188/07.CJON.119-124

Barnoy, S., Levy, O., & Bar-Tal, Y. (2010). Nurse or physician: Whose recommendation influences the decision to take genetic tests more? *Journal of Advanced Nursing, 66,* 806–813. doi:10.1111/j.1365-2648.2009.05239.x

Beery, T., & Hern, M. (2004). Genetic practice, education, and research: Overview for advanced practice nurses. *Clinical Nurse Specialist, 18,* 126–132. doi:10.1097/00002800-200405000-00012

Bennett, R.L., French, K.S., Resta, R.G., & Doyle, D.L. (2008). Standardized human pedigree nomenclature update and assessment of the recommendations of the National Society of Genetic Counselors. *Journal of Genetic Counseling, 17,* 424–433. doi:10.1007/s10897-008-9169-9

Berger, S.L., Kouzarides, T., Shiekhattar, R., & Shilatifard, A. (2009). An operational definition of epigenetics. *Genes and Development, 23,* 781–783. doi:10.1101/gad.1787609

Burke, W. (2002). Genetic testing. *New England Journal of Medicine, 347,* 1867–1874. doi:10.1056/NEJMoa012113

Calzone, K., Lea, D.H., & Masny, A. (2006). Non-Hodgkin's lymphoma as an exemplar of the effects of genetics and genomics. *Journal of Nursing Scholarship, 38,* 335–343. doi:10.1111/j.1547-5069.2006.00124.x

Caris Life Sciences. (2012). Caris Target Now™ molecular profiling. Retrieved from http://www.carislifesciences.com/oncology-target-now

Chang, E.T., Smedby, K.E., Hjalgrim, H., Porwit-MacDonald, A., Roos, G., Glimelius, B., & Adami, H.O. (2005). Family history of hematopoietic malignancy and risk of lymphoma. *Journal of the National Cancer Institute, 97,* 1466–1474. doi:10.1093/jnci/dji293

Chapman, D.D. (2007). Cancer genetics. *Seminars in Oncology Nursing, 23,* 2–9. doi:10.1016/j.soncn.2006.11.002

Crockett-Maillet, G. (2010). Know the red flags of hereditary cancers. *Nurse Practitioner, 35,* 39–43. doi:10.1097/01.NPR.0000383660.45156.40

Eggert, J., & Kasse, M. (2010). Biology of cancer. In K.A. Calzone, A. Masny, & J. Jenkins (Eds.), *Genetics and genomics in oncology nursing practice* (pp. 13–45). Pittsburgh, PA: Oncology Nursing Society.

Esteller, M. (2008). Epigenetics in cancer. *New England Journal of Medicine, 358,* 1148–1159. doi:10.1056/NEJMra072067

Evans, W.E., & McLeod, H.L. (2003). Pharmacogenomics—Drug disposition, drug targets, and side effects. *New England Journal of Medicine, 348,* 538–549. doi:10.1056/NEJMra020526

Genomic Health, Inc. (n.d.). Oncotype DX breast cancer assay. Retrieved from http://www.oncotypedx.com/en-US/Breast.aspx

Habel, L.A., Shak, S., Jacobs, M.K., Capra, A., Alexander, C., Pho, M., … Quesenberry, C.P. (2006). A population-based study of tumor gene expression and risk of breast cancer death among lymph node-negative patients. *Breast Cancer Research, 8,* R25. doi:10.1186/bcr1412

Hamilton, R. (2009). Nursing advocacy in a postgenomic age. *Nursing Clinics of North America, 44,* 435–446. doi:10.1016/j.cnur.2009.07.007

Hampel, H., Sweet, K., Westman, J.A., Offit, K., & Eng, C. (2004). Referral for cancer genetics consultation: A review and compilation of risk assessment criteria. *Journal of Medical Genetics, 41,* 81–91. doi:10.1136/jmg.2003.010918

Issa, J. (2008). Cancer prevention: Epigenetics steps up to the plate. *Cancer Prevention Research, 1,* 219–222. doi:10.1158/1940-6207.CAPR-08-0029

Kang, D., Rice, M., Park, N., Turner-Henson, A., & Downs, C. (2010). Stress and inflammation: A biobehavioral approach for nursing research. *Western Journal of Nursing Research, 32,* 730–760. doi:10.1177/0193945909356556

Kirk, M., Lea, D., & Skirton, H. (2008). Genomic health care: Is the future now? *Nursing and Health Sciences, 10,* 85–92. doi:10.1111/j.1442-2018.2008.00374.x

Myriad Genetic Laboratories. (2012). Etiology and clinical features of hereditary breast and ovarian cancer (HBOC). Retrieved from https://www.myriadpro.com/test-offerings/genetic-testing/bracanalysis

National Cancer Institute. (2008). Surveillance, Epidemiology, and End Results. Retrieved from http://seer.cancer.gov/csr/1975_2008/index.html

National Cancer Institute. (2012, January 18). Genetics of breast and ovarian cancer (PDQ®) [Health professional version]. Retrieved from http://www.cancer.gov/cancertopics/pdq/genetics/breast-and-ovarian/healthprofessional

National Institutes of Health Biomarkers Definition Working Group. (2001). Biomarkers and surrogate endpoints: Preferred definitions and conceptual framework. *Clinical Pharmacology and Therapeutics, 69,* 89–95. doi:10.1067/mcp.2001.113989

National Institutes of Health National Human Genome Research Institute. (2010). Glossary of genetic terms. Retrieved from http://www.genome.gov/glossary

Payne, J.K. (2006). The trajectory of biomarkers in symptom management for older adults with cancer. *Seminars in Oncology Nursing, 22,* 31–35.

Pelchat, M.L., Bykowski, C., Duke, F.F., & Reed, D.R. (2010). Excretion and perception of a characteristic odor in urine after asparagus ingestion: A psychophysical and genetic study. *Chemical Senses, 36,* 9–17. doi:10.1093/chemse/bjq081

Petrucelli, N., Lazebnik, N., Huelsman, K.M., & Lazebnik, R.S. (2002). Clinical interpretation and recommendations for patients with variants of uncertain significance in BRCA1 or BRCA2: A survey of genetic counseling practice. *Genetic Testing, 6,* 107–113. doi:10.1089/10906570260199357

Richards, J.E., & Hawley, R.S. (2011). *The human genome: A user's guide* (3rd ed.). Burlington, MA: Elsevier Academic Press.

Rodriguez-Paredes, M., & Esteller, M. (2011). Cancer epigenetics reaches mainstream oncology. *Nature Medicine, 17,* 330–339. doi:10.1038/nm.2305

Silviera, M.L., Smith, B.P., Powell, J., & Sapienza, C. (2012). Epigenetic differences in normal colon mucosa of cancer patients suggest altered dietary metabolic pathways. *Cancer Prevention Research, 5,* 374–384. doi:10.1158/1940-6207.CAPR-11-0336

Skirton, H., & Patch, C. (2002). The family history. In A. Bosher (Ed.), *Genetics for healthcare professionals* (pp. 15–21). Oxford, UK: BIOS Scientific Publishers Ltd.

Tavernier, D. (2009). The genogram: Enhancing student appreciation of family genetics. *Journal of Nursing Education, 48*, 222–225. doi:10.3928/01484834-20090401-10

U.S. Department of Energy Genome Program. (2008, September 19). How many genes are in the human genome? Retrieved from http://www.ornl.gov/sci/techresources/Human_Genome/faq/genenumber.shtml

U.S. Department of Energy Genome Program. (2011, September 19). Medicine and the new genetics. Retrieved from http://www.ornl.gov/sci/techresources/Human_Genome/medicine/medicine.shtml

Zhang, Y., Lan, Q., Rothman, N., Zhu, Y., Zahm, S.H., Wang, S.S., … Zheng, T. (2005). A putative exonic splicing polymorphism in the BCL6 gene and the risk of non-Hodgkin lymphoma. *Journal of the National Cancer Institute, 97*, 1616–1618. doi:10.1093/jnci/dji344

CHAPTER 7

Nursing in Genetics

Kristi L. Wiggins, MSN, RN, ANP-BC, AOCNP®, CCRC

Introduction

The art of nursing practice involves genetics. Although they may not be aware of it, nurses use genetics every day to obtain family histories, review diagnoses, and educate patients on treatment plans. Nurses and advanced practice registered nurses (APRNs) are expected to recognize and classify a patient's cancer risk, develop treatment strategies based on risk, and apply individualized prevention measures. This brave new world forces us to consider the patient as an individual in more intricate ways than we ever dreamed. The future of genetics is now.

Academic Programs and Continuing Education

The expectation for nurses to apply genetic knowledge to their practice is growing. Keeping up with advances is complicated. How does one start when few nursing programs offer a distinctive focus in genetics education (Beery & Hern, 2004)?

Nursing professionals focus on formal education, not just training. Training typically applies to short-term, focused learning. Education, on the other hand, contributes to formal learning that leads to changes in practice behaviors. Formal nursing education applies evidence-based models to structure learning based on performance standards. Nurses need to apply and practice what they know, as well as implement effective clinical research. For the future health of patients and the success of the healthcare system, nurses must examine the gaps in knowledge and begin to bridge them. The application of genetic knowledge will strengthen nursing practice as nurses collaborate with scientists, clinicians, and laypersons to move toward more successful care. Nurses are in a strategic position to be the thought leaders in their respective institutions. Knowledge of genetics will grow in everyday clinical practice as nurses are educated and subsequently provide proactive training to those with whom they work (Stolovich & Keeps, 2002).

Curriculum changes in nursing historically have been slow. Consider the discovery of the DNA double helix in 1953. More than 40 years ago, it was recommended that nurses have genetic education. Twenty years elapsed before Wendy J. Fibison, PhD, published a review (Fibison, 1983) of the role of nursing in genetics. She denoted the clinical activities of a clinical nurse specialist in genetics, including patient care, research, education of healthcare professionals, and implementing change in nursing practice related to genetics. In 2005, only about 15% of nursing programs offered basic genetics education. Education has improved since that time, but it still lags far behind what is expected of nurses in the genomic era. A survey conducted in 2005 showed that genetics and genomics curricula was only offered in about one-third of all nursing programs in the United States, and there was marginal increase in the genomic content of nursing courses over the previous nine years (Jenkins & Calzone, 2007).

A significant amount of literature is now available to support the necessity of genetics knowledge in nursing and advanced clinician education. Growth in this area is vital to improving patient outcomes as technologic advances rapidly march forward (Burke & Kirk, 2006). Nursing school faculty are expected to include genetics and genomics content into nursing programs at all levels. The Essential Nursing Competencies and Curricula Guidelines for Genetics and Genomics currently include data applicable to doctoral, master's, and baccalaureate programs. These Essentials were published in 2006, 2008, and 2010, respectively. However, research is necessary to evaluate the effectiveness of genetics education strategies to substantiate the successful integration of genetics and genomics education in undergraduate and graduate nursing curricula in the United States (American Association of Colleges of Nursing, 2008, 2011; Consensus Panel on Genetic/Genomic Nursing Competencies, 2009).

Today, nearly all academic nursing programs have some genetic component, usually in the form of focused lectures, but few have a genetics course, and even fewer have a genetics focus as part of a degree program. Genetic and pharmacogenomic discoveries are being brought to light daily as research moves forward. So, why has the development of nursing education in genetics been so difficult? Nursing education is demanding, and it seems nearly impossible to attain the necessary requisite courses to complete a degree program. Therefore, inserting yet another course seems overwhelming. Focus is often placed on improving the current core curricula, so a genomics-related course may be perceived as less important. Most schools of nursing lack faculty that have the genetics/genomics knowledge to teach a full course on the subject. It is difficult to find placement for clinical genetics experiences (Horner, 2004; Horner, Abel, Taylor, & Sands, 2004; Williams, 2002).

Despite the aforementioned difficulties, some schools of nursing have excelled at implementing genetics into their curricula. For instance, the University of Pittsburgh developed and incorporated the first genetics course offered as part of their baccalaureate degree program in 2001. Since that time, schools have begun to offer genetics as part of their undergraduate and graduate programs, mostly by integrating the biology of genetics into their existing science courses. Others have risen to the occasion by offering post-graduate certificates in genetics and making genetics a key focus in advanced practice nursing programs (Beery & Hern, 2004). The National Institute of Nursing Research (NINR), as part of the National Institutes of Health (NIH), made a landmark decision to provide funding to support the first post-doctoral nursing fellowship in clinical genetics nursing research at the University of Iowa. The program emphasizes collaboration between nursing and health science researchers to further genetics scholarship and research (University of Iowa College of Nursing, 2011). See Table 7-1 for many of the well-established "genetics in nursing" programs currently being offered in the United States.

Schools of nursing are now being expected to implement genetics information into their curricula. If it is not possible to develop a completely genetics-based course, then at minimum, schools are being asked to incorporate genetics principles within

Table 7-1. Nursing Genetics Programs Offered in the United States

Academic Program	Education Level	Focus
Clemson University www.clemson.edu/hehd/ departments/nursing/academics/ degrees/phd.html	Doctoral degree	The first interdisciplinary PhD, with core courses in genetics, healthcare genetics, psychology, political science, and policy. Three tracks are available: Intervention- ists, Bench Science, and Ethics and Health Policy.
Columbia University http://sklad.cumc.columbia.edu/ nursing/academics/genAdvPrac .php	Master's degree	Genetics in Advanced Practice Sub-Spe- cialty is designed for nurses in a master's program in nursing who wish to develop expertise in working with families at risk for or with genetic disorders.
University of California, San Francisco http://nurseweb.ucsf.edu/www/ genomic.htm	Master's degree	Centered on accelerated translation of discoveries in basic genetic science into clinical practice. Three dual-specialty programs are available in advanced prac- tice nursing: Cardiovascular/Genomics, Oncology/Genomics, and Gerontology/ Genomics.
University of Iowa www.medicine.uiowa.edu/ humangenetics/postdoc	Doctoral fellowship	Psychosocial aspects of genetic testing, biobehavioral research, population-based surveillance, ethics, and minority popula- tion use of genetic services
	Doctoral degree	Genetics PhD program individualized to the academic goals of the student
University of Pittsburgh www.nursing.pitt.edu	Doctoral fellowship	Focal area of research includes genetics applications in nursing care focusing on molecular genetics and psychosocial implications.
	Post-master's DNP	Standard DNP program is expanded upon through cognates within selected areas of focus.
University of Washington http://nursing.uw.edu/academic -services/degree-programs.html	Doctoral degree Master's degree	Both degrees allow students to create their own research interest.

existing science courses (Read, Dylis, Mott, & Fairchild, 2004). To grow in genetics knowledge, nurses must also be provided with genetics resources, such as local agen- cies and genetics counselors who are involved in genetic screening and care. Students are beginning to request clinical experiences to incorporate their genetics knowl- edge in the clinical setting (Hetteburg & Prows, 2004). So, how does a nursing school begin to make this necessary knowledge available to all nurses in their programs?

In addition to integrating genetics into core curriculum courses, an elective course in genetics is a logical strategy. Undergraduate and graduate nurses should be taught basic genetic science, patterns of inheritance, pedigree construction, genetic risk as- sessment, and how to conduct and/or refer for genetic testing. Students will apply these concepts to identify common genetic-based disorders, consider pharmacoge nomic implications, and think critically about the ethical, legal, and social issues related to genetic testing and protected health information (Horner et al., 2004). Teaching strategies may include the following: didactic presentations, case studies, educational videos, examination of past and current research, discussion of clinical applications, and guest lectures by genetics experts. Web-based modules or digitally saved course materials provide additional formats for class interaction and learning online. Formal presentations and papers developed by individual students allow for the synthesis of literature on various genetic topics (Horner, 2004; Williams, 2002). Williams (2002) recommends that schools offer a post-master's certification in ge netics and encourage advanced practice nurses to attend the Summer Genetics In stitute at NIH geared toward doctoral scholars.

For new curricula to function well, interesting subject matter is essential. Pro grams must have educated and engaging instructors and provide adequate support and positive reinforcement, as many of the students involved in this area of study are new to the material. Students must be encouraged to interact with one another and seek out genetics resources. They must also be allowed autonomy and provided with opportunities for clinical application and practice (Horner, 2004; Seibert, 2008).

The road to successful implementation of new genetics education includes use ful practice guidelines. The effectiveness of genetic information must be evaluated and validated. As care providers, nurses will examine how genomics technology, in formation, and interventions influence patient and healthcare outcomes. In 2010, the American Nurses Association (ANA) updated its *Scope and Standards of Nursing Practice* by which all nurses are to engage in consistent professional role activities. *Es sentials of Genetic and Genomic Nursing: Competencies, Curricula Guidelines, and Outcome Indicators* (referred to hereafter as the Essentials) regarding genetics and genomics was updated in 2009. These essentials provide guidelines to measure the success of implementing genetic information that impacts nursing practice (Consensus Panel on Genetic/Genomic Nursing Competencies, 2009). See Figure 7-1 for an outline of the professional responsibilities and professional practice domains.

Professional Responsibilities

All registered nurses are expected to engage in professional role activities that are consistent with *Nursing: Scope and Standards of Practice* (2004) by the American Nurses Association. In addition, competent nursing practice now requires the incorporation of genetic and genomic knowledge and skills in order to:

• Recognize when one's own attitudes and values related to genetic and genomic science may affect care provided to clients.
• Advocate for clients' access to desired genetic/genomic services and/or resources including sup port groups.
• Examine competency of practice on a regular basis, identifying areas of strength, as well as areas in which professional development related to genetics and genomics would be beneficial.
• Incorporate genetic and genomic technologies and information into registered nurse practice.
• Demonstrate in practice the importance of tailoring genetic and genomic information and services to clients based on their culture, religion, knowledge level, literacy, and preferred language.
• Advocate for the rights of all clients for autonomous, informed genetic- and genomic-related deci sion-making and voluntary action.

Figure 7-1. Consensus Panel on Genetic/Genomic Nursing Competencies Essential Competencies

---

(Continued on next page)

Professional Practice Domain
Nursing Assessment: Applying/Integrating Genetic and Genomic Knowledge
The registered nurse:
- Demonstrates an understanding of the relationship of genetics and genomics to health, prevention, screening, diagnostics, prognostics, selection of treatment, and monitoring of treatment effectiveness.
- Demonstrates ability to elicit a minimum of three-generation family health history information.
- Constructs a pedigree from collected family history information using standardized symbols and terminology.
- Collects personal, health, and developmental histories that consider genetic, environmental, and genomic influences and risks.
- Conducts comprehensive health and physical assessments which incorporate knowledge about genetic, environmental, and genomic influences and risk factors.
- Critically analyzes the history and physical assessment findings for genetic, environmental, and genomic influences and risk factors.
- Assesses clients' knowledge, perceptions, and responses to genetic and genomic information.
- Develops a plan of care that incorporates genetic and genomic assessment information.

Identification
The registered nurse:
- Identifies clients who may benefit from specific genetic and genomic information and/or services based on assessment data.
- Identifies credible, accurate, appropriate, and current genetic and genomic information, resources, services, and/or technologies specific to given clients.
- Identifies ethical, ethnic/ancestral, cultural, religious, legal, fiscal, and societal issues related to genetic and genomic information and technologies.
- Defines issues that undermine the rights of all clients for autonomous, informed genetic- and genomic-related decision-making and voluntary action.

Referral Activities
The registered nurse:
- Facilitates referrals for specialized genetic and genomic services for clients as needed.

Provision of Education, Care, and Support
The registered nurse:
- Provides clients with interpretation of selective genetic and genomic information or services.
- Provides clients with credible, accurate, appropriate, and current genetic and genomic information, resources, services, and/or technologies that facilitate decision-making.
- Uses health promotion/disease prevention practices that:
  - Consider genetic and genomic influences on personal and environmental risk factors.
  - Incorporate knowledge of genetic and/or genomic risk factors (e.g., a client with a genetic predisposition for high cholesterol who can benefit from a change in lifestyle that will decrease the likelihood that the genetic risk will be expressed).
- Uses genetic- and genomic-based interventions and information to improve clients' outcomes.
- Collaborates with healthcare providers in providing genetic and genomic health care.
- Collaborates with insurance providers/payers to facilitate reimbursement for genetic and genomic healthcare services.
- Performs interventions/treatments appropriate to clients' genetic and genomic healthcare needs.
- Evaluates impact and effectiveness of genetic and genomic technology, information, interventions, and treatments on clients' outcome.

Figure 7-1. Consensus Panel on Genetic/Genomic Nursing Competencies Essential Competencies *(Continued)*

Note. From *Essentials of Genetic and Genomic Nursing: Competencies, Curricula Guidelines, and Outcome Indicators* (2nd ed., pp. 11–13), by the Consensus Panel on Genetic/Genomic Nursing Competencies, 2009, Bethesda, MD: American Nurses Association. Copyright 2009 by the American Nurses Association. Reprinted with permission.

In October 2008, Thompson and Brooks (2010) performed a convenience sample survey (N = 47) at a national nursing conference to estimate the number of nurses who had knowledge of the Essentials. The majority of those who responded to the survey were nursing school faculty. Their findings revealed that only 36% of respondents knew what the Essentials were and had read them. Less than 30% had received any kind of genetics/genomics continuing education. Those who had knowledge of the Essentials had a direct correlation with those who have had recent continuing genetics education. Although the sample size was small, the results demonstrated that most nurses are not familiar with the competencies related to genetics information. Educators may not be passing this information on to their students. The more genetics/genomics information is disseminated, the more nurses will begin to comprehend the guidelines, incorporate the knowledge into practice, and become more confident in providing genomic information to others. The complexities of our current healthcare delivery system require nurses, even at the baccalaureate level, to be highly educated. Nurses at all education and practice levels are expected to provide competent care incorporating genomics that will improve patient safety and health outcomes in the clinical setting.

Competencies

Recognizing the need for competent clinical genomic care, ANA, the American Medical Association, and the National Human Genome Research Institute (NHGRI) created an initiative to promote professional education about advances in genetics beginning in 1996. They created an organization called the National Coalition for Health Professional Education in Genetics (NCHPEG). Today, more than 100 professional organizations participate in the vision of NCHPEG. One of the primary goals of this initiative is to recommend and establish core competencies for all healthcare professionals (NCHPEG, 2001). NCHPEG strongly believes that anyone working in a health-related field should have a basic understanding of genetics and genomics (NCHPEG, 2007). Additional goals of NCHPEG are to (Consensus Panel on Genetic/Genomic Nursing Competencies, 2009; Greco & Salveson, 2009)
- Influence integration of genetics into certification and licensing examinations
- Develop useful and accessible Web information
- Develop potential clinical tools such as a family history collection tool
- Influence the availability of useful genetic resources.

Credentialing

Heralding the importance of genetics and genomics in nursing is the International Society of Nurses in Genetics (ISONG). ISONG has continued to be instrumental in fostering collaboration across all disciplines in health care with NCHPEG while being a strong advocate for nurses in genetics. ISONG developed the Genetic Nursing Credentialing Commission (GNCC) to provide the first credentialing examination for nurses in the specialty of genetics. Credentialing was developed to prove that an individual has the minimum level of genetic knowledge, performance, and interdisciplinary collaboration, as well as adherence to client privacy.

Nurses holding a baccalaureate degree with genetics nursing experience may qualify for the Genetics Clinical Nurse (GCN) credential. Those with a master's degree or higher may qualify for the Advanced Practice Nurse in Genetics (APNG) credential. GNCC grants these respective credentials based upon a portfolio of evidence, including genetics-related experiences of the applicant. Details pertaining to these portfolios can be found online at www.geneticnurse.org. For additional options in genetics nursing certification and continuing education, see Figure 7-2.

American Nurses Association (ANA)
Scope and Standards: "The International Society of Nurses in Genetics (ISONG) and ANA publish newly revised *Genetics/Genomics Nursing: Scope and Standards of Practice":* www.nursingworld .org/FunctionalMenuCategories/MediaResources/PressReleases/2006/pr1121068570.aspx
ANA Nursing World: www.nursingworld.org
American Society of Clinical Oncology
The Genetics of Cancer
www.cancer.net/patient/All+About+Cancer/Genetics/The+Genetics+of+Cancer
American Society of Human Genetics
Professional organization for human genetics specialists
www.ashg.org
Atlas of Genetics and Cytogenetics in Oncology and Haematology
Peer-reviewed online journal
http://atlasgeneticsoncology.org
Centers for Disease Control and Prevention National Office of Public Health Genomics Human Genome Project HuGENeT™ (Human Genome Epidemiology Network)
Epidemiologic aspects of human genes
www.cdc.gov/genomics/hugenet/default.htm
EthnoMed
Cultural and social factors affecting health in selected ethnic groups
http://ethnomed.org
Gene Test Organization
An advertising-supported resource for consumers regarding the availability of genetic testing
www.genetest.org
Genetic Alliance
Nonprofit health advocacy organization that promotes health through genetics
www.geneticalliance.org
HUM-MOLGEN (Germany)
Interactive international Listserv promoting collaboration, news, literature reviews, biotechnology
www.hum-molgen.de
International Society of Nurses in Genetics
International professional organization for nurses who specialize in genetics
www.isong.org
National Cancer Institute
www.cancer.gov
Genetics Gateway: www.cancer.gov/cancertopics/genetics
Risk Assessment Information: www.cancer.gov/cancertopics/pdq/genetics/risk-assessment-and-counseling/HealthProfessional
National Coalition for Health Professional Education in Genetics
An "organization of organizations" that promotes health education
www.nchpeg.org
National Conference of State Legislatures Genetics Overview
Addresses technologies and law
www.ncsl.org/IssuesResearch/Helaht/GeneticTechnologiesProject/tabid/14524/Default.aspx

---

Figure 7-2. Genetics Nursing Resources

(Continued on next page)

National Genetics Education and Development Centre (United Kingdom)
Learners and educators resource for activities to undertake in clinical practice; videos, PowerPoint®, case presentations)
www.geneticseducation.nhs.uk

National Institutes of Health
Genetics/Genomics Competency Center for Education: www.g-2-c-2.org
Bioethics Resources on the Web: http://bioethics.od.nih.gov
Genetics Home Reference (Contains general information about genetic counseling, genetic testing, gene therapy, and the Human Genome Project): http://ghr.nlm.nih.gov
National Human Genome Research Institute (NHGRI): www.genome.gov
Online Mendelian Inheritance in Man (OMIM) (This database is a catalog of human genes and genetic disorders): www.ncbi.nlm.nih.gov/omim
Secretary's Advisory Committee on Genetics, Health, and Society (archived material): http://oba.od.nih.gov/sacghs/sacghs_home.html

National Society of Genetic Counselors
Professional association
www.nsgc.org

Oncology Nursing Society
www.ons.org
Genetics Clinical Resource Area: www.ons.org/ClinicalResources/Genetics
Cancer Genetics 101 Web course: www.ons.org/CourseDetail.aspx?course_id=98
Genetics and Genomics in Oncology Nursing Practice: The latest text by editors Kathleen Calzone, Agnes Masny, and Jean Jenkins and a group of expert authors broadens the topic of genetics from a discussion of risk assessment to encompass such issues as cancer biology, clinical applications of genetic study, and the scope of oncology nursing practice. Order online at http://esource.ons.org/ProductDetails.aspx?sku=INPU0585

Thomas, The U.S. Library of Congress on the Internet
www.thomas.gov

University of Kansas Medical Center
Clinical, research, and educational resources for genetic counselors, clinical geneticists, and medical geneticists
www.kumc.edu/gec/geneinfo.html

U.S. Department of Energy (DOE) Genomics Web Sites
http://genomics.energy.gov
DOE Joint Human Genome Institute: www.jgi.doe.gov
Human Genome Project Information: www.ornl.gov/sci/techresources/Human_Genome/home.shtml

U.S. Surgeon General's Family History Initiative
www.hhs.gov/familyhistory

Figure 7-2. Genetics Nursing Resources *(Continued)*

Training and Continuing Education in Genetics

In addition to providing credentialing for nurses with a specialty in genetics, ISONG provides resources on human genetics for anyone in nursing practice. ISONG "is a global nursing specialty organization dedicated to fostering the scientific and professional growth of nurses in human genetics and genomics worldwide. The ISONG vision is: caring for people's genetic and genomic health" (ISONG, 2010).

ISONG provides continuing education and research activities. The organization also provides forums for professional networking and discussions, as well as open access to all of the educational materials offered online. The ISONG Web site contains links to professional practice, research, research grants, and educational resources.

The Oncology Nursing Society (ONS) is the largest professional oncology group in the United States composed of more than 35,000 nurses and other allied health professionals. ONS promotes excellence in oncology nursing and quality health care to individuals affected by cancer. As part of its mission, ONS upholds a strong commitment to advocacy for the public good.

Because of the impact of genetics and genomics in oncology, ONS has made a concerted effort to provide educational opportunities for oncology nurses in genetics. Oncology continues to be the flagship for genetics knowledge, testing, and technology. ONS embraced this concept and began preparing for the genomic era more than 20 years ago.

To address the continuing advancement of genetic science and the increased responsibility of the oncology nurse, ONS developed position statements regarding oncology genetics: Cancer Predisposition Genetic Testing and Risk Assessment Counseling, and The Role of the Oncology Nurse in Cancer Genetic Counseling. These and other informative position statements can be found online at www.ons.org/Publications/Positions (ONS, 2010a).

Current educational offerings include an online genetics education series that reviews the following: basic introduction to genetics, DNA mutations and DNA repair, chromosome abnormalities, patterns of inheritance, genetic basis of cancer, gene regulation, genetic testing, therapies based on genetic information, and current uses of DNA technologies. In 2010, ONS published an updated comprehensive genetics book titled *Genetics and Genomics in Oncology Nursing Practice.* Current ONS disease-specific publications include genetic information for the basis of respective cancers and indications for genetic testing. The Oncology Nursing Certification Corporation includes a genetic component in all oncology nursing certification examinations.

The ONS Cancer Genetics Special Interest Group (SIG) is an extensive resource for oncology nurses with a specialty in genetics, or those with an earnest desire to learn more about genetic science in the world of oncology. Membership in the SIG is free with the ONS national membership. Many tools are available on the Cancer Genetics SIG page on the ONS Web site (www.ons.org), including research articles, genetic testing resources, posting of healthcare-related activities in Washington, DC, informational videos, and links to other professional genetics organizations. ONS leads the way in promoting oncology nursing professionalism and continues to take us forward into the exciting era of genetics and genomics (ONS Cancer Genetics SIG, 2011).

NIH, in collaboration with the Human Genome Project, has developed a wide range of Web site resources, not just for scientists but for the general public, educators, and healthcare providers. The NIH Genetics Home Reference page (http://ghr.nlm.nih.gov/Resources/education) has links to references for online education kits, basic information on understanding the human genome, and tips for giving presentations on genetics (NIH, 2011a). The Human Genome Project provides online access to an extensive glossary of genetic-related terms, instructions on how to take a family history, and free PowerPoint® presentations for educators (www.genome.gov/10000002). Topics including forensics, behavioral genetics, and genetic diseases and disorders are also covered. NHGRI is motivated to share genetic information, most of which can be accessed through their site map at www.genome.gov/sitemap.cfm (NHGRI, 2011b). They also have a glossary, as well as a webinar series and information on careers in genetics.

Future Trends in Oncology Practice

Nurses are on the front lines using genetic information every day. Current roles are already being challenged with the transformations in the way treatments are prescribed, how efficacy is evaluated, and how risk for toxicity is predicted. Future jobs in clinical practice, healthcare education, and research will continue to grow and change as the climate for personalized medicine responds to the necessity of individualized care.

The majority of nurses currently involved in genetics clinical care are advanced practice or advanced degree nurses. This trend is likely to continue, but expected competencies in genetics are being implemented at every level of nursing education and practice setting (Lea et al., 2006). Although oncology is a primary forerunner of genetic research and personalized therapy, soon it will be the expectation of every healthcare specialty to be well versed in genetics. Ample opportunities already exist in the current job market for nurses in genetics.

The non-oncology specialties of school nursing and family practice benefit from genetic nursing expertise by performing health screenings and evaluating family histories to identify potential genetic-related health concerns. Being aware of common genetic syndromes and finding trends in family health issues provides the first step in providing individualized care (National Cancer Institute, 2011). Educating the public through this type of interaction is paramount. Most people are not aware of the role genes play in most diseases, how genes are shared between parents and siblings, and the limitations of current genetic testing. With genetic awareness, nurses working in these specialties will be able to make the appropriate referrals for genetics counseling and testing as well as provide valuable education and guidance as to necessary screening and health maintenance activities (Christianson et al., 2010).

Perinatal and pediatric nurses are involved in genetics in a variety of ways. They provide genetic screening before, during, and after a child's birth. Expectant families are evaluated for possible genetic syndromes through family history. Knowledge of genetics is key in identifying potential genetic mutation carriers that need additional screening and potential testing. This knowledge also provides an opportunity for the nurse to discuss potential risks for the parent and for the offspring (Cook, 2003). In addition to a family history, nurses gather important information regarding maternal age, tobacco use, diet, alcohol consumption, illicit drug use, medications, chemical exposures, and immunizations. These items exclusively, or in addition to a known genetic risk, can impact the genetic development of a fetus as well as offspring throughout childhood. These nurses are responsible for providing the appropriate education regarding these risk factors and making a referral for genetic counseling when deemed appropriate (Dolan, Biermann, & Damus, 2007).

Industry and private companies already employ the expertise of nurses. Consider the benefit of having a highly skilled genetics nurse who could serve as a liaison or case manager for insurance companies, managed care, and health systems auditors. As health care in the United States adjusts to legal reforms, nurses who embrace the business culture may opt to take their clinical skills to the world of managed care to provide a unique perspective on oncology nursing and genetics to navigate reasonable care for patients (Pulcini, Mason, Cohen, Kovner, & Leavitt, 2000). Pharmaceutical and biotechnology companies have benefited from nurses as educators and as an integral connection with health systems, providers, and the public. This practice is likely to continue, but with the upsurge in targeted therapies, nurses will need genetics knowledge to provide optimal education and leadership in this role. Nurses desiring to conduct research may appeal to pharmaceutical companies for funding to support clinical trials in genetics. However, nurses acting as the principal investigator on privately sponsored research protocols must apprise themselves of potential conflicts of interest in this type of venture (Rosenzweig, Bender, & Brufsky, 2005).

The traditional oncology roles of home care and hospice nursing are also changing. Home care provides the prime opportunity to perform risk assessments on the patient and family. Encouraging routine cancer screenings should be an integral part of every patient visit. Even a patient being seen for a nonmalignant condition may benefit by having a nurse that can identify at-risk individuals. People receiving the appropriate education and interventions are given an opportunity to lessen their risk for cancer and other diseases (Smith-Stoner & Veitz, 2008). For instance, a patient is seen in the home for postoperative wound care. The patient is a smoker. The nurse understands that genetic changes occur when lung tissue is exposed to tobacco smoke, increasing the risk of lung cancer. It is also known that smoking increases the risk of deep vein thrombosis postoperatively. By providing education and promoting smoking cessation, the nurse potentially can help the patient avoid future lung cancer, as well as other pulmonary and cardiovascular complications.

Hospice nurses are highly skilled in providing psychosocial support along with clinical care. This unique position provides opportunities to discuss genetics with hospice patients and family members by providing psychosocial support. Education on the etiology of cancer, with or without a known genetic abnormality, can provide useful knowledge to families. Often, families seek to clarify known and suspected risks and how this might impact surviving family members as it relates to their state of health and health maintenance. Promoting routine cancer screening for family and friends of the patient should be a part of this role. Hospice nurses understand the importance of genetic information in this setting but are not confident in taking the lead on explaining genetics or implementing genetics-oriented care (Metcalf, Pumphrey, & Clifford, 2010; Smith-Stoner & Veitz, 2008).

With the increasing healthcare demands of an aging population and a decreasing number of medical school graduates choosing oncology as a specialty, nurse practitioners and clinical nurse specialists in oncology are finding themselves with growing responsibilities. Opportunities to cultivate the genetic nurse role in disease-specific specialty clinics are emerging. Nurses and APRNs working in these clinics are already exposed to genetic testing and genetically directed therapies. As in primary care, nurses should evaluate the family history, perform cancer risk screening, genetic screening, conduct high-risk surveillance, make referrals for genetic counseling, and provide cancer prevention education (Kelly, 2009).

Often, APRNs also provide genetic counseling and facilitate genetic testing when indicated. They provide education regarding the need for testing, how the results may be interpreted, and the psychosocial and clinical implications for the patient, as well as other family members. They must be prepared to discuss the impact of genetic results on potential offspring (Lea et al., 2006).

Individuals with advanced knowledge in clinical genetics will be the leaders that provide specialized genetic information to nurses (Lea et al., 2006). Nurses educate patients and families as well as each other. Academic nursing education is still sorely lacking in genetic information, but this is changing. As noted previously, more and more nursing programs are integrating genetics into existing courses, creating new courses, and in some cases developing programs with a specialty in genetics for nurses. As these programs continue to grow, there will be an increasing demand for educators on the academic playing field. Nursing schools in the United States are already experiencing a shortage of faculty (Calzone et al., 2010). Motivated nurses must seek education, and in turn, educate.

Whether in academics or clinical practice, ample opportunity exists for nursing research in genetics. There is a great need to study education, the content and methods for nurses, so that genomic practice guidelines can be established. Research is needed to provide effective ways to promote and manage genetic nursing practice. Proof is needed to support the notion that genetic knowledge in nursing practice improves patient outcomes and patient safety. Guidelines are also needed for education of interdisciplinary staff, patients, families, and the general public. Nurses need to explore how to best connect with individuals interested in genetic testing and those who are not interested but would benefit from it (Calzone et al., 2010).

Research involves clinical trials. Nurses with a specialty in genetics are in a unique position to manage clinical trials involving targeted therapeutic agents. Clinical trials responsibilities in the genomic era include providing genetic education for families and patients; understanding and teaching the indications, risks, and benefits of targeted agents; possible clinical outcomes; and managing patients' care as they proceed with treatment. Nurses excel in supportive care. New research projects may be built around symptom etiology and treatment based on personalized genomic information. A need also exists for psychosocial research on decision making related to genetic testing, to do it or not, and the impact of test results (Burns & Grove, 2009). Further examination is needed on how the general public views genetic information and how they use it. Some assume that genetic information may change patient behavior, but clinical trials have not yet proven this theory. Research can provide insight into how to best approach genetics with patients to optimize their health and affect future healthcare goals. Behavioral research is an integral facet of research complementing the basic science of genetics. There is a world of possibilities in genetic nursing research.

Basic science research is where some genetics nurses and APRNs are finding their niche. Basic genetic science includes direct analysis of gene arrays to look for mutations or patterns in sequencing. Basic genetic science also evaluates the uniqueness of one's genome by looking for the single nucleotide polymorphisms (SNPs) that affect metabolism of medications or nutrients and how these affect symptoms or individual treatment outcomes. A few examples of the types of basic genetic research in which nurses are involved include inflammatory and cardiovascular markers that identify risk for cardiovascular events, the impact of gene expression in solid organ transplant recipients and risk of rejection, and epigenetics involving breast cancer (Loescher & Merkle, 2005).

Epigenetics is a growing field in basic genetic science. Literally translated, *epigenetics* means "above the genes." This type of gene research evaluates changes in phenotype, or appearance, of an organism. However, there is no change in genotype. More scientists are attempting to find out how these changes occur without observable genetic changes. Genes are "expressed" differently at different times, without a change in the gene sequence. Most scientists agree that this change in expression is influenced by environmental factors. Consider identical human twins, almost indistinguishable in early life. As they age, they may begin to look different from each other, and often develop different health problems, but continue to have identical DNA. These differences are attributed to epigenetic influences (Davis & Milner, 2004).

Proteomics is the combined study of proteins and genomics. Study involves the entire complement of proteins existing or produced by an organism. Scientists are researching ways to identify proteins produced by normal and abnormal cells. This technology is already being used and is continuing to grow. One common example is immunohistochemistry that is used in staining for positive cancer cells. Proteins expressed by malignant cells take up specific stains in a pathology specimen. Other examples are the Western blot test and mass spectrometry. Oncology researchers use proteins to look for new targets in cancer cell protein production and try to develop new methods for halting the growth of cancer cells (Davis & Milner, 2004).

Nutrigenomics is the combined study of nutrition or nutrients and the genome. The purpose of this field is to take a closer look at the molecular activities of the body and how nutrients are used. All individuals differ somewhat in how they absorb, metabolize, and eliminate different nutrients. This goes back to how SNPs create differences within a specific genome, even though the differences are often not harmful. Some scientists are focusing on how to tailor individual diets to fight disease, such as how certain foods reduce cholesterol. Epidemiology and physiology are still key in monitoring the prevalence and incidence of diseases, but nutrigenomics hopes to provide insight from within the genome. As nurses, we often counsel patients on how diet modification may be needed during cancer therapy, how certain foods or supplements affect medications, or simply counseling on diet for health maintenance. Nutrigenomics will likely play a large role on how future counseling is conducted, based on an individual's genomic information (Davis & Milner, 2004).

In the current clinical model, individuals are proactively treated for risk factors related to type II diabetes and cardiovascular disease. At part of the interdisciplinary oncology team, nurses should work toward the same paradigm in cancer care.

Collaboration Versus Controversy in Genetic Counseling

The increasing demand for genetic services in clinical practice will increase the need to develop new models of care to expand and provide genetic-based care. Nurse practitioners with clinical genetics and oncology backgrounds will be sought after as these services grow.

There are not enough genetic clinicians to support the demand for genetic-focused care. On one hand is a lack of clinicians with in-depth knowledge of genetics to perform the necessary care. On the other hand is an issue of the financial commitment to support such clinicians. Even though nurse practitioners can bill for their services, they are often reimbursed at a lower fee than what a third-party contractor will pay. Medicare and Medicaid continue to reimburse for only 85% of what a medical doctor is reimbursed for the same care provided (Buppert, 2007). In community settings it is often the physician who bills for genetic counseling services. At larger centers, oncology genetic counselors often perform the genetic counseling and testing under the auspices of an attending physician, an oncology clinic, and/ or a hereditary cancer clinic. Thus, the salary for genetics counselors is taken from revenue generated by the physician billing for genetic services. Genetic counseling was not fully recognized as a subspecialty until after the year 2000. In 2006, the National Society of Genetic Counselors collaborated with the American Medical Association to develop a Medical Genetics and Genetic Counseling Services CPT® code. Therefore, genetic counseling has only been a billable service since January 1, 2007 (Harrison et al., 2010).

The National Nursing Centers Consortium has estimated that more than 50% of insurance companies now recognize nurse practitioners as primary care providers, and the number is growing. Before genetic counselors were allowed to bill for their services, this was seen as a potential threat to trained genetics counselors. Today's nurse practitioners can bill for clinical services, as well as genetics counseling, if they have the experience to perform this service. Even though more insurance companies are recognizing advanced practice nurses, allowing for equal reimbursement, the change is clearly not occurring quickly enough. Nurse practitioners provide comprehensive patient education and typically see their patients twice as often as physician providers. Research has proven that this type of care increases patient satisfaction, decreases patient visits to the emergency department, increases patient compliance, and thus, decreases hospitalizations and overall costs to the healthcare system (Mundinger et al., 2000).

Equal payment for equal work remains a point of contention with non-physician healthcare providers. Although different types of providers may do the work, the goals and outcomes are the same, if not often improved, compared to the traditional medical model of care. Recently approved healthcare legislation includes provisions for increased funding for nursing education, grants for advanced practice nurses, and funding for nurse-managed health centers (Donelan, Buerhaus, DesRoshes, & Burke, 2010). Nurse practitioners have historically worked with underserved populations in the community setting. With increased funding in this area, there are abundant opportunities to impact genetic education and counseling in this setting. Pilot programs are already under way to implement genetics services in rural areas (Buchanan et al., 2009). Patient demographics may be different in the rural setting, but their need for genetic information and care should be the same as those individuals being seen at metropolitan centers.

All providers in the genetic clinical world should work toward collaborative care for the most comprehensive plan for the individual patient. This is the only way personalized health care will thrive.

Ethical, Legal, and Social Issues

This exciting new era of genetics in nursing brings many opportunities and responsibilities. With the advent of new technology and discovery of new information, an abundance of ethical issues must be considered. As nurses' genetic knowledge grows, they will become expert patient educators and learn to efficiently interpret genetic information as it relates to the individual. They will also be expected to attain a higher level of ethical judgment (Kirk, 2000). In addition, genetics nurses will need to be able to interpret and apply healthcare policy appropriately. As a guideline for the genetic nursing professional, consider the precepts set forth by ISONG. These principles include but are not limited to patient privacy, informed consent, ethical practice guidelines, and gaining familiarity with legislation that affects clinical practice as it relates to genetic information. Detailed information is available on the ISONG Web site (www.isong.org/ISONG_PS_privacy_confidentiality.php).

All individuals are entitled to the right to privacy. Healthcare information for a patient cannot be shared without his or her written permission. This concept was incorporated in a proposed law as part of the Health Insurance Portability and Accountability Act of 1996 (HIPAA) (Williams, Skirton, & Masny, 2006). Having a law with set statutes provides clear guidance as to a patient's privacy and confidentiality rights, right? Well, it depends.

Effective July 1, 1997, the HIPAA law established that no one could be denied healthcare insurance based on preexisting medical and genetic conditions. It requires that insurance companies provide continuous coverage for an individual as long as continuous premiums are being paid, a guarantee for insurance policy renewal. It also provides coverage provisions for people who are changing employment, otherwise known as continuity and portability of insurance coverage. However, the law does not establish caps on premiums, so continuing to pay the premiums can become cost-prohibitive for a great number of patients. HIPAA does not protect patients who were enrolled in their current healthcare policy prior to July 1, 1997. HIPAA also does not protect policies that are provided to individuals by large, multistate, self-insured insurance companies (HIPAA, 1996; U.S. Department of Health and Human Services [DHHS], 2011).

Healthcare providers need to be apprised of the protections as well as gaps in the laws that are meant to protect and bear in mind these facts when conducting genetic risk assessment and counseling. This practice requires a good grasp of the ethical, legal, and social implications (often referred to as ELSI) that accompany the complexities of genetic information. How clinicians view genetics as well as their view of ethics affect how genetic information will be conveyed. Clinicians must consider the precepts of beneficence, nonmaleficence, autonomy, and justice. These ethical principles were set forth by the Belmont Report in 1974 to protect human research subjects (U.S. Food and Drug Administration, 2005).

This report not only guides the practices of institutional review boards in the United States but also can be applied to any clinical setting. Each tenet of the Belmont Report is important to ethical clinical practice. Beneficence is to show kindness. One must consider a patient's state of mind, education level, perception, expectations, and values associated with genetic information. Next is nonmaleficence, or "to do no harm." Clinicians must provide genetic information in a way that evaluates the risks and benefits of genetic testing and potential discovery of genetic abnormalities. Autonomy is to allow patients the freedom to choose and to make their own decisions. Genetic testing must be voluntary. Justice refers to equality. All individuals should have the right to genetic testing and to have the opportunity made available to them (NIH, 2011a).

Committing genetic information to memory is only the start. Knowing something is one thing, but choosing what to do with it becomes much more important. Try on your patient's shoes for a moment. What does the patient know about genetics and what does it mean to him or her? How interested is he or she in genetic information? Is the patient aware of the impact of results, for himself and for the family? Does the patient have access to and financial coverage for genetic testing? Does he or she fear discrimination from an employer or health insurance providers?

Providers of genomic care also have a duty to consider the potential ensuing ethical implications. Will patients be privy to all of their genetic information, even if we are uncertain of its current utility? Will genetic data be private or shared for the benefit of others? "Others" could be family members that may also be affected by a genetic finding, or "others" could be unrelated families that might benefit from research of a particular genetic finding. Will the individualized therapies be patented by companies, owned by patients, or regulated by healthcare providers?

With knowledge and compassion, we have a duty to provide genetic information to individuals whose health care is affected by this knowledge. Providers can no longer be complacent about learning and sharing genetic information with their patients. Although laws to protect genetic information lag far behind the technologic advances in genetics, lawmakers are focusing more and more on genetics. Eventually, providers will be held liable for not disclosing and incorporating genomic discoveries in the clinical setting that impact a patient's care (Calzone et al., 2010).

Direct-to-Consumer Marketing

One area of controversy related to the advance in personal genetic information is direct-to-consumer (DTC) marketing for genome testing. DTC marketing began in September 2008 when Myriad Genetics first opened the availability of *BRCA1/ BCRA2* gene tests for breast cancer to the general public. Although only 5%–10% of the population will use these tests, the demand will largely come from the low-risk populations. Most often the consumers will be curious individuals with the money to spend on such a test. Autonomy is an ethical precept, but with autonomy comes responsibility.

Consider the good that could come from DTC genetic testing. Results of such testing in the hands of knowledgeable healthcare providers could open up honest dialogue with patients. Providers could discuss the patient's current health, known risks, and health maintenance issues. Some patients may become more compliant with therapy if they think they are at higher risk for a certain problem, and if not, at least they have been informed of a potential risk and provided tools in which to combat that risk. Healthcare providers may be motivated more to educate themselves on the topic of genetic testing. However, responsibility with limited knowledge sets the stage for a multitude of harms (Loud, 2010).

Private companies such as deCODE, Progenix, 23andMe, and Navigenics are available to the public to perform a full genomic analysis for individuals, for a price. Consumers select themselves for testing without appropriate genetic counseling, predisposing them to confusion or false hope depending on their results. Each company has developed its own assay to do the genomic analysis. This presents issues with the objective versus subjective analysis of results. Individuals expect care providers to apply the answers each analysis may provide to their personal risk, diagnosis, screening, and treatment of known or anticipated diseases. Technology is amoral; it is we, the humans, who assign value to it. As healthcare providers, we must be aware of the value our patients assign to independent genetic testing (Lee & Crawley, 2009).

A great number of these tests have no clinical utility. They may over- or underestimate risk. Nurses must be aware that these tests are available and the possible implications for the information that is provided to patients. As the methods for genomic testing become easier, the cost will likely decrease, and more of the general public may opt to have this type of testing performed. On these assays, genes are often looked at as single entities to predict disease risk. Current science has proven that most genes work in concert to function properly and to cause genetic abnormalities that lead to disease, especially cancer. The function of genes is multifactorial. The American Society of Clinical Oncology (ASCO), ONS, the Society of Gynecologic Oncology, and the National Society of Genetic Counselors recommend pre- and post-gene testing counseling to address these issues. Patients need to be educated that knowledge is a moving target. Genome-wide testing assays are limited. The methodology for performing the tests will change; thus, the implications for the results of testing will change as technology progresses (ASCO, 2003). What may be true today will change tomorrow.

DTC genetic testing eliminates the opportunity for some individuals to be tested under the auspices of clinical trials by which standards of care could be developed for the future utilization of genetic testing. Most genetic testing is not regulated because of lack of third-party surveillance to ensure quality. An extra burden is placed upon healthcare providers to address unconfirmed tests, of which the risks and benefits are principally unknown. We are responsible for assessing our patients' risks, but this pushes assessment into a realm that currently has little clinical utility (Loud, 2010).

Policy and Protections

Policy cuts across all elements of the genetics and genomics field: resources, technology development, training, ELSI, and education. Policy also impacts how basic and applied research is prioritized. Policies govern legal issues, economics, education, and the acceptance and implementation of new technologies. Despite all this involvement and legislators' efforts to write laws to provide protections for patients, healthcare disparities continue to exist.

Privacy, Confidentiality, and the Duty to Warn

It is understood that genomic information affecting an individual's health must be shared with that individual. However, what if that information impacts the health care of other individuals? Is it ever ethical to disclose personal genetic information?

There are no strict laws at the federal level that govern disclosure of genetic information. However, HIPAA allows disclosure of any health information without the consent of the individual if the public is at risk as a result of withholding the information. HIPAA allows exceptions to the nondisclosure policy for the following reasons: "There is serious or imminent threat to the health or safety of a person or the public. The threat constitutes an imminent, serious threat to an identifiable third party. The physician has the capacity to avert significant harm" (DHHS, 2002).

Some individual states have case law pertaining to the duty to warn. States have the right to hear and make judgment on individual privacy cases related to disclosing health information. For instance, the Florida state court judged that a physician had the duty to warn a patient that her children were at risk of developing thyroid cancer so that the disease could have been detected and cured at an earlier age. This is an example of "duty to warn" family members when a patient has a hereditary risk of cancer that could affect the health of the other family members. In the United States, the consensus among care providers is that confidentiality be upheld regardless of the situation. What would you do if you had a patient who tested positive for a genetic mutation, and this person has an identical twin that will have the mutation as well? If patients are unwilling to share their genetic information with family members, and there is a known risk to others, nurses have an obligation to continue an open dialogue with the patient regarding the risks and benefits of disclosure. The goal is to encourage, not coerce. If the risk is imminent, the clinician has a duty to warn; however, there are no federal mandates on the issue, so the patient also has the right to sue (Offit, Groeger, Turner, Wadsworth, & Weiser, 2004). In state case law, thus far, the duty to warn has won out. ASCO has also taken a stand to support informing family members affected by genetic information so that they may benefit from genetic counseling and testing as well as the patient (DHHS, 2002).

When individuals participate in research that involves screening for genetic diseases, they are afforded the rights of privacy and confidentiality. Researchers are provided with a "Certificate of Confidentiality" through NIH. This exempts the researcher from revealing any research subject's identity (Offit, 1998).

Patients fear discrimination from their employer when considering genetic testing. There have been reports of employers using an employee's positive test for a genetic abnormality as grounds for termination or to deny life insurance (Lapham, Kozma, & Weiss, 1996). Patients considering testing must fully understand the risks and benefits of genetic testing and the potential implications before proceeding. Discrimination is still a factor that influences healthcare providers without a genetics specialty when referring patients for genetic testing (Lowstuter et al., 2008).

Genetic Information Nondiscrimination Act of 2008

The Genetic Information Nondiscrimination Act (GINA) is a federal law passed in May 2008 to provide patients protection against genetic discrimination regarding health insurance and employment. It extends the protections offered by HIPAA. The goal is to protect individuals desiring to take advantage of genetic testing, clinical trials, and targeted treatments in the hopes of attaining personalized medicine without fear of discrimination. It protects the privacy of those individuals undergoing genetic testing who may be at an increased risk for developing a genetically linked disease, such as colon cancer or Alzheimer disease. It also covers any pharmacogenomic testing, such as CYP450 analysis. GINA also protects any family history information a patient provides. However, GINA does not cover those individuals who may already be sick with a genetically linked disease. It does not protect those enlisted in the U.S. military, veterans obtaining care at a Veteran's Administration facility, or those receiving care through the Indian Health Service. GINA does not afford protection from genetic discrimination to obtain disability insurance, life insurance, or long-term care insurance. However, some individual states have passed laws that protect individuals regarding these other healthcare policies not covered by GINA (Genetics and Public Policy Center, 2008; Hudson, Holohan, & Collins, 2008). See Figure 7-3 for GINA details.

When considering our healthcare protection laws, "'one size fits all' genetic health policies might not work" (Feetham, Thompson, & Hinshaw, 2005, p. 106). Even with anticipated improvements in policies and protections, no real change will occur unless our society is committed to change. In the world of genomics, what we consider "race" is only skin deep. Education requires a focus on genetics and genomics, but the nursing profession must not lose sight of the disparities affected by demographics such as race, socioeconomic status, education level, lifestyle, and environmental exposures. The gaps in protection and access to care are wide and diverse. All individuals have the right to look forward to a healthier future. This will happen with educated and determined healthcare providers leading the way. Providers should lead the way to personalized healthcare. Policy makers should work in tandem to provide guidelines for protection, consistency, and availability of genetic information for all citizens (Abel, Horner, Tyler, & Innerarity, 2005; Haga & Willard, 2006). For more about health disparities, please see Chapter 14.

GINA protects the provision of health insurance and employment against discrimination based on genetic information as follows:
- Prohibits access to individuals' personal genetic information by insurance companies and employers.
- Prohibits insurance companies from requesting that applicants for group or individual health coverage plans be subjected to genetic testing or screening and prohibits them from discriminating against health plan applicants based on individual genetic information.
- Does not mandate coverage for medical tests or treatments.
- Does not interfere with or limit treating healthcare providers, including those employed by or affiliated with health plans, from requesting or notifying individuals about genetic tests.
- Prohibits employers from using genetic information to refuse employment and prohibits them from collecting employees' personal genetic information without their explicit consent.
- Prohibits employment agencies from failing or refusing to refer a candidate on the basis of genetic information.
- Prohibits labor organizations from refusing membership based on a member's genetic makeup.
- Does not prohibit occupational testing for toxic monitoring programs, employer-sponsored wellness programs, administration of federal and state family and medical leave laws, and certain cases of inadvertent acquisition of genetic information.

Figure 7-3. The Genetic Information Nondiscrimination Act of 2008 (GINA)

Note. Based on information from Long, 2008.

Law Making

Before making plans to march on Capitol Hill, we need to be honest with ourselves. As a whole, healthcare providers know very little about the laws that govern their practice and how these laws are implemented. Consider this brief primer on state law compared to federal law and the types of guidelines and laws implemented at those levels.

State law is similar to the federal legislative process, but less involved. Genetics state legislation currently includes newborn testing, DTC testing, and genetic testing.

Federal law includes legislation that is written, enforceable law. Both the U.S. House of Representatives and Senate must approve all bills and proposals. This is the most difficult means of creating policy, and it is very labor intensive. Federal law is necessary in governing rules related to intellectual property. In other words, federal law decides who can claim genes and genetic information "ownable" as property. Updates on current and past laws affecting health care and genetic information can be found at www.federalregister.gov.

Rules and regulations are precepts open for public comment, but most people are completely unaware of the proposed issues that may affect them. As science evolves and merges into the public sector, it would be ideal to have rules open to public comment. No formal rules have been set forth thus far for the education of healthcare professionals. However, NHGRI (2012) created the Education and Community Involvement Branch, part of the Office of Policy, Communications, and Education, as a move in that direction.

Guidelines provide structure by which professional organizations conduct themselves. This is not law. This type of structure allows for "gray zones" as to how deviations in the guidelines should be handled. For example, one may make the assumption that individuals will be more willing to make lifestyle changes regarding controllable risk factors if they are aware of the genetic implications. No compelling research has been conducted to substantiate this claim. Researchers should move forward to examine the role of personal choice with the input of experts and the public. This information affects the acceptance and implementation of genetic information and care (NHGRI, 2011a).

Advisory committees are composed of a group of experts, as well as public and industry representatives. It is often difficult to find willing participants to fill patient and consumer positions on such committees. NIH uses this method to be visible in the prioritization of research areas. All stakeholders affected by policies should have input, but again, most people are unaware that these activities are open for participation (NHGRI, 2011a).

Case law is when the law is applied to a unique set of circumstances. Each case is treated individually. For instance, this type of law has been instrumental in the "duty to warn" in certain states (DHHS, 2011; NHGRI, 2011a).

DHHS is 1 of 15 departments governed under the executive branch of the U.S. government. Five centers under the purview of DHHS affect the outcomes of genetics: Center for Food Safety and Applied Nutrition, Center for Drug Evaluation and Research, Center for Veterinary Medicine, Center for Devices and Radiological Health, National Center for Toxicological Research, and Center for Biologics Evaluation and Research (FDA, 2010).

Nurses in Politics

Nurses can no longer afford the luxury of trusting someone else to take care of their practice act and the policy that affects their patients' care. Nurses are involved in politics in a number of ways. ONS developed ONStat, a legislative action center that aims to advance oncology healthcare policy at the national level. ONS apprises nurses of healthcare policy priorities and provides current information on news and events in Washington, DC. Tools are also available online for making steps toward legislative advocacy. These tools include advice for writing or calling Congress, collaborating with other organizations on policy, and advocating for health care with the media. ONStat also provides the latest updates on healthcare reform. The Web site can be accessed at www.ons.org/LAC/getinvolved/ONStat (ONS, 2010b).

The Nursing Organizations Alliance (2009) is "a coalition of nursing organizations united to create a strong voice for nurses" (para. 1). This organization offers a Nurse in Washington Internship (NIWI). The objectives of NIWI include demonstrating how nurses can be involved and influence policy at the local and national level, how to work with legislative staff, how to make an impact on the legislative process, and how to identify political and economic forces driving healthcare policy. The internship usually occurs over a four-day period on Capitol Hill. On the last day of the internship, nurses meet and network with their legislators to discuss issues affecting nursing practice and patient care. As nurses become more politically savvy, they will be able to hold legislators accountable to their goals and to the needs of their constituents (Nursing Organizations Alliance, n.d.).

Goals of Our Government

DHHS, in cooperation with the NIH, have set forth goals to support personalized health care by linking clinical and genetic information. To accomplish this task,

DHHS wishes to protect individuals from discrimination and unauthorized use of genetic information. They plan to ensure the accuracy and clinical validity of genetic tests that are used in medical care, and develop policies for access to genomic databases for federally sponsored programs (DHHS, 2010).

Conclusion

As the genomic era progresses, we should engage in professional interdisciplinary collaboration throughout our nursing careers. It is not the amount of information or memorized facts that make nurses intelligent care providers. Instead, it is the application of knowledge and the ability to access and manage our resources. Every individual has a unique genetic signature. Sequencing idiopathic genetic disorders will soon become a way of the past. We are on the precipice of discovering what is normal-unique and what is pathologic-unique. Whether in academics, clinical practice, or research, nurses are the key leaders in the interdisciplinary genetic present and future. Florence Nightingale said, "Nursing is a progressive art in which to stand still is to have gone back" (Cook, 1914, p. 367). From bench to bedside and from ethics to politics, nurses will move genetic science forward.

References

Abel, E., Horner, S.D., Tyler, D., & Innerarity, S.A. (2005). The impact of genetic information on policy and clinical practice. *Policy, Politics, and Nursing Practice, 6,* 5–14. doi:10.1177/1527154404272143

American Association of Colleges of Nursing. (2008, October). The essentials of baccalaureate education for professional nursing practice. Retrieved from http://www.aacn.nche.edu/Education/pdf/BaccEssentials08.pdf

American Association of Colleges of Nursing. (2011, March). The essentials of master's education in nursing. Retrieved from http://www.aacn.nche.edu/education-resources/MastersEssentials11.pdf

American Society of Clinical Oncology. (2003). American Society of Clinical Oncology policy statement update: Genetic testing for cancer susceptibility. *Journal of Clinical Oncology, 21,* 2397–2406. doi:10.1200/JCO.2003.03.189s

Beery, T., & Hern, A. (2004). Genetic practice, education, and research: Overview for advanced practice nurses. *Clinical Nurse Specialist, 18,* 126–132. doi:10.1097/00002800-200405000-00012

Buchanan, A., Skinner, C.S., Calingaert, B., Schildkraut, J.M., King, R.L., & Marcom, P.K. (2009). Cancer and genetic counseling in rural North Carolina oncology clinics. *Community Oncology, 6,* 70–77. Retrieved from http://www.communityoncology.net/co/journal/articles/0602070.pdf

Buppert, C. (2007). Billing for nurse practitioner services—Update 2007: Guidelines for NPs, physicians, employers, and insurers. Retrieved from http://www.medscape.com/viewarticle/422935

Burke, S., & Kirk, M. (2006). Genetics education in the nursing profession: Literature review. *Journal of Advanced Nursing, 54,* 228–237. doi:10.1111/j.1365-2648.2006.03805.x

Burns, N., & Grove, S. (2009). Genetics for advanced practice nursing. *Nurse Practitioner, 33*(11), 10–18.

Calzone, K.A., Cashion, A., Feetham, S., Jenkins, J., Prows, C.A., Williams, J.K., & Wung, S.F. (2010). Nurses transforming health care using genetics and genomics. *Nursing Outlook, 58,* 26–35. doi:10.1016/j.outlook.2009.05.001

Christianson, C.A., Powell, K.P., Hahn, E.S., Bartz, D., Roxbury, T., Blanton, S.H., ... Henrich, V.C. (2010). Findings from a community education needs assessment to facilitate the integration of genomic medicine into primary care. *Genetics in Medicine, 12,* 597–593. doi:10.1097/GIM.0b013e3181ed3f97

Consensus Panel on Genetic/Genomic Nursing Competencies. (2009). *Essentials of genetic and genomic nursing: Competencies, curricula guidelines, and outcome indicators* (2nd ed.). Retrieved from http://www.genome.gov/Pages/Careers/HealthProfessionalEducation/geneticscompetency.pdf

Cook, E.T. (1914). *The life of Florence Nightingale: 1982–1910* (Vol. 2). London, UK: Macmillan.

Cook, S. (2003). Deconstructing DNA: Understanding genetic implications on nursing care. *AWHONN Lifelines, 7,* 140–144. doi:10.1177/1091592303253867

Davis, C.D., & Milner, J. (2004). Frontiers in nutrigenomics, proteomics, metabolomics, and cancer prevention. *Mutation Research, 551,* 51–64. doi:10.1111/j.1547-5069.2007.00136.x

Dolan, S., Biermann, J., & Damus, K. (2007). Genomics for health in preconception and prenatal periods. *Journal of Nursing Scholarship, 39,* 4–9. doi:10.1111/j.1547-5069.2007.00136.x

Donelan, K., Buerhaus, P.I., DesRoshes, C., & Burke, S.P. (2010). Health policy thoughtleaders' views of the health workforce in an era of health reform. *Nursing Outlook, 58,* 175–180. doi:10.1016/j.outlook.2010.06.003

Feetham, S., Thompson, E.J., & Hinshaw, A.S. (2005). Nursing leadership in genomics for health and society. *Journal of Nursing Scholarship, 37,* 102–110. doi:10.1111/j.1547-5069.2005.00021.x

Fibison, W.J. (1983). The nursing role in the delivery of genetic services. *Issues in Health Care of Women, 4,* 1–15. doi:10.1080/07399338309510806

Genetics and Public Policy Center. (2008). Information from the Genetic Information Nondiscrimination Act (GINA). Retrieved from http://www.dnapolicy.org/resources/WhatGINAdoesanddoesnotdochart.pdf

Greco, K., & Salveson, C. (2009). Identifying genetics nursing competencies among published recommendations. *Journal of Nursing Education, 48,* 557–565. doi:10.3928/01484834-20090716-02

Haga, S., & Willard, II (2006). Defining the spectrum of genome policy. *Nature Reviews Genetics, 7,* 966–972. doi:10.1038/nrg2003p966-972

Harrison, T.A., Doyle, D.L., McGowan, C., Cohen, L., Repass, E., Pfau, R.B., & Brown, T. (2010). Billing for medical genetics and genetic counseling services: A national survey. *Genetic Counseling, 19,* 38–43. doi:10.1007/s10897-009-9249-5

Health Insurance Portability and Accountability Act of 1996, Pub. L. No. 104-191 (1996). Retrieved from http://aspe.hhs.gov/admnsimp/pl104191.htm

Hetteburg, C., & Prows, C.A. (2004). A checklist to assist in the integration of genetics into nursing curriculum. *Nursing Outlook, 52,* 85–88. doi:10.1016/j.outlook.2004.01.007

Horner, S. (2004). A genetics course for advanced clinical nursing practice. *Clinical Nurse Specialist, 18,* 194–199. doi:10.1097/00002800-200407000-00010

Horner, S., Abel, E., Taylor, K., & Sands, D. (2004). Using theory to guide the diffusion of genetics content in nursing curricula. *Nursing Outlook, 52,* 80–84. doi:10.1016/j.outlook.2003.08.008

Hudson, K.L., Holohan, M.K., & Collins, F.S. (2008). Keeping pace with the times—The Genetic Information Nondiscrimination Act of 2008. *New England Journal of Medicine, 52,* 2661–2663. doi:10.1056/NEJMp0803964

International Society of Nurses in Genetics. (2010). Privacy and confidentiality of genetic information: The role of the nurse. Retrieved from http://www.isong.org/ISONG_PS_privacy_confidentiality.php

Jenkins, J., & Calzone, K. (2007). Establishing the essential nursing competencies for genetics and genomics. *Journal of Nursing Scholarship, 39,* 10–16. doi:10.1111/j.1547-5069.2007.00137.x

Kelly, P. (2009). The clinical nurse specialist and essential genomic competencies: Charting the course. *Clinical Nurse Specialist, 23,* 145–150. doi:10.1097/NUR.0b013e3181a42356

Kirk, M. (2000). Genetics, ethics, and education: Considering the issues for nurses and midwives. *Nursing Ethics, 7,* 215–226.

Lapham, E.V., Kozma, C., & Weiss, J.O. (1996). Genetic discrimination: Perspectives of consumers. *Science, 274,* 621–624. doi:10.1126/science.274.5287.621

Lea, D.H., Williams, J.K., Cooksey, J.A., Flanagan, P.A., Forte, G., & Blitzer, M.G. (2006). U.S. genetics nurses in advanced practice. *Journal of Nursing Scholarship, 38,* 213–218. doi:10.1111/j.1547-5069.2006.00105.x

Lee, S.S., & Crawley, L. (2009). Research 2.0: Social networking and direct-to-consumer marketing. *American Journal of Bioethics, 9*(6–7), 35–44. doi:10.1080/15265160902874452

Loescher, L.J., & Merkle, C.J. (2005). The interface of genomic technologies and nursing. *Journal of Nursing Scholarship, 37,* 111–119. doi:10.1111/j.1547-5069.2005.00022.x

Long, K. (2008, April 24). Genetic scientists applaud U.S. Senate passage of the Genetic Information Nondiscrimination Act: American Society of Human Genetics supports important new legislation [Press release]. Retrieved from http://www.ashg.org/pdf/GINAPressRelease4.24.08.pdf

Loud, J.T. (2010). Direct-to-consumer genetic and genomic testing: Preparing nurse practitioners for genomic healthcare. *Journal for Nurse Practitioners, 6,* 585–594. doi:10.1016/j.nurpra.2010.06.007

Lowstuter, K.J., Sand, S., Blazer, K.R., MacDonald, D.J., Banks, K.C., Lee, C.A., … Weitzel, J.N. (2008). Influence of genetic discrimination perceptions and knowledge on cancer genetics referral practice among clinicians. *Genetics in Medicine, 10,* 691–698. doi:10.1097/GIM.0b013e3181837246

Metcalf, A., Pumphrey, R., & Clifford, C. (2010). Hospice nurses and genetics: Implications for end-of-life care. *Journal of Clinical Nursing, 19,* 192–207. doi:10.1111/j.1365-2702.2009.02935.x

Mundinger, M.O., Kane, R.L., Lenz, E.R., Totten, A.M., Tsai, W., Cleary, P.D., … Shelanski, M.L. (2000). Primary care outcomes in patients treated by nurse practitioners or physicians. *JAMA, 283,* 59–68. doi:10.1001/jama.283.1.59

National Cancer Institute. (2011). Genetic risk assessment and counseling (PDQ®). Retrieved from http://www.cancer.gov/cancertopics/pdq/genetics/risk-assessment-and-counseling/HealthProfessional/page6

National Coalition for Health Professional Education in Genetics. (2001). Recommendations of core competencies in genetics essential for all health professionals. *Genetics in Medicine, 3,* 155–159. doi:10.1097/00125817-200103000-00011

National Coalition for Health Professional Education in Genetics. (2007). Core competencies in genetics for health professionals (3rd ed.). Retrieved from http://www.nchpeg.org/core/Core_Comps_English_2007.pdf

National Human Genome Research Institute. (2011a). Legislation database glossary of terms. Retrieved from http://www.genome.gov/15014431

National Human Genome Research Institute. (2011b). NHGRI site map. Retrieved from http://www.genome.gov/sitemap.cfm

National Human Genome Research Institute. (2012, February 6). Education and Community Involvement Branch. Retrieved from http://www.genome.gov/11008538

National Institutes of Health. (2011a). Genetics home reference. Retrieved from http://ghr.nlm.nih.gov

National Institutes of Health. (2011b). NIH bioethics resources on the Web. Retrieved from http://www.nih.gov/sigs/bioethics

Nursing Organizations Alliance. (n.d.). Nurse in Washington Internship (NIWI). Retrieved from http://www.nursing-alliance.org/content.cfm/id/niwi

Nursing Organizations Alliance. (2009). The Alliance: Nursing Organizations Alliance. Retrieved from http://www.nursing-alliance.org/index.cfm

Offit, K. (1998). Psychological, ethical, and legal issues in cancer risk counseling. In K. Offit (Ed.), *Clinical cancer genetics: Risk counseling and management* (pp. 287–315). New York, NY: Wiley.

Offit, K., Groeger, E., Turner, S., Wadsworth, E.A., & Weiser, M.A. (2004). The "duty to warn" a patient's family members about hereditary disease risks. *JAMA, 292,* 1469–1473. doi:10.1001/jama.292.12.1469

Oncology Nursing Society. (2010a). Oncology Nursing Society positions. Retrieved from http://www.ons.org/publications/positions

Oncology Nursing Society. (2010b). ONS Legislative Action Center. Retrieved from http://www.ons.org/LAC/getinvolved/ONStat

Oncology Nursing Society Cancer Genetics Special Interest Group. (2011). Cancer genetics SIG virtual community. Retrieved from http://cancergenetics.vc.ons.org

Pulcini, J., Mason, D.J., Cohen, S.S., Kovner, C., & Leavitt, J.K. (2000). Health policy and the private sector: New vistas for nurses. *Nursing and Health Care Perspectives, 21,* 22–28.

Read, C.Y., Dylis, A.M., Mott, S.R., & Fairchild, N.J. (2004). Promoting integration of genetics core competencies into entry-level nursing curricula. *Journal of Nursing Education, 43,* 376–380.

Rosenzweig, M.Q., Bender, C.M., & Brufsky, A.M. (2005). The nurse as principal investigator in a pharmaceutically sponsored drug trial: Considerations and challenges. *Oncology Nursing Forum, 32,* 293–299. doi:10.1188/05.ONF.293-299

Seibert, D.C. (2008). Secrets to creating effective and interesting educational experiences: Tips and suggestions for clinical educators. *Journal of Genetic Counseling, 17,* 152–160. doi:10.1007/s10897-007-9141-0

Smith-Stoner, M., & Veitz, A.L. (2008). Home healthcare nurses in high-risk cancer screening. *Home Healthcare Nurse, 6,* 96–101. doi:10.1097/01.NHH.0000311027.33894.c1

Stolovich, H.D., & Keeps, E.J. (2002). *Telling ain't training.* Alexandria, VA: Society for Training and Development Press.

Thompson, H.J., & Brooks, M.V. (2010). Genetics and genomics in nursing: Evaluating *Essentials* implementation. *Nurse Education Today, 31,* 623–627. doi:10.1016/j.nedt.2010.10.023.

University of Iowa College of Nursing. (2011). Center for genetics: Postdoc in nursing genetics research. Retrieved from http://www.nursing.uiowa.edu/excellence/genetics/postdoc.htm

U.S. Department of Health and Human Services. (2002). OCR privacy brief: Summary of the HIPAA privacy rule. Retrieved from http://www.hhs.gov/ocr/privacy/hipaa/understanding/summary/privacysummary.pdf

U.S. Department of Health and Human Services. (2010). Personalized health care. Retrieved from http://www.hhs.gov/myhealthcare/goals/index.html

U.S. Department of Health and Human Services: Office of the Secretary. (2011). 45 CFR Parts 160 through 164. Rin: 0991-AB08. Standards for privacy of individually identifiable health information. Retrieved from http://aspe.hhs.gov/admnsimp/nprm/pvc00.htm

U.S. Food and Drug Administration. (2005). *The Belmont report: Ethical principles and guidelines for the protection of human subjects of research.* Retrieved from http://www.fda.gov/ohrms/dockets/ac/05/briefing/2005-4178b_09_02_Belmont%20Report.pdf

Williams, J.K. (2002). Education for genetics and nursing practice. *AACN Clinical Issues, 13,* 492–500. doi:10.1097/00044067-200211000-00003

Williams, S., Skirton, H., & Masny, A. (2006). Ethics, policy, and educational issues in genetic testing. *Journal of Nursing Scholarship, 38,* 119–125. doi:10.1111/j.1547-5069.2006.00088.x

CHAPTER 8

Systems and Safety in the Oncology Practice Environment

Regina S. Cunningham, PhD, RN, AOCN®

Introduction

Healthcare systems refers to the organization of people, institutions, and resources required to deliver healthcare services to meet the health needs of specific populations. Clinical practice organization, information management, research, education, and professional development are *interdependent* and must be considered as such in planning for the delivery of healthcare services. Aspects of the system cannot be viewed in isolation. *Systems thinking* is a way of viewing things as a whole and considering interactions and relationships rather than isolated events. "Systems thinking is a discipline for seeing wholes. It is a framework for seeing interrelationships rather than things, for seeing patterns of change rather than static 'snapshots'" (Senge, 2006, p. 68). It is through this lens that we must consider the delivery of oncology care.

Systems, Complexity, and Healthcare Delivery

Over the past several decades, the delivery of services within healthcare systems across all disciplines, at all levels, and throughout the world has become more complex (Plsek & Greenhalgh, 2001); this is especially true in the area of cancer care delivery. Cancer care is typically highly specialized and fragmented, leaving patients to navigate a complex maze of services often delivered in different settings across their trajectory of illness. As a result, patients may experience what we think of as the healthcare "system" as more of a "non-system." Comprehensive cancer care needs to be reconceptualized along a continuum that spans from prevention through survivorship. As individuals navigate this continuum, diverse providers with appropriate expertise render care. Transitions between care settings and providers are complex, multidimensional processes that will require closely fitted communication and collaboration in order to avoid "quality chasms." Ensuring patient safety across the cancer care continuum is an essential goal of contemporary cancer care delivery.

Patient Safety as a Theme in Healthcare Delivery

The landmark Institute of Medicine (IOM) report *To Err Is Human: Building a Safer Health System* (Kohn, Corrigan, & Donaldson, 2000) alerted the healthcare community and the public that as many as 98,000 patients die each year in U.S. healthcare institutions as a result of medical errors. The report indicated that more than 7,000 of these instances may be related specifically to medication errors (Kohn et al., 2000). Although some of the methods used to calculate the error-related deaths in this report have been questioned, since its publication in 2000, keeping patients safe has become a major focal point for healthcare institutions, health delivery systems, regulatory agencies, and payers. The IOM committee that developed the report explicitly recommended that healthcare organizations make developing a culture of safety within the practice environment a top priority that is driven by the highest levels of leadership within the organization. Other recommendations emanating from this report included the need to

- Establish a national focus to create leadership, research, tools, and protocols to advance the knowledge of patient safety
- Raise expectations for improvements in safety through the action of oversight organizations, group purchasers, and professional groups
- Identify and learn from errors with the aim of ensuring that the system continues to be made safer for patients
- Create safety systems within healthcare organizations through the implementation of safety practices *at the delivery level.*

One important aspect of the recommendations was the focus on care systems and the need to make system-wide improvements that lead to the delivery of safer patient care. The notion that systems and system issues, rather than individual practitioners' poor performance, cause the majority of errors is crucial to advancing safety and providing a foundation for the improvement of healthcare delivery. Blaming individuals is, in most instances, both unfair and ineffective (Leape & Berwick, 2005).

Building a Culture of Safety

What is a culture of safety? An organization's safety culture has been defined as the "product of individual and group values, attitudes, perceptions, competencies, and patterns of behavior that determine the commitment to and the style and proficiency of an organizations' health and safety management" (Health and Safety Commission Advisory Committee on the Safety of Nuclear Installations, 1993, as cited in Sammer, Lykens, Singh, Mains, & Lackan, 2010, p. 156).

Sammer and colleagues (2010) conducted a review of the literature to investigate what constitutes a patient safety culture. Investigators used qualitative techniques to develop a typology of the patient safety culture literature and create a conceptual framework. This analysis revealed seven subcultures: (a) leadership, (b) teamwork, (c) use of an evidence base, (d) communication, (e) learning, (f) justice, and (g) patient-centeredness. Senior leadership's role has been identified as a key variable in establishing a viable culture of safety.

Leaders drive the safety culture by designing strategy, building the structure, and providing resources to ensure that safe practices can happen throughout the organization. Once the stage is set, everyone within the organization needs to contribute to creating a safe culture. Teamwork among all members and all ranks of the organization is essential. The complexity of patient care often requires the engagement of personnel with different types of expertise. All groups involved in the delivery of patient services need to work in concert to achieve optimal patient outcomes. This is especially true in the oncology-specific setting, where multidisciplinary care represents the gold standard (Jacobson, 2010; Taylor et al., 2010).

The use of evidence to guide clinical practices was also identified as an important component of a patient safety culture. Using research findings to develop best practices or establish standards or guidelines is an effective means of decreasing variation and ensuring that quality is consistent in care delivery. Several specialty organizations have developed clinical practice guidelines (CPGs) that can be adopted by healthcare agencies. For example, the American Society of Clinical Oncology (ASCO) and the Multinational Association of Supportive Care in Cancer developed CPGs that provide a summary of evidence-based interventions for the management of chemotherapy-induced nausea and vomiting. The Oncology Nursing Society (ONS) Putting Evidence Into Practice (PEP) initiative also provides quick reference guidelines for practicing nurses on the management of symptoms that commonly occur in the oncology population. Healthcare organizations can use these CPGs to develop policies and procedures that govern specific clinical practices.

A culture of learning within organizations is also essential to patient safety. A culture that promotes learning exists when organizations are open to reviewing their performance and learning from mistakes, staff is comfortable reporting adverse events, frontline workers' observations are welcome, and no one fears retaliation for identifying mishaps (Weingart et al., 2007). A key approach to effectively instilling a culture of learning is identifying fundamental variables that reflect quality care, collecting data on the performance of these variables, reporting on them, and correcting issues that reflect potential quality concerns. No national consensus exists regarding a specific set of variables that reflect quality cancer care. Selected indicators will vary from specialty to specialty, and the determination of what to measure should be made with input from multiple disciplines within a given specialty. For example, ASCO developed the Quality Oncology Practice Initiative (QOPI), a practice-based system of quality self-assessment designed with the goal of promoting high-quality cancer care. This initiative identified disease-, modality-, and supportive care–specific variables that reflect quality cancer care. Physician practices and larger healthcare organizations offering cancer services can use the QOPI variables to collect data on their individual practice patterns and then compare themselves to other practices or benchmarks (ASCO, n.d.; Neuss et al., 2005). Many oncology programs have developed dashboards of variables that report on selected metrics that reflect quality of care. Increasingly, data of this type will be used by payers to select providers for their constituents (Blayney et al., 2009; Jacobson et al., 2008; Neuss et al., 2009).

Systematic data collection and trend analysis on specific indicators is a strategy for identifying potential patient safety issues. Once issues are identified, an organization must take action to make improvements.

Oncology-Specific Patient Safety Issues

Oncology care is associated with a number of high-risk activities, such as administering chemotherapy, biotherapy, and radiation therapy, as well as handling blood and blood products. Oncology nurses play a pivotal role in keeping patients safe, preventing errors, and ensuring quality cancer care delivery. The ONS (2009) position on quality cancer care specifically identifies the importance of professional oncology nurses in creating a culture of accountability and safety.

A variety of factors contribute to the risk associated with the delivery of cancer therapeutics: patients are often quite ill, many patients have comorbidities, the therapeutic agents used in cancer care are associated with a high degree of toxicity, the margin between cure and potential harm can be very narrow, and chemotherapy/ biotherapy regimens often involve multiple agents of varying doses administered on different days. Moreover, cancer is a major area of drug development, so both investigational and novel agents contribute to care complexity and error potential in the therapeutic setting. Any error in the delivery of these interventions can have catastrophic implications, resulting in significant toxicity, loss of function, and death. The effects reach far beyond the individual patient and are often devastating to the family, the institution, and the professionals involved.

Ensuring Safety in the Oncology Clinical Practice Environment

Some of the safety measures commonly used in clinical oncology practice today developed as a result of serious errors that occurred in the oncology-specific setting. One of the most notable cases occurred in 1994 and involved Betsy Lehman, a 39-year-old *Boston Globe* health reporter who died from complications of an overdose of cyclophosphamide, a chemotherapeutic agent she received to treat breast cancer. The error involved breakdowns in standard processes and raised questions of trainee supervision, nursing competence, and order execution. As a result of this incident, the Dana-Farber Cancer Institute developed a major focus on medical errors and iatrogenic injury. Nurses were required to double-check high-dose chemotherapy orders and to complete specialized training in new chemotherapeutic treatment protocols. Details of this case were widely publicized; the media reported on the event intensively, with 28 front-page headlines over the three-year period following the event.

The majority of chemotherapy and biotherapy prescribed for patients with cancer is administered in the ambulatory care oncology setting. Yet, relatively little is known about medication errors that occur in this context. The American Society for Blood and Marrow Transplantation conducted an anonymous national survey to identify the rate of errors in the administration of high-dose chemotherapy. Of the 170 transplantation centers in the United States, 68% (n = 115) completed the survey. The overall chemotherapy error rate reported was 0.06%, or 6 cases per 10,000 transplants. The errors were related to chemotherapy overdoses and infusion errors. Rates of error were lower among more experienced transplantation centers (Chen et al., 1997).

Gandhi and colleagues (2005) assessed the rate of medication errors in three (two adult and one pediatric) outpatient chemotherapy infusion units at a National Cancer Institute–designated Comprehensive Cancer Center. The adult unit used an electronic computer ordering system that included drug allergy and drug interaction checklists as well as automatic dose limitations for chemotherapy orders. The pediatric infusion center was using a paper medical record and chemotherapy ordering process. The researchers reviewed 8,008 adult and 2,104 pediatric orders, representing 1,380 adults and 225 children and found that the overall error rate was 3%. Gandhi et al. (2005) found that 82% of chemotherapy errors in the adult units and 60% of the errors in the pediatric unit had the potential to cause harm. In approximately one-third of the pediatric cases, the potential for harm was serious. Pharmacists and nurses intercepted 45% of potential adverse events before they reached the patients. These findings, which reflected the organization's ability to monitor its processes and learn from them, led to a number of process changes within the organization.

Higher error rates related to chemotherapy have also been reported. In a more recent retrospective review of 1,262 adult ambulatory oncology clinic visits involving the administration of close to 11,000 medications, 7.1% were associated with a medication error (Walsh et al., 2009). Of the pediatric cases reviewed (n = 117 visits) involving the administration of 913 medications, 18.8% were associated with an error. Among all cases analyzed, 57% of the errors had the potential to cause harm and 15 resulted in injury to the patient. Most of the errors were related to the therapy administration and were specifically attributable to confusion over two sets of orders (Walsh et al., 2009). The chemotherapy and biotherapy ordering process is complex, and systematic approaches to reviewing these documents are necessary to ensure patient safety.

Strategies to Systematically Build Safety Into the Practice Environment

A number of strategies have been identified to improve the safety of the practice environment. Those that will be discussed in this chapter include the use of checklists; standardization, including the use of standards, guidelines, policies, and procedures; the use of technology; "handoffs" at points of transfer; the use of medical event reporting systems; and patients' and families' roles in ensuring patient safety.

Checklists

Checklists were first introduced in aviation in 1935 to mitigate the risks of flying the B299 bomber and are commonly used throughout the aviation industry today as a means of ensuring safety (Winters, Aswani, & Pronovost, 2011). A checklist is a "formal list used to identify, schedule, compare, or verify a group of elements or . . . used as a visual or oral aid that enables the user to overcome the limitations of short-term memory" (Federal Aviation Administration, 2007). Popularized by Atul Gawande's (2009) best-selling book *The Checklist Manifesto*, the use of checklists in healthcare settings has been identified as a practical strategy to improve quality and safety. Checklists may seem like an extraordinarily simple solution, but they have been used effectively to improve the safety of care delivery in a number of clinical settings.

Pronovost and colleagues (2006) conducted a collaborative cohort study to assess the effectiveness of an intervention to decrease the incidence of catheter-related bloodstream infections in 108 intensive care units (ICUs) in Michigan. The intervention included identifying a physician and a nurse to serve as team leaders on each of the participating units. These individuals received education and training in the science of patient safety and disseminated this information to staff and faculty caring for patients on the units. The intervention also involved using five evidence-based procedures recommended by the Centers for Disease Control and Prevention for central venous catheter insertion and care. These included hand washing, using full barrier protection during the central venous catheter insertion, cleaning the skin with chlorhexidine, avoiding femoral sites if possible, and removing unnecessary catheters. A checklist was used to ensure that infection control practices were endorsed.

The analysis was completed using data from a total of 1,981 ICU-months and 375,757 catheter-days. The median rate of catheter-related bloodstream infections decreased from 2.7 infections per 1,000 catheter-days to 0 at three months. Overall, the intervention resulted in a significant and sustained reduction in the rates of catheter-related bloodstream infections over the entire 18-month study period.

Drawing on lessons from the aviation experience with checklists, the World Health Organization (WHO) Patient Safety Program developed an initiative to improve surgical practices around the world. To accomplish this, the program team developed a checklist of actions that should be accomplished in all settings where surgery takes place. This checklist was subsequently tested in several settings. In a prospective study, Haynes et al. (2009) demonstrated lower rates of complications and death among a large sample of patients (N = 3,955) undergoing noncardiac surgical procedures in diverse geographic locations across the world. The intervention involved using a 19-item Surgical Safety Checklist that was based on the WHO safe surgical practice recommendations and designed to facilitate communication and improve the consistency of care. Members of the surgical team completed the Surgical Safety Checklist at three specific points: before anesthesia was initiated, immediately prior to the incision, and prior to discharging the patient from the operating room. Examples of checklist elements included confirmation of identity, introduction of all surgical team members and identification of their roles, a review of patient allergies, the procedure to be performed, site, anticipated complications, estimated blood loss, and the availability of essential imaging results for the correct patient. Members of the surgical team must verbally confirm these and other items. Statistically significant differences were reported in the primary outcome variables once the checklist was implemented. Inpatient complication rates fell from 11% to 7% (p < 0.001), and the death rate declined from 1.5% to 0.8% (p = 0.003) following implementation of the Surgical Safety Checklist (Haynes et al., 2009).

Checklist usage has also been associated with decreased healthcare costs. Semel and colleagues (2010) performed a decision analysis of the implementation and use of the WHO Surgical Safety Checklist in a U.S. hospital over a one-year period. These investigators found that for every complication averted using the checklist, a savings of $8,652 was appreciated (costs were adjusted for inflation to 2008 dollars based on the Consumer Price Index and the Medical Care Price Index). In order for these cost savings to be appreciated, at least five major complications would need to be averted using the checklist. Additional work in the area is warranted, but this study demonstrates that the adoption of the WHO Surgical Safety Checklist represents a potential cost-saving safety strategy for organizations (Semel et al., 2010).

Why do checklists work? Checklists assist with memory recall and make explicit the minimum expected steps in complex processes (Gawande, 2007). The evidence suggests that checklists are *part* of an intervention. When used within a context of safety education and behavioral change, they have led to dramatic change in specific outcomes. Communication and teamwork were also important aspects of the interventions tested. The importance of knowing the fellow team members, understanding their unique roles, and ensuring that communication among team members is open were all components that contributed to the outcomes. The five essential steps in the development of a checklist are (a) content and format, (b) timing, (c) trial and feedback, (d) formal testing and evaluation, and (e) local modification (Weiser et al., 2010).

Empirical evidence on the use of checklists in the oncology population was not specifically identified; however, it stands to reason that the interventions employed in the central venous catheter studies would be applicable to patients with cancer. Moreover, several areas of oncology practice would be appropriate to consider studying the effect of a checklist and the associated safety behaviors that were taught to those clinicians who took part in the checklist studies. These might include the administration of chemotherapy and biotherapy or the administration of blood and blood products.

Standards, Guidelines, Policies, and Procedures

Standardization of care can decrease variability in care delivery, minimize the risk of errors, improve efficiency, and provide a framework for ensuring quality practice. ASCO and ONS initiated a collaborative project in 2008 to develop standards for safe chemotherapy administration to adult patients with cancer. Initially, these standards were focused on patients receiving chemotherapy in the ambulatory care setting. However, in January 2011 a group of experts convened to review and revise the original standards as necessary. The most significant change recommended at that time was that the standards should be expanded in scope to include patients being treated in the inpatient setting (ASCO & ONS, 2011). This change was important in ensuring a uniform standard for patients receiving these agents regardless of setting.

The chemotherapy and biotherapy standards encompass eight domains: (a) review of clinical information and selection of a treatment regimen, (b) treatment planning and informed consent, (c) treatment ordering, (d) drug preparation, (e) assessment of treatment compliance, (f) administration and monitoring, (g) assessment of response, and (h) toxicity monitoring. These standards indicate that policies, procedures, and guidelines explicating the education and training process for staff involved in chemotherapy administration should be in place.

Chemotherapy and biotherapy prescribing, dispensing, and administration require a distinct knowledge base and specialized skills. All professionals involved in prescribing, dispensing, or administering chemotherapy or biotherapy must be knowledgeable about their mechanism of action, side effects and toxicity, dosage range, rate and route of excretion, potential responses, and interactions with other medications and foods. This knowledge will facilitate the safe and effective management of patients receiving chemotherapy and biotherapy.

ASCO and ONS (2011) specifically indicated that only qualified personnel administer chemotherapy and that the practice or setting where these agents are administered has a comprehensive educational program for all new personnel who will be involved with chemotherapy administration. A description of how competency will be assessed, maintained, and documented is a necessary component. An example of a comprehensive chemotherapy and biotherapy education program is the ONS Chemotherapy and Biotherapy Course. This ONS program was used as one of the components in the development of a comprehensive interdisciplinary policy at the Mount Sinai Medical Center in New York City. This document specifically outlined the education, training, and competency assessment requirements for all professionals who were responsible for prescribing, dispensing, or administering chemotherapeutic and biotherapeutic agents within the organization. Representatives from medicine, patient safety, pharmacy, nursing, and the Office of the Chief Medical Officer were involved in the development of this policy. Because it was interdisciplinary in nature, the document was reviewed and approved by the organization's medical board. Developing this type of policy ensures a consistent level of quality and safety in the management of patients receiving these agents. Policies clearly outlining all aspects of care for patients receiving chemotherapy and biotherapy should be available to staff managing these patients.

The development of CPGs has proliferated over the past several decades. The surge of interest in the development and use of these tools has been promulgated by the discovery of inappropriate variations in patient care, the need to base clinical practice on outcomes and evidence, and the thrust to contain healthcare costs (Larson, 2003). Understanding how CPGs are utilized and the effects of their implementation on outcomes is an important safety goal.

The purpose of guidelines is to help ensure that patients receive recommended interventions; however, studies have demonstrated that they are not used as consistently in clinical practice as we would like them to be. Moreover, when they are used, it has been difficult to demonstrate that they change outcomes. Reasons for guideline underuse are diverse and include lack of user-friendliness, clinician barriers, lack of knowledge about or agreement with the evidence, lack of access to resources to carry out guidelines as published, or implementation barriers (resistance) (Cunningham, 2006; Lashoher & Pronovost, 2010). If guidelines are in place within an organization, then they should be as straightforward as possible so that they are readily usable by end users, and periodic measurement of adherence is suggested.

Using Technology to Keep Patients Safe: Electronic Medical Records

Along with the use of standardized and preprinted order sets, the use of computerized physician order entry (CPOE) has been identified as a strategy to minimize medication errors and adverse drug events. Another approach to standardization in the oncology clinical setting is the use of standardized chemotherapy and biotherapy order sets. Defining standard chemotherapeutic regimens by diagnosis and providing clinical parameters, rationale for dose adjustments, and appropriate references have been identified as key components of minimizing errors in the chemotherapy prescribing, dispensing, and administration processes. The ASCO-ONS (2011) Standards for Safe Chemotherapy Administration recommend the use of standardized, regimen-level, preprinted or electronic order forms for both oral and parenteral chemotherapeutic and biotherapeutic agents. Preprinted order sets should include the ASCO-ONS defined complete chemotherapy/biotherapy order elements, which include important information about the patient and the treatment. Patient elements include

- Patient's full name and second patient identifier (e.g., birth date, medical record number)
- Date
- Diagnosis
- Height, weight, and any other variables used to calculate dose
- Allergies.
   Elements related to the treatment include
- Date of treatment
- Regimen name and cycle number
- Protocol name and number (if applicable)
- Appropriate criteria to treat (e.g., based on relevant laboratory results and toxicities)

- Reference to the methodology of dose calculation or standard practice equations (e.g., calculation of creatinine clearance)
- Dosage route and rate (if applicable) of administration
- Schedule
- Duration
- Cumulative lifetime dose (if applicable)
- Supportive care treatments appropriate for the regimen (including premedications, hydration, growth factors, and hypersensitivity medications)
- Sequence of drug administration (if applicable).

Note that dosage orders do not include trailing zeros, and a leading 0 should be used for doses less than 1 milligram. Also, orders for parenteral and oral chemotherapy should be written with a time limitation to ensure appropriate evaluation at predetermined intervals. Furthermore, ASCO and ONS (2011) recommend that preprinted or electronic order forms contain a list of the full regimen using generic drug names and follow the Joint Commission (TJC) standards on abbreviations. Although this strategy clearly has great potential to facilitate safety, it can also have unintended consequences. It is critical when implementing these systems to ensure that the proofing process is comprehensive and multidisciplinary. Any inaccuracies during the development of these documents can introduce the risk of systematic error.

Handoffs at Point of Transfer

The transfer of essential information and the responsibility for care of the patient from one healthcare provider to another is an essential component of communication in health care (Friesen, White, & Byers, 2008). This critical point is termed a *handoff*. The handoff is defined as the "transfer of information (along with authority and responsibility) during transitions in care across the continuum; to include an opportunity to ask questions, clarify, and confirm" (King, Hohenhaus, & Sailsbury, 2007, slide 26). Handoff communication is a complex process that includes multiple types of interactions between and among providers at all transition points in care. Handoffs typically occur at the change of shift, when a patient is transferred from one level of care to another, when a patient's service is changed, or when a physician transfers on-call responsibility. This communication should include up-to-date information about the patient's condition, care, treatment, medications, services, and any recent changes in clinical status. When key information is omitted or inaccurate, it can lead to near misses or adverse events. In a study of post-call handoffs, researchers found that pediatric interns overestimated the effectiveness of their communications post-call (Chang, Arora, Lev-Ari, D'Arcy, & Keysar, 2010).

Clinical environments are complex and present numerous challenges for effective communication among healthcare providers, patients, and families (Hendrich, Fay, & Sorrells, 2004). Interruptions during handoff communication should be minimized to reduce the possibility of information failures. A method to verify the information received, including read-back or repeat-back techniques, should be incorporated into the process. Handoffs routinely occur in all types of settings and across the entire healthcare continuum. TJC introduced a national safety goal on handoffs that became effective in January 2006. The patient safety goal raised awareness about the importance of the handoff and required healthcare organizations to implement a standardized approach to handoffs, including an opportunity to ask and respond to questions (TJC, 2008). Handoffs may include the use of electronic medical records

(EMRs), pagers, and other handheld devices. However, the human factor, such as how humans interact with those around them and the application of knowledge to safe, efficient designs, is an area of much-needed research.

Medical Event Reporting Systems and Analysis

Patient safety event reporting systems are now common in hospitals and represent a mainstay of efforts to detect patient safety events and quality problems. Patient safety reporting systems are a method of capturing information about near misses and adverse events. An event that causes harm is typically called an *adverse event*, whereas one that is not associated with harm is referred to as a *near miss*. Reports are generated by frontline personnel who are directly involved in the event or the actions leading up to the incident. Because they are voluntary, medical event reporting systems are subject to selection bias. An effective reporting system requires four key components, including a supportive environment for reporting, the ability to have a broad range of personnel complete the report, dissemination of summary data within a timely period, and a structured approach to event analysis and action planning (Agency for Healthcare Research and Quality [AHRQ], n.d.). Investigations of event reporting systems have demonstrated that patient falls and medication errors are the most frequent type of events reported in these systems.

The Role of the Patient and Family in Patient Safety

The inclusion of patients and family members in ensuring patient safety has been identified as an important strategy. Patients who know more about their disease and treatment plan may be less likely to experience a medication error. TJC has developed Speak Up™ initiatives (www.jointcommission.org/speakup.aspx) to help decrease errors in care. This campaign includes both written and video educational materials to increase patient awareness and provide information about how they can increase the involvement in their care. These educational materials contain specific information about paying attention to the medications they are receiving. Patients are instructed to be aware of the medication type, the time of administration, and the importance of having their identification verified prior to taking any medication. Patients are strongly encouraged to ask questions about their medications and instructed not to take a medication without knowing the rationale for its administration.

While media reports have increased public awareness about the issue of medical errors, little is known about patients' ability to recognize such events in the clinical setting. Weingart et al. (2007) conducted a study to determine the extent to which patients recognize medical errors. In this investigation, volunteer "patient safety liaisons" interviewed patients who were receiving treatment on a chemotherapy infusion unit and asked them to identify possible instances of medical errors or injuries. Using qualitative methods, the researchers categorized responses into four categories: (a) adverse events (injuries due to medical care versus the course of illness), (b) close calls, (c) medical errors with minimal risk of harm, and (d) service quality issues. Twenty-two percent of patients interviewed reported having a "recent unsafe experience." Further analysis of the data indicated that only 1% of reported instances actually represented a medical injury, and only 2% represented a close call. Instead, most of the events were identified as being related to service quality, including complaints about parking, delays, security, and emotional distress.

Impediments to Patient Safety

In 2008, TJC issued a sentinel event alert titled "Behaviors That Undermine a Culture of Safety." Intimidating or disruptive behaviors such as verbal outbursts, condescending tone of voice, or more passive activities such as exhibiting uncooperative attitudes can undermine patient safety and create risk for organizations. The delivery of safe and effective patient care relies on effective communication, teamwork, and a collaborative work environment. TJC (2008) has indicated that organizations that fail to address unprofessional behavior are indirectly promoting it. Concern over the role of such behaviors on the delivery of safe and effective care led TJC to implement new leadership standards that require organizations to have a process in place that clearly defines and manages disruptive behaviors. A number of suggested actions have been advanced by TJC to support adherence to this standard; these include providing education on what constitutes appropriate professional behavior as defined by the organization's code of conduct, holding all team members accountable to model expected behaviors, providing skills-based training and coaching for all leaders and managers on working collaboratively, building relationships, having difficult conversations, and providing appropriate feedback on unprofessional behaviors (TJC, 2008).

TJC has established a number of other standards that help organizations to develop safe and accountable practices. One excellent example of this was the institution of the National Patient Safety Goals (NPSGs). NPSGs went into effect in 2003 and were established specifically to help organizations to address specific areas of concern with regard to patient safety. Initially, these goals were developed by a multidisciplinary group of professionals (physicians, nurses, safety experts, clinical engineers, risk managers, and other professionals) who had hands-on experience with safety issues within healthcare settings. Although not designed for any particular patient population, each of the NPSGs outlined is germane in caring for the patient with cancer. The 2011 Ambulatory Care NPSGs, for example, include stipulations about correct identification of patients, using medications safely, preventing infections, and preventing mistakes in surgery. TJC adds new NPSGs each year. For 2012, a goal focused on catheter-associated urinary tract infections (CAUTIs) will be implemented. This is to address the fact that CAUTI is the most frequent type of healthcare-acquired infection. When considered within the oncology-specific context, this goal has particular relevance (TJC, 2012).

Implications for Nursing Practice and Research

More health services research is needed in order to develop strategies aimed at improving quality of care. In 2001, the U.S. Congress appropriated $50 million annually for patient safety research. Congress identified the AHRQ as the lead federal agency for patient safety research. Since that time, AHRQ has established a Center for Quality Improvement and Safety and has become a leader in education, measurement, and standard setting in this area (Leape & Berwick, 2005).

Nurses have a substantive role in identifying how to effectively lead, design, test, and change safety structures and processes in health systems. A research focus is needed to create and sustain organizational cultures aimed toward safe and high-quality care. This includes altering power gradients in clinical settings to ensure free flow of information and testing approaches to educating teams of health providers and professional students to maximize communication (IOM, 2004). Nurses are a vital component and need to have an equal voice in planning and implementation meetings. Research targeting quality improvement continues to be supported and implemented by various stakeholders, ranging from health professional organizations to federal agencies to health providers themselves (IOM, 2004).

Although not all-inclusive, health services research is needed on the delivery of health care, safety issues, workforce planning, education and ongoing training, evidence-based practice, translational science, staff competencies for health professionals, and implementation of patient care.

Conclusion

Limitations in access to health care continue to be a problem and frequently coincide with lower socioeconomic status. The homeless population is increasing at an alarming rate. These individuals often opt for no care or use emergency facilities in response to health problems. However, the unemployed and their families are a growing portion of the population seeking access to health care. Transitional care is a major issue in our current state of healthcare delivery, and more research is needed in this area. For those families who have jobs, individuals are working longer hours. Our healthcare system does not yet have an effective mechanism to bridge the accommodation of patients, such as patients with cancer, who are being discharged from the hospital and who are not yet able to care for themselves. Finally, with a focus toward developing evidence and measurement, as well as linking payment with quantifiable performance, substantial work remains in both practice and academic settings. Although Florence Nightingale was the first nurse to identify and attend to the issues of safety and quality, we have an opportunity again to take the lead in creating a safe environment and providing quality care for our patients.

References

Agency for Healthcare Research and Quality. (n.d.). Patient safety primers: Voluntary patient safety event reporting (incident reporting). Retrieved from http://psnet.ahrq.gov/primer. aspx?primerID=13

American Society of Clinical Oncology. (n.d.). ASCO quality programs. Retrieved from http:// qopi.asco.org

American Society of Clinical Oncology & Oncology Nursing Society. (2011, November 15). ASCO-ONS standards for safe chemotherapy administration [2011]. Retrieved from http://www.asco.org/ ASCOv2/Practice+%26+Guidelines/Quality+Care/Quality+Measurement+%26+Improvement/ ASCO-ONS+Standards+for+Safe+Chemotherapy+Administration+%5B2011%5D

Blayney, D.W., Stella, P.J., Ruane, T., Martin, J., Lavasseur, B., Leyden, T., & Malloy, M. (2009). Partnering with payers for success: Quality Oncology Practice Initiative, Blue Cross Blue Shield of Michigan, and the Michigan Oncology Quality Consortium. *Journal of Oncology Practice, 5,* 281–284. doi:10.1200/JOP.091043

Chang, V.Y., Arora, V.M., Lev-Ari, S., D'Arcy, M., & Keysar, B. (2010). Interns overestimate the effectiveness of their hand-off communication. *Pediatrics, 125,* 491–496. doi:10.1542/ peds.2009-0351

Chen, C.S., Seidel, K., Armitage, J.O., Fay, J.W., Appelbaum, F.R., Horowitz, M.M. ... Sullivan, K.M. (1997). Safeguarding the administration of high-dose chemotherapy: A national practice survey by the American Society for Blood and Marrow Transplantation. *Biology of Blood and Marrow Transplantation, 3,* 331–340.

Cunningham, R.S. (2006). Clinical practice guideline use by oncology advanced practice nurses. *Applied Nursing Research, 19,* 126–133. doi:10.1016/j.apnr.2005.06.003

Federal Aviation Administration. (2007, September 13). FAA Order 8900.1 Flight standards information management system. Retrieved from http://fsims.faa.gov/WDocs/8900.1/V03%20Tech%20Admin/Chapter%2032/03_032_012.htm

Friesen, M.A., White, S., & Byers, J. (2008). Handoffs: Implications for nurses. In R.G. Hughes (Ed.), *Patient safety and quality: An evidence-based handbook for nurses* (pp. 1–48). Rockville, MD: Agency for Healthcare Research and Quality.

Gandhi, T.K., Bartel, S.B., Shulman, L.N., Verrier, D., Burdick, E., Cleary, A., … Bates, D.W. (2005). Medication safety in the ambulatory chemotherapy setting. *Cancer, 104,* 2477–2483. doi:10.1002/cncr.21442

Gawande, A. (2007, December 10). The checklist. *The New Yorker, 83*(39), 86–95.

Gawande, A. (2009). *The checklist manifesto.* New York, NY: Metropolitan Books.

Haynes, A.B., Weiser, T.G., Berry, W.R., Lipsitz, S.R., Breizat, A.H., Dellinger, E.P., … Safe Surgery Saves Lives Study Group. (2009). A surgical safety checklist to reduce morbidity and mortality in a global population. *New England Journal of Medicine, 360,* 491–499. doi:10.1056/NEJMsa0810119

Hendrich, A.L., Fay, J., & Sorrells, A.K. (2004). Effects of acuity-adaptable rooms on flow of patients and delivery of care. *American Journal of Critical Care, 13,* 35–45. Retrieved from http://ajcc.aacnjournals.org/content/13/1/35.full.pdf+html

Institute of Medicine. (2004). *Patient safety: Achieving a new standard for care.* Retrieved from http://books.nap.edu/openbook.php?record_id=10863

Jacobson, J.O. (2010). Multidisciplinary cancer management: A systems-based approach to deliver complex care. *Journal of Oncology Practice, 6,* 274–275. doi:10.1200/JOP.2010.000164

Jacobson, J.O., Neuss, M.N., McNiff, K.K., Kadlubek, P., Thacker, L.R., II, Song, F., … Simone, J.V. (2008). Improvement in oncology practice performance through voluntary participation in the Quality Oncology Practice Initiative. *Journal of Clinical Oncology, 26,* 1893–1898. doi:10.1200/JCO.2007.14.2992

Joint Commission. (2008, July 9). Sentinel event alert: Behaviors that undermine a culture of safety. Retrieved from http://www.jointcommission.org/assets/1/18/SEA_40.PDF

Joint Commission. (2012). National patient safety goals effective January 1, 2012. Retrieved from http://www.jointcommission.org/assets/1/6/NPSG_Chapter_Jan2012_HAP.pdf

King, H., Hohenhaus, S., & Salisbury, M. (2007, May 21–22). Team-STEPPS™ strategies and tools to enhance performance and patient safety. (Slide number 26). Slide presentation given at the New York State Department of Public Health Patient Safety Conference. Retrieved from http://www.health.state.ny.us/professionals/patients/patient_safety/conference/2007/does/toimplementing_a_teamworkinitiative.pdf

Kohn, L.T., Corrigan, J.M., & Donaldson, M.S. (Eds.). (2000). *To err is human: Building a safer health system.* Washington, DC: National Academies Press.

Larson, E. (2003). Status of practice guidelines in the United States: CDC guidelines as an example. *Preventive Medicine, 36,* 519–524. doi:10.1016/S0091-7435(03)00014-8

Lashoher, A., & Pronovost, P. (2010). Creating a more efficient healthcare knowledge market: Using communities of practice to create checklists. *Quality and Safety in Health Care, 19,* 471–472. doi:10.1136/qshc.2010.047308

Leape, L.L., & Berwick, D.M. (2005). Five years after *To Err Is Human*: What have we learned? *JAMA, 293,* 2384–2390. doi:10.1001/jama.293.19.2384

Neuss, M.N., Desch, C.E., McNiff, K.K., Eisenberg, P.D., Gesme, D.H., Jacobson, J.O., … Simone, J.V. (2005). A process for measuring the quality of cancer care: The Quality Oncology Practice Initiative. *Journal of Clinical Oncology, 23,* 6233–6239. doi:10.1200/JCO.2005.05.948

Neuss, M.N., Jacobson, J.O., McNiff, K.K., Kadlubek, P., Eisenberg, P.D., & Simone, J.V. (2009). Evolution and elements of the quality oncology practice initiative measure set. *Cancer Control, 16,* 312–317.

Oncology Nursing Society. (2009, January). Quality cancer care. Retrieved from http://www.ons.org/Publications/Positions/Quality

Plsek, P., & Greenhalgh, T. (2001). Complexity science: The challenge of complexity in health care. *BMJ, 323,* 625–628. doi:10.1136/bmj.323.7313.625

Pronovost, P., Needham, D., Berenholtz, S., Sinopoli, D., Chu, H., Cosgrove, S., … Goeschel, C. (2006). An intervention to decrease catheter-related bloodstream infections in the ICU. *New England Journal of Medicine, 355,* 2725–2732. doi:10.1056/NEJMoa061115

Sammer, C.E., Lykens, K., Singh, K.P., Mains, D.A., & Lackan, N.A. (2010). What is patient safety culture? A review of the literature. *Journal of Nursing Scholarship, 42,* 156–165. doi:10.1111/j.1547 -5069.2009.01330.x

Semel, M.E., Resch, S., Haynes, A.B., Funk, L.M., Bader, A., Berry, W.R., … Gawande, A.A. (2010). Adopting a surgical safety checklist could save money and improve the quality of care in U.S. hospitals. *Health Affairs, 29,* 1593–1599. doi:10.1377/hlthaff.2009.0709

Senge, P.M. (2006). *The fifth discipline: The art and practice of the learning organization* (2nd ed.). New York, NY: Currency Doubleday.

Taylor, C., Munro, A.J., Glynne-Jones, R., Griffith, C., Trevatt, P., Richards, M., & Ramirez, A.J. (2010). Multidisciplinary team working in cancer: What is the evidence? *BMJ, 340,* c951. doi:10.1136/ bmj.c951

Walsh, K.E., Dodd, K.S., Seetharaman, K., Roblin, D.W., Herrinton, L.J., Von Worley, A., … Gurwitz, J.H. (2009). Medication errors among adults and children with cancer in the outpatient setting. *Journal of Clinical Oncology, 27,* 891–896. doi:10.1200/JCO.2008.18.6072

Weingart, S.N., Price, J., Duncombe, D., Connor, M., Sommer, K., Conley, K.A., … Reid Ponte, P. (2007). Patient-reported safety and quality of care in outpatient oncology. *Joint Commission Journal on Quality and Patient Safety, 33,* 83–94.

Weiser, T.G., Haynes, A.B., Lashoher, A., Dziekan, G., Boorman, D.J., Berry, W.R., & Gawande, A.A. (2010). Perspectives in quality: Designing the WHO Surgical Safety Checklist. *International Journal for Quality in Health Care, 22,* 365–370. doi:10.1093/intqhc/mzq039

Winters, B.D., Aswani, M.S., & Pronovost, P.J. (2011). Commentary: Reducing diagnostic errors: Another role for checklists? *Academic Medicine, 86,* 279–281. doi:10.1097/ACM.0b013e3182082692

CHAPTER 9

Ethics

Carlin A.M. Callaway, MSN, MS, RN, ACNP-BC, ACNS-BC, OCN®
Jeanne M. Erickson, PhD, RN, AOCN®

Introduction

Ethics, ethical dilemmas, and moral distress are woven into everyday oncology nursing practice. However, nurses may not sense how these dynamics impact their professional relationships with patients and colleagues and how these dynamics affect their own personal feelings and well-being. Oncology nurses often experience ethics in personal ways. Oncology nurses work in a variety of clinical settings to achieve optimal patient outcomes and overcome challenges related to the alleviation of human suffering, adequate and appropriate use of resources and technology, and attainment of professional satisfaction within complex healthcare systems. In ethically challenging situations, nurses may feel frustration, anger, sorrow, and distress. Furthermore, nurses may not articulate ethical dilemmas or unmet ethical principles as the source of these uncomfortable and intense responses.

While the field of ethics refers to the systematic contemplation of right and wrong (Beauchamp & Childress, 2009), a basic understanding of ethics in nursing practice provides foundations for nurses to use in critical thinking, decision making, and conflict resolution (Myser, Donehower, & Frank, 1999). Understanding ethical principles and theories may be helpful but not sufficient for nurses. In order for nurses to be effective advocates for patients and to help nurses manage their own moral distress when trying to determine the best course of action in ethically challenging situations (Wocial, Hancock, Bledsoe, Chamness, & Helft, 2010), nurses need to be comfortable with their own moral values. Nurses also need to use ethical language to articulate ethical conflicts and dimensions inherent in many clinical situations where the right courses of action, available resources, or acceptable outcomes are not obvious. Furthermore, nurses seek to work in supportive, professional environments with compassionate colleagues. Nurses strive to cultivate positive climates and team relationships that enable them to act in accordance with their own per-

The views expressed in this chapter are those of the authors and do not necessarily reflect the official policy or position of the Department of the Navy, the Department of Defense, or the United States government.

sonal and professional values. Positive ethical climates yield feasible and acceptable solutions to ethical problems in practice (Park, 2009).

Personal and Professional Ethics

Each nurse brings a unique set of morals to the professional role—personal beliefs and values about what is right and good that have developed over a lifetime of experience, education, maturity, and environment (Ham, 2004). These individual sets of beliefs and values influence personal conduct as well as how nurses think, reason, and make decisions in the clinical setting. With a sense of mindfulness and self-reflection, nurses should be able to identify these conscious and subconscious beliefs in themselves and recognize when their beliefs come in conflict with a patient's choice, a colleague's actions, or an organization's priorities.

Frameworks for Professional Ethics

Despite different personal belief systems, nurses are expected to adhere to professional values established in nursing codes and guidelines. *Code of Ethics for Nurses With Interpretive Statements* (American Nurses Association [ANA], 2001), with its nine provisions, is the ethical cornerstone for nurses and establishes a social contract between nurses and society. The code outlines the nurse's obligations to individual patients, to the profession, to the community, and to self (see Figure 9-1).

Provision 1: The nurse, in all professional relationships, practices with compassion and respect for the inherent dignity, worth, and uniqueness of every individual, unrestricted by considerations of social or economic status, personal attributes, or the nature of health problems.

Provision 2: The nurse's primary commitment is to the patient, whether an individual, family, group, or community.

Provision 3: The nurse promotes, advocates for, and strives to protect the health, safety, and rights of the patient.

Provision 4: The nurse is responsible and accountable for individual nursing practice and determines the appropriate delegation of tasks consistent with the nurse's obligation to provide optimum patient care.

Provision 5: The nurse owes the same duties to self as to others, including the responsibility to preserve integrity and safety, to maintain competence, and to continue personal and professional growth.

Provision 6: The nurse participates in establishing, maintaining, and improving health care environments and conditions of employment conducive to the provision of quality health care and consistent with the values of the profession through individual and collective action.

Provision 7: The nurse participates in the advancement of the profession through contributions to practice, education, administration, and knowledge development.

Provision 8: The nurse collaborates with other health professionals and the public in promoting community, national, and international efforts to meet health needs.

Provision 9: The profession of nursing, as represented by associations and their members, is responsible for articulating nursing values, for maintaining the integrity of the profession and its practice, and for shaping social policy.

Figure 9-1. American Nurses Association Code of Ethics for Nurses

---

Note. From *Code of Ethics for Nurses With Interpretive Statements*, by the American Nurses Association, 2001. Retrieved from http://www.nursingworld.org/MainMenuCategories/EthicsStandards/CodeofEthicsforNurses/Code-of -Ethics.pdf. Copyright 2001 by the American Nurses Association. Adapted with permission.

In addition to ANA's code of ethics, the International Council of Nurses created a Code of Ethics for Nurses in 1953. Most recently revised in 2006, this international code states that nurses have four fundamental responsibilities in the profession. These responsibilities include health promotion, illness prevention, health restoration, and the minimization of suffering. The international code emphasizes the obligations of nurses to maintain a global perspective of healthcare needs and disparities and to respect the basic rights and needs of all human persons (International Council of Nurses, 2006). The International Code is available at www.icn.ch/about -icn/code-of-ethics-for-nurses.

Several principles form the underlying structure for ethical theories, frameworks, and professional codes. Beauchamp and Childress (2009) provided an overview of a principle-based ethics model that often guides patient care. The principles of autonomy, beneficence, nonmaleficence, and justice provide general and comprehensive guidance for nurses and other healthcare professionals. Additional ethical rules related to confidentiality, fidelity, privacy, and veracity provide more specific directions for action (see Figure 9-2).

Jameton (1984) developed an original framework that outlines three types of ethical encounters that nurses may experience: (a) moral uncertainty, (b) moral or ethical dilemmas, and (c) moral distress. In situations of moral uncertainty, the nurse senses that something is not right or good but is incapable of identifying conflicting principles and values. The nurse also may be unsure of which ethical principles and rules apply to the situation. As an example, an oncology nurse may experience moral uncertainty when he or she wonders how a young patient with cancer will cope with chemotherapy-associated infertility.

Ethical Dilemmas and Moral Distress

Ethical dilemmas are characterized by more apparent conflicts between two or more ethical principles. Because the principles suggest opposing courses of action, nurses are confronted with moral dilemmas (Beauchamp & Childress, 2009). While both actions may be ethically justified, members of the healthcare team must select actions based on one ethical principle or rule. Such selection then violates other principles and rules. Oncology nurses frequently face ethical dilemmas when therapeutic interventions intended to benefit patients cause pain and discomfort.

In situations of moral distress, nurses comprehend the correct ethical actions. Notably, nurses are prevented from implementing such actions because of inherent limitations. Oncology nurses may experience moral distress, for example, when

---

Autonomy—an individual's right to form thoughts, make decisions, and take action
Beneficence—striving to achieve goodness
Nonmaleficence—striving not to impose harm or cause suffering
Justice—treating people fairly
Confidentiality—an individual's right to control disclosure of information about self
Fidelity—faithfulness of one person to another
Privacy—an individual's right to control access
Veracity—obligation to act with integrity and truthfulness

Figure 9-2. Definitions of Common Ethical Principles and Rules

---

Note. Based on information from Beauchamp & Childress, 2009.

they discharge uninsured patients to home settings with little or no social support or resources.

Moral distress, the most complex of the three ethical encounters, perpetuates powerlessness (Epstein & Hamric, 2009). In morally distressing situations, nurses are prevented or prohibited from taking appropriate actions. Moral distress is influenced by internal and external factors. Internally, nurses may doubt themselves and their abilities to intervene in situations. Externally, actual or perceived interdisciplinary power imbalances may prevent nurses from voicing their views and participating in active decision-making processes to address ethical concerns. Ultimately, nurses may fear repercussions of expressing their views. Nurses may choose to avoid confrontation for fear of losing their jobs (Hamric, Davis, & Childress, 2006).

Moral distress may be more prominent in organizations that emphasize cost-containment, situations threatened by potential legal action, and events with limited communication leading to compromised patient care (Epstein & Delgado, 2010). Situations associated with high moral distress frequently include cases where nurses are concerned about deception, futility, or inadequate or inappropriate information conveyed to families (Rice, Rady, Hamrick, Verheijde, & Pendergast, 2008).

The crescendo effect model, as first described by Epstein and Hamric (2009), describes long-term effects of moral distress. Although troubling situations eventually end, some amount of moral distress lingers. This lingering distress, known as *moral residue*, has unique properties that will escalate after numerous morally distressing situations. Without interventions, moral residue will continue to silently escalate or crescendo. Familiarity, futility, and predictability ensue (Epstein & Delgado, 2010) (see Figure 9-3).

The crescendo effect has three deleterious effects on nurses and other healthcare professionals. First, healthcare professionals risk losing their moral sensitivities; such loss prevents them from identifying and participating in ethically troubling situations. Second, healthcare professionals may begin to oppose future morally distressing situations. Opposition may be demonstrated positively by initiating ethics consultations. However, opposition may also be apparent in hostile conversations or documenta-

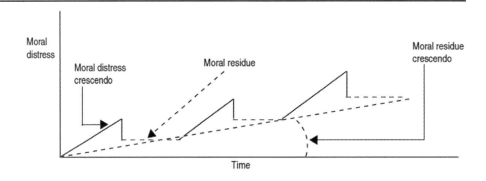

Solid lines indicate moral distress; dotted lines indicate moral residue.

Figure 9-3. The Crescendo Effect

Note. From "Moral Distress, Moral Residue, and the Crescendo Effect," by E.G. Epstein and A.B. Hamric, 2009, *Journal of Clinical Ethics, 20,* p. 333. Copyright 2009 by University Publishing Group, Incorporated. Reprinted with permission.

tion (Epstein & Hamric, 2009). Third, and most concerning, moral residue leads to burnout. Hamric and Blackhall (2007) noted that moral distress may be associated with nurses leaving their jobs and, ultimately, their profession.

Epstein and Delgado (2010) warn of breaking points following multiple episodes of moral distress. To halt the crescendo effect, interventions to reduce moral distress and residue are imperative.

Ethical Issues in Oncology Nursing Practice

Regardless of practice setting, oncology nurses constantly encounter ethical issues. Ethical dilemmas often originate from the ever-changing and increasingly complex healthcare system (de Casterlé, Izumi, Godfrey, & Denhaerynck, 2008). Fry and Duffy (2001) categorized ethical issues that nurses experience in practice into three categories: (a) patient care issues, (b) human rights issues, and (c) end-of-life treatment decisions. Patient care issues incorporate concerns about the health care that patients receive. Human rights issues encompass issues related to rights of nurses, patients, families, and healthcare providers. End-of-life issues include matters of death and dying.

Park (2009) reviewed recent empirical studies about the types of ethical issues that hospital-based nurses experience. Park discovered that the most frequently occurring ethical issues involved patient care issues and human rights issues. Although less common, end-of-life issues were the most disturbing (see Figure 9-4).

Oncology nurses encounter ethical issues when providing care for patients across the continuum of cancer care to include diagnosis, treatment, survivorship, and death. New and reconstituted dilemmas and concerns will emerge because of an aging population, complex and costly treatments, technology advances, and increas-

---

Patient care issues
- Inadequate staffing patterns and resources
- Colleagues' irresponsible or incompetent behavior
- Unclear treatment orders
- Conflict with colleagues
- Dealing with difficult patients

Human rights issues
- Providing care that puts the nurse at risk
- Patient abuse and neglect
- Informed consent to treatment
- Acting against the nurse's personal views
- Patient confidentiality and privacy

End-of-life issues
- Prolonging life with aggressive or heroic measures
- Unclear do-not-resuscitate orders
- Quality of life at the end of life
- Pain management at the end of life
- Abortion

Figure 9-4. Examples of Ethical Issues Frequently Reported by Hospital-Based Nurses

---

Note. Based on information from Fry & Duffy, 2001; Park, 2009.

ing survivor longevity. The nursing shortage, the globalization of cancer care, and the ongoing and unresolved debates about healthcare economics will also impact nurses' ethical practice environment for years to come.

The following paragraphs discuss specific ethical issues that may be especially challenging for oncology nurses in today's healthcare climate. Healthcare costs, evidence-based practice and quality improvement, research, genetics, survivorship, futility, end-of-life care, electronic health records, and social networking will be discussed.

Healthcare Costs

Rising healthcare costs create ethical issues and dilemmas. Today, many cancer treatments cost thousands of dollars per treatment cycle. Normally, such treatments are given multiple times. Throughout disease continuums, the costs of cancer treatment may have deleterious effects on families. In 2006, nearly one-fourth of American families affected by cancer used the majority or all of their savings to pay for cancer treatments (Elkin & Bach, 2010). Furthermore, ethnic, racial, and socioeconomic disparities adversely impact survival rates (Hughes, Gudmundsdottir, & Davies, 2007).

At the June 2011 American Society of Clinical Oncology meeting, Zafar et al. (2011) announced results from their study of 127 patients with cancer who received financial assistance from the Healthwell Foundation. Although all participants had health insurance (64% with Medicare) and 83% had prescription coverage, study participants still lost more than $700 each month because of copays, medications, transportation, and lost wages. In some cases, patients had to choose between groceries and medications. Other patients did not attend their treatment appointments or receive requested tests. These examples of "financial toxicities" illustrate real dilemmas for patients with cancer and oncology professionals.

Oncology providers need to discuss the high cost of cancer care and possible consequences of such care with their patients. In 2008, Americans spent approximately $90 billion for cancer care. This figure (adjusted for inflation) represents a two-fold increase from the $27 billion spent in 1990 (Elkin & Bach, 2010). Despite the costs, research has shown that some patients receive chemotherapy during their last three months and one month of life (McCabe & Storm, 2008). Patients are unable to receive simultaneous treatment and hospice services because of restrictions imposed by the Medicare Hospice Benefit (Centers for Medicare and Medicaid Services, 2011). Consequently, these patients with advanced cancer receive delayed hospice referrals (McCabe & Storm, 2008). When oncology providers discuss financial matters and implications, they demonstrate beneficence and nonmaleficence.

Additionally, some healthcare organizations have engaged in unethical behavior to lower their operating costs and increase their profits. Some organizations have compromised infection control standards to save money, and others have performed needless but profitable procedures, such as heart surgery. Notably, many organizations bill their patients unethically. Examples include billing Medicare inappropriately, billing uninsured patients more than insured patients, and hostilely pursuing past-due payments (Deshpande, 2009).

Evidence-Based Practice and Quality Improvement

Oncology nurses are ethically obligated to engage in evidence-based practice. Evidence-based practice is now the standard and norm for safe patient care (Baily, Bottrell, Lynn, & Jennings, 2006). Such duty is complicated by the overwhelming quantity of publications and sources of information available in today's world (Mayer, 2011).

Nurses also have responsibilities to participate in quality improvement (QI) activities. Such participation yields safe, timely, and cost-effective care that benefits patients and their families (Lynn et al., 2007). QI activities and research conducted on human subjects are distinct concepts, as human subject research requires approval and oversight from institutional review boards. Regardless, QI activities and projects must be conducted in accordance with ethical standards, such as patient confidentiality and sound methodology. Examples of QI activities include observing and auditing hand washing, medication administration, and specific procedures (Lynn et al., 2007).

Nationwide, nurses audit and report nurse-sensitive indicators findings to the National Database of Nursing Quality Indicators (NDNQI). Examples of nurse-sensitive indicators include falls, IV infiltrations, pressure ulcers, and restraint use (NDNQI, n.d.). Such broad reporting enables units and organizations to compare their results with national averages. Nurses may then prioritize and set goals accordingly to improve patient outcomes directly influenced by nursing care.

Once nurses identify and agree to implement new recommendations that incorporate evidence-based practice or QI strategies, nurses often encounter many obstacles. Lack of authority, autonomy, knowledge, and time pose serious threats to advances (Brown, Wickline, Ecoff, & Glaser, 2009). Regardless, oncology nurses must do their best to learn and incorporate new interventions and treatments into their practices.

Research

Oncology nurses have made remarkable contributions to research efforts, which have led to advances in cancer care and support. As integral members of research teams, nurses assume principal investigator, project coordinator, and data manager roles. In such roles, nurses are ideally positioned to ensure ethical conduct of research. However, mandatory ethics education and oversight from institutional review boards will not eliminate misconduct. Misconduct may occur at any point along the research continuum.

Research studies must offer potential for discovering valuable knowledge, be methodically rigorous, and offer favorable benefit-to-risk ratios to participants. To prevent study participants from receiving known inadequate treatments, clinical trials must possess equipoise. *Equipoise,* or professional uncertainty, serves as the foundation for randomized controlled trials (Miller & Joffe, 2011). Interim data analyses of therapeutic trials should be conducted to discover possible treatment variances. Such variances could reduce trial durations.

Conflicts routinely exist between research and clinical goals (Lidz et al., 2009). Such conflicts affect eligibility requirements. Clinical trials strive to produce valid results to benefit future patients but require scientific rigor to ensure quality results. Clinical care strives to improve the lives of current patients. Healthcare providers may be tempted to enroll patients into specific studies despite patients' failing to meet eligibility requirements. By doing so, providers hope to provide potentially beneficial interventions and treatments not otherwise available.

Although participants volunteer to take part in clinical trials, misconduct may occur during recruitment phases. Participants may not understand the purposes of trials because informed consent may be inadequate. The seven elements of informed consent, as outlined by Beauchamp and Childress (2009), must be present to ensure autonomy (see Figure 9-5).

Despite the strict regulation of actual informed consent, many study participants do not understand the purposes of their clinical trials (Cohn & Larson, 2007). Although the intention of phase I trials is to determine maximum tolerated dosages (versus therapeutic efficacy), many phase I trial participants believe that they may benefit from their participation (Kohara & Inoue, 2010). Safeguards are necessary to protect vulnerable patient populations who may not be able to act with autonomy or make informed decisions, such as children and people with cognitive disabilities.

Participants may also feel obligated to participate. Clinical research nurses must remain neutral during consent processes, and they must use easy-to-understand language. Ultimately, oncology nurses must respect individual patient choices with regard to clinical trial participation.

Research misconduct may also occur throughout data management processes and result dissemination. Because of lengthy time requirements and limited resources, data may be misrepresented or falsified. Oncology nurses must remain vigilant to ensure ethical management of trial data.

Genetic and Genomic Health Care

Since the completion of the human genome sequencing in 2003, gene-based technologies have emerged. These technologies assist with cancer prevention, screening, diagnosis, and treatment (Lea, 2008). Unlike with nutrition and personal behavior, individuals are incapable of modifying their unique genetic codes (Lowrey, 2004). Accordingly, genetic discoveries have created ethical issues regarding cost, discrimination, equal access, personal impact, privacy, and confidentiality (Lea, 2008). The National Institutes of Health and the U.S. Department of Energy are collaborating to address ethical, legal, and social issues. The "grand challenges" for such issues include (a) cultural and religious views, (b) diversity as it relates to genomics, (c) implications of new discoveries, (d) intellectual property issues, (e) research conduct, and (f) the use of genetic information for non–healthcare-related matters (Lea, 2008).

Many ethical issues now center on confidentiality and privacy. Oncology nurses are encouraged to explain history and information gathering processes prior to obtaining consent for genetic testing. When patients test positive for potentially damaging genes and choose not to share such information with others who may be directly affected, nurses face ethical dilemmas. Also, discrimination may be possible if genetic testing is required for employment or insurance coverage.

- Patient is competent to make a decision about research participation.
- Patient is willing to make a decision about research participation.
- Patient has adequate information to make the decision about research participation.
- Patient receives a plan about research participation.
- Patient demonstrates understanding about the research participation plan.
- Patient makes a decision to participate in the research.
- Patient gives permission to participate in the research.

Figure 9-5. Seven Elements of Informed Consent

Note. Based on information from Beauchamp & Childress, 2009.

Many unanswered questions have also emerged. Will patients have equitable access to genomic technologies? If so, how might expensive genomic science and treatments be made available to those with limited resources? Who will fund treatment development for rare genetic conditions? Lowrey (2004) also identified inconclusive findings and associated psychosocial consequences as concerns.

Oncology nurses fully participate in genetic-based and genomic-based practice activities. Oncology nurses collect family histories, obtain informed consent for genetic testing and treatment, and administer gene-based therapies. Accordingly, they have critical roles and responsibilities to advocate on behalf of, counsel, educate, and support patients as they make gene-based decisions.

Survivorship Issues

Although evidence-based guidelines exist for childhood cancer survivors, only a small percentage of survivors actually receive appropriate follow-up care. Much less is known about the late effects and needs of adult cancer survivors. Additional challenges include lacking survivorship research designed to inform practice and shortages of providers trained to care for survivors.

Despite the number of cancer survivors increasing in recent years, the quality of their health care has not improved as quickly. Consequently, the 2005 Institute of Medicine report *From Cancer Patient to Cancer Survivor: Lost in Transition* (Hewitt, Greenfield, & Stovall, 2006) recommended survivorship care plans for each of the nation's 10 million cancer survivors. Such individualized plans should communicate previous treatments and their potential long-term effects, appropriate follow-up intervals and studies, health maintenance and lifestyle tips, and psychosocial needs (Hewitt et al., 2006). The goals of these plans are to ultimately improve communication between primary care providers and oncologists and improve overall outcomes for cancer survivors.

Oncology nurses and other healthcare professionals have ethical responsibilities to ensure patients may access care and understand their conditions. Patients also need to understand associated short-term and long-term treatment complications. Such complications include late comorbidities, organ dysfunction, and secondary malignancies. Patients' abilities to comprehend such crucial information may be negatively affected by the associated shock and adjustment periods following cancer diagnoses.

Specifically, fertility is affected by cancer treatment. Reproductive technology will continue to assist survivors to conceive children. Yet, such technology will have its own dilemmas associated with availability, awareness, cost, and timing. Many young men and women affected by chemotherapy-related infertility will struggle with the costs associated with such options and their unknown risks (Jukkala, 2009; King et al., 2008).

Futility

Futility generally describes actions that serve no meaningful purpose. When determining futility, McCabe and Storm (2008) encouraged healthcare providers to consider (a) treatment goals, (b) the likelihood of achieving such goals, (c) associated risks, benefits, and costs for pursuing treatment versus associated risks, benefits, and costs for not pursuing treatment, and (d) needs of individual patients.

Understandably, patients and families may want to receive treatment. Patients believe in their rights to seek aggressive care or decline palliative care interventions.

Many patients with advanced malignancies want to do everything possible to survive and live (Rousseau, 2002; von Gruenigen & Daly, 2005a). According to patients, treatment is often linked to hope (Schonwetter, 2006, as cited in von Gruenigen & Daly, 2005a; Weissman, 2003). Because treatment may slow disease progression, many healthcare providers strive to maintain hope and respect patients' self-determination and autonomy by offering treatment.

von Gruenigen and Daly (2005b) expressed that when treatment serves no meaningful purpose or fails to achieve goals related to quality of life, treatment should be considered futile. Futile treatment does not impact overall survival, as the treatment will not reverse or halt disease progression. Although providers are ethically obligated to respect patient autonomy, patient autonomy does not obligate providers to offer treatment to all patients. Providers, according to von Gruenigen and Daly (2005b), are obligated to avoid causing harm (nonmaleficence).

Moratti (2009) noted that professional nursing and medical standards are violated when futile treatments are administered. According to Moratti (2009), providers must follow two rules to adhere to professional standards. First, providers should carefully use core nursing and medical skills to perform their professional duties. Second, providers need to know the appropriate criteria listed in clinical and professional guidelines prior to offering treatment. Such guidelines combine evidence from clinical trials and medical-ethical considerations to ensure consistency. Consistency, in turn, promotes fairness. When providers offer futile treatments, providers may be violating professional standards and ignoring principles of justice.

Howard and Pawlik (2009) also described futile treatments as violations of professional ethics. Despite clinical and ethical consequences of labeling treatments *futile*, Howard and Pawlik believe that providers are not ethically obligated to provide such treatments. Ultimately, in cases of futility, Howard and Pawlik believe that providers are ethically obligated to transition patients to palliative care. To minimize clinical and ethical dilemmas, Howard and Pawlik favor nonmaleficence and beneficence by encouraging providers to develop and maintain open communication with their patients and families. Ultimately, providers need to be clear to minimize misunderstandings and unrealistic expectations.

Although many families may be unprepared for frank discussions about diagnosis and prognosis, David (as cited in King & Quill, 2006) noted that "terminal candor" is necessary for families to process life-limiting illnesses. Also, research has demonstrated that patients and their families want to know the truth about their conditions. Truth, even when difficult to hear, allows patients to discuss their end-of-life options in terms of (a) anticipated success, (b) costs, (c) projected effect on length of life, and (d) quality of life (Rodriguez & Young, 2006).

Rather than use the term *futile*, other experts support an obligation to be honest and objective (Marik, 2007; Rodriguez & Young, 2006; Rousseau, 2002). Citing data from multiple studies, Marik (2007) explained that patients with advanced cancer do not do well in critical care settings. Essentially, patients may be harmed in critical care settings. Rodriguez and Young (2006) acknowledged that honesty requires effort, patience, and time. By not abandoning their patients, providers will gain the respect and trust of all patients and families (Rousseau, 2002). Such actions demonstrate commitments to justice. Also, providers may facilitate positively perceived deaths. Ultimately, patients will have the autonomy to choose how they die.

End-of-Life Care

Healthcare providers should also be educated about conducting goals-of-care conversations and consulting palliative care. Such crucial conversations help to address issues associated with unclear or incomplete advance directives (Nishimura et al., 2007). Such conversations also address surrogates' influences (Vig, Starks, Taylor, Hopley, & Fryer-Edwards, 2007). Prior to hospitalizations, providers should encourage patients and families to discuss goals based on possible scenarios (Emanuel, 2008). When patients with chronic illnesses desire all interventions, healthcare professionals should explore the wishes of these patients (Quill, Arnold, & Back, 2009). Notably, administrators may choose to support palliative care efforts because reduced healthcare costs are associated with achieved goals of care (Freeman, 2010; Hanchate, Kronman, Young-Zu, Ash, & Emanuel, 2009).

Electronic Health Records

Electronic health records (EHRs) offer numerous benefits. Such benefits include increased access to healthcare information, enhanced communication among healthcare providers, and built-in safeguards to prevent errors and promote evidence-based practice (Richards, 2009). As EHRs become more prevalent throughout health care, their abilities to store and communicate healthcare data raise many ethical issues for nurses and other healthcare providers. Ethical concerns associated with the use of EHRs relate to violations of patient privacy and confidentiality as well as the quality and quantity of data in the record.

EHRs assimilate information from various healthcare providers as well as from patients themselves. Although central databases for healthcare data offer tremendous advantages, challenges may arise from excessive information (Wynia & Dunn, 2009). Healthcare providers assume some degree of liability and responsibility for content not easily located. Also, EHRs require maintenance and attention to detail to minimize errors that may be quickly duplicated.

Many patients would like their sensitive information restricted from general view within their EHRs. Such sensitive information may include infectious diseases, genetic issues, mental illnesses, psychological issues, and substance abuse (Dunlop, 2010). For example, adolescents have rights to withhold sensitive information from their parents and legal guardians. Conversely, parents and legal guardians have rights to the healthcare information of their children (Sittig & Singh, 2011).

Although violations of patient confidentiality are not unique to EHRs, private information from EHRs may be leaked with greater speed and depth than private information from written records. Unfortunately, information from electronic records may be easily accessed by unauthorized users. Nurses may unintentionally forget to close computer screens within public viewing areas. Also, employees within healthcare organizations may attempt to view private information for non-professional purposes.

The widespread use of EHRs also creates disparities. Older, low-income, and undereducated patients may not have access to computers. Also, patients who live in rural or remote areas may not have access to high-speed or reliable Internet access. Such patients may experience deficits compared to those who have rapid electronic interactions enhanced by EHRs.

Finally, although EHRs may facilitate more efficient and timely communication, Internet communication decreases face-to-face and telephone communication between patients and providers. When less time is spent directly interacting with patients and families, oncology nurses may miss subtle cues and nonverbal behaviors that are important contributors to the development of therapeutic nurse-patient relationships.

Social Networking and Social Media

Internet-based and mobile communication sites such as Facebook, Twitter, and YouTube are effective tools for entertainment and professional and personal networking. However, social media poses challenges for oncology nurses related to confidentiality and appropriate professional boundaries. Oncology nurses must use social media appropriately and maintain professional boundaries.

Because information disseminated across the Internet becomes immediately and (usually) permanently available to others, oncology nurses need to be sensitive to potential consequences associated with posting professional and personal content. When posting professional content including photographs and stories of clinical incidents, oncology nurses clearly violate patients' and colleagues' rights to privacy and confidentiality. When oncology nurses connect with patients and families on social networking sites, essential professional boundaries between patients and providers may be crossed (Bressler, 2010).

Professional boundaries safeguard nurse-patient relationships. Ultimately, the primary commitment of nurses is to act on behalf of patients' best interests. Online networking with patients may lead to inappropriate interactions and sharing of information. Such sharing may not serve the best interests of patients. Invitations and opportunities to network with patients may be particularly problematic with younger patients, who are more likely to rely on electronic communication.

Although oncology nurses are free to post photographs and other content that reflect their personal values and lifestyles outside of work settings, they must understand that employers, patients, and families also have access to these sites. Any negative or controversial personal information posted and viewed reflects poorly upon the professional values of individuals. Such postings may erode credibility within work settings. Ultimately, nurses need to be cautious about what content they choose to self-disclose on social media sites (McBride & Cohen, 2009).

Developing and Maintaining Ethical Nursing Practice

Given the abundance of ethical dilemmas in daily practice, oncology nurses need to know where to turn for assistance. Nurses should acknowledge the importance of ethical climates, cultivate moral courage, build moral communities within their work settings, and promptly address ethical dilemmas with interdisciplinary colleagues. Furthermore, ethics education is critical for all nurses. Ethics education should be incorporated into nursing school curriculum, and ongoing initiatives should be pursued for novice and experienced nurses to strengthen their ethics knowledge and expertise.

The Importance of Ethical Climates

Ulrich et al. (2007) found that increased ethics-related stress is associated with decreased job satisfaction. According to the survey results of more than 1,200 nurses and social workers, roughly two-thirds of those surveyed felt exhausted, frustrated, and helpless with various ethical issues. When the respondents perceived that they did not have support from their organizations, they reported that they considered seeking alternative employment. One-fourth of the respondents acknowledged that they did not want to continue their current job because of excess stress and lack of respect and satisfaction. These unfortunate results should cause alarm for organizational leaders and managers. In order to improve job satisfaction and retain qualified and capable nurses, leaders and managers need to acknowledge and improve their ethical climate, dedicate resources to their ethical climate, and strive to reduce ethics-related stress.

Combating Moral Distress and the Crescendo Effect

Nurses need to identify and acknowledge the repetitive nature of moral distress in their practice (Epstein & Delgado, 2010). Because moral distress may not realistically be eliminated (Epstein & Hamric, 2009), nurses have moral imperatives to ultimately collaborate with other healthcare professionals (Hamric et al., 2006). Furthermore, moral distress must be reduced to ensure employee retention and satisfaction (Rice et al., 2008).

According to Epstein and Hamric (2009), oncology nurses should confront moral distress. To do so, they recommended that oncology nurses (a) identify moral distress by using proper terminology, (b) address root causes in institutional or unit culture that foster moral distress, (c) adopt policies that enable all healthcare providers to identify ethical concerns and initiate ethics consultations, (d) develop unified support networks, (e) foster interdisciplinary collaboration, (f) implement change to maintain moral integrity, (g) incorporate mentoring and institutional resources such as moral distress consultation services, (h) make conscious decisions, and (i) provide and join educational offerings and discussions.

Considerable support and resources are necessary to identify, process, and decrease moral distress. Nurses need to seek value clarification once they understand their individual healthcare organizations (Epstein & Delgado, 2010). In addition, nurses need to enhance their communication skills to improve communication with multiple healthcare disciplines (Epstein & Delgado, 2010). Oncology nurses require supportive advanced practice nurses and administrators who support ethical climates and foster interdisciplinary collaboration. Such staff should encourage rotating staffing assignments to relieve individual nurses. Rounds, in-services, and case studies should strive to educate oncology nurses about ethical dilemmas. Nursing support groups may also lend support and stimulate discussion. Survivor celebrations enable oncology nurses to reconnect with their patients (Shepard, 2010).

To reduce the negative effects of moral distress, the American Association of Critical-Care Nurses (n.d.) recommended that nurses adopt the "4As." Essentially, nurses should ask, affirm, assess, and act. First, nurses should question whether they are experiencing moral distress. Next, they should affirm their feelings and acknowledge their threatening moral integrity. Third, they should assess the origins of their moral distress and their possible actions. Finally, nurses should act to reduce moral distress.

Ethics committees also have the potential to decrease moral distress. As such, oncology nurses should also volunteer to serve on ethics committees. Patients, oncology nurses, and ethics committees benefit when oncology nurses volunteer in this capacity (Shepard, 2010). Furthermore, ethics consultation services should understand the crescendo effect. Although professionals with moral distress may initiate ethics consultations, ethics consultants should assess for moral distress. Also, moral distress originates from individual cases and leaps into the lives of units, teams, and healthcare systems (Epstein & Hamric, 2009).

Many possible outcomes may result when moral distress is confronted. Notably, interventions can expose a true liability to healthcare professionals when moral distress is identified. Also, threats to providers' moral integrity can be reduced. Such reduction may decrease the moral distress and residual crescendo slopes. Such reduction may also keep healthcare professionals working in health care. Furthermore, individuals in less powerful positions will be able to have their voices heard. These actions strengthen moral integrity and sensitivity (Epstein & Delgado, 2010). Several nursing experts believe that the identification and management of moral distress is essential to retaining competent nurses for years to come (Rice et al., 2008).

Moral Courage

With an understanding of moral distress, oncology nurses may wonder how to demonstrate moral courage. LaSala and Bjarnason (2010) noted that ethical foundations are essential for developing ethical values and stimulating ethical practice. Oncology nurses, however, should be cautioned that such incorporations do not guarantee moral courage.

What is moral courage? Lachman (2007) defined *moral courage* as "the individual's capacity to overcome fear and stand up for his or her core values" (p. 131). Lachman explained that individuals who display moral courage have the ability to confront and reduce fear by voicing their core values. Their willingness to speak and act for righteousness enacts ethical principles and concepts. To resolve ethical dilemmas, nurses with moral courage are able to incorporate conflict resolution skills into their ethical conversations. Individuals with moral courage seek to act correctly and properly and accept the consequences of their actions. Furthermore, such courage may also foster self-confidence and confessions as appropriate. Nurses with moral courage reflect positively for their patients, themselves, and their profession.

Nurses demonstrate moral courage when they voice concerns about premature discharges for patients with limited resources or do not give medications with unknown dosages and efficacy (LaSala & Bjarnason, 2010). Moral courage, integral for ethical behavior, enables individuals to act in challenging situations. Individuals with moral courage incorporate ethical principles into their practice (Murray, 2010).

Acting with moral courage may have undesired consequences and risks. Such oncology nurses may encounter rejection and humiliation (Lachman, 2007). Potentially, they may become victims of lateral violence or lose their jobs (Lachman, 2007; LaSala & Bjarnason, 2010). However, nurses who publically display moral courage tend to experience internal peace for discussing ethical issues and dilemmas (Lachman, 2007).

Because moral courage is not always apparent, it needs to be cultivated. Moral courage development should begin in associate and baccalaureate nursing programs. Clinics, organizations, healthcare systems, and professional organizations should continue to develop moral courage through policy development, educational offerings, and professional literature. Ethical principle-based discussions, case studies, and role modeling will promote moral courage (Murray, 2010). Moral courage may also be developed through shared governance, which favors collaborative decision making and shared responsibility (LaSala & Bjarnason, 2010).

Lachman (2010) believes moral courage to be virtuous. Moral courage incorporates knowledge and reasoning acquired over time through education and situations. Although professionals who demonstrate moral courage perceive fear, they continue to act. Oncology nurses should consider using cognitive reframing and self-soothing techniques to alleviate some of their fear. They should also consider practicing assertive and negotiation skills. Such techniques may reduce fear and make risk more tolerable. In time, oncology nurses will develop self-confidence.

When nurses assert themselves, Lachman (2010) recommended that they incorporate the following four factors into their communication. First, nurses should discuss the desired behavior to be changed. Nurses should communicate this change in nonjudgmental, objective, and nonthreatening manners. Second, nurses should discuss their personal feelings. Third, nurses should discuss the behavior implications in the situation. Finally, nurses should reveal their desired action or intervention. Lachman (2010) gave an example of this type of assertion in the following passage:

> When you refuse to talk to the family about the patient's prognosis, I feel upset because they now believe he will be going home. I would like you to spend time with them and help them understand that this will not happen. (p. 7)

Murray (2010) listed many organizations committed to developing moral courage. These organizations include the ANA Center for Ethics and Human Rights, the American Society for Bioethics and Humanities, the Foundation for Moral Courage, the Institute for Global Ethics, and the Moral Courage Project.

The American Organization of Nurse Executives believes that all nurses should work in healthy environments that promote moral courage. Because nurse leaders impact patient care and make decisions that influence healthcare organizations, nurse leaders are strongly encouraged to adapt shared governance concepts. Yet, nursing leaders must also display moral courage to act justly and have impact. Moral courage will transform patient care situations, units, and healthcare systems (Edmonson, 2010).

Although developing nurse leaders with moral courage is quite challenging, Edmonson (2010) recommends the following four interventions. First, nurse leaders need to understand the degree of moral distress currently experienced by their nurses. Second, nurse leaders should allow moral courage to develop within the professional culture. Third, nurse leaders should increase moral courage by choosing a model that fosters a healthy professional environment. Finally, nurse leaders should learn about ethical concepts, theories, and decision making.

Oncology nurses are encouraged to use methodical processes to manage ethical issues in clinical settings. Purtillo (as cited in Cohen & Erickson, 2006) suggested that nurses collaborate with members of the interdisciplinary team using a six-step method similar to the nursing process. Specifically, Purtillo encouraged nurses to (a) assess situations, (b) identify ethical issues, (c) analyze ethical issues, (d) weigh potential solutions, (e) act, and (f) evaluate the effects. When nurses use the "SBAR" process, they communicate with structure and purpose: **S**ituation,

Background, **A**ssessment, and **R**ecommendation discussions improve communication (Rice et al., 2008).

Building Moral Communities and Ethical Climates

According to Hamric (1999), nurses who perceive that they may positively influence their work environment are more likely to respond to ethical dilemmas. To increase nurses' capacity for ethical action, nurses should feel professionally empowered to respond in ethically appropriate ways (de Casterlé et al., 2008).

Canadian nurses Rodney, Doane, Storch, and Varcoe (2006) defined *moral climate* as "the implicit and explicit values that drive healthcare delivery and shape the workplaces in which care is delivered" (p. 24). They acknowledged the negative impact of autocratic organization decision-making styles, intradisciplinary and interdisciplinary team conflict, reductions in clinical leadership, and staffing cutbacks on moral climates. In order to strengthen moral climates, direct care nurses should be engaged and supported (Rodney et al., 2006). Advanced practice nurses, managers, and administrators are encouraged to promote and maintain collaboration, as well as opportunities for direct care nurses to reflect on their work environments and nursing practice. The authors also concluded that all nurses must incorporate ethical language into their professional conversations, as correct language lends credibility. Notably, Rodney et al. (2006) emphasized that strong moral climates cultivate and enhance safe patient care.

The American Association of Critical-Care Nurses has recognized the importance of healthy work environments. The organization identified six standards for creating and maintaining healthy work environments: (a) skilled communication, (b) true collaboration, (c) effective decision making, (d) appropriate staffing, (e) meaningful recognition, and (f) authentic leadership (American Association of Critical-Care Nurses, 2005). The American Association of Critical-Care Nurses continues to develop resources and tools to assist nurses and healthcare organizations.

By incorporating ethical conversations into practice, oncology nurses may support each other and members of the interdisciplinary team. Such support may reduce feelings of betrayal, loneliness, and misunderstanding. Such support may also foster shared decision making (Austin, 2007).

Shirey (2005) identified 22 strategies to create ethical climates. Some of those strategies include (a) incorporate ANA position statements and resources into practice, (b) determine baseline and periodically assess ethical climates, (c) disclose climate results, (d) hold all organizational leaders accountable for developing and maintaining ethical climates, (e) create and maintain ethical leadership programs, (f) evaluate organizational rewards for leaders, (g) encourage direct care nurses to learn about ethical decision making and participate in ethical decision-making forums such as educational opportunities, ethics committees, and rounds, (h) ensure ethical consistency throughout organizations by periodically conducting audits, and (i) create forums that enable all nurses to celebrate their caring accomplishments.

Ethics Consultation Services

Well-known cases such as Karen Quinlan and Nancy Cruzan focused the nation's attention on ethical issues. Ethics committees were created because of simultaneous professional, regulatory, and legal forces. Ethics committees were thought to serve as alternatives to possible legal action. The President's Commission for the Study of Ethical Problems in Medicine and Biomedical Research, the American Medical Association, and the Joint Commission encouraged ethics committees to be created and maintained. Ethics committees were also created to enable healthcare decisions to be made objectively according to ethical frameworks and to provide opportunities for individual rights to be acknowledged (Aulisio & Arnold, 2008).

Today, ethics committees enable clinicians to discuss morally conflicting views and concepts with individuals who have likely had some degree of ethics training. Ethics committees may also promote education and policy development for healthcare providers and community members. When consulted, ethics committees receive requests to assist with challenging cases. Ethics committees are composed of administrators, chaplains, lawyers, nurses, physicians, and social workers (Aulisio & Arnold, 2008). Often, community members with no medical knowledge are invited to join ethics committees. The authors of this chapter feel that nursing representation on ethics committees is essential and that ethics committees should not confuse ethical issues with legal issues.

Aulisio and Arnold (2008) discussed ethics in relation to palliative care, as ethics and palliative care have many similarities. Many palliative care clinicians have studied clinical ethics. By nature of their specialty, palliative care clinicians often provide care to patients and families in critical care settings and end-of-life situations. By nature of the associated complexities, ethics committees often discuss critically ill patients nearing the end of their lives. Furthermore, many studies have demonstrated that ethics consults and palliative care consults improve patient satisfaction, decrease length of stay in critical care environments, and promote goals of care (Aulisio & Arnold, 2008).

However, ethics experts who consult when requested and palliative care providers are fundamentally different. Ethics consultants consider conflicts and uncertainties in complex issues. Often, such issues are value laden. Ethics consultants will attempt to identify and review conflicts. Ethics consultants will also recommend moral options based on committee consensus. Palliative care providers holistically manage symptoms for patients with life-limiting illnesses. Oncology nurses, therefore, are encouraged to familiarize themselves with available ethics and palliative care consult teams.

Although evidence supports ethics consultations, ethical experts may not be frequently consulted. Gordon and Hamric (2006) surveyed 504 nurses and then interviewed 83 of them. Many nurses did not know how to obtain ethics consultations. Assuming nurses knew about ethics consultations, many feared repercussions stemming from power imbalances. Such repercussions negatively affected nurses. Because of diverging views, nurses encountered moral dilemmas when they took necessary steps to discuss ethical issues with physicians. Ethics consultations were perceived to signal communication breakdowns. Consequently, physicians became angry when nurses sought ethics consultations prior to discussing their concerns with physicians. Ultimately, nurses avoided discussing moral situations because of physicians' responses. Those surveyed also expressed concern about the potential of negatively impacting other professional relationships and losing their jobs if they requested ethics consultations. Eventually, such communication failures perpetuate medical hierarchies and inhibit moral community development. Such failure calls for collaborative dialogue, interdisciplinary education, and continued professional education.

Unit-Based Ethics Conversations

Because research has shown that nurses have difficulties expressing their concerns to other healthcare professionals, one healthcare system developed a unit-based ethics conversations (UBEC) program (Wocial et al., 2010). Nurses may use UBECs as a method to discuss ethical issues. UBECs ultimately create moral openness and safe environments. UBECs also enable nurses to process their personal emotions associated with ethical dilemmas. Over time, nurses who participated in such conversations were more capable and felt more confident to deal with ethical dilemmas (Wocial et al., 2010).

During UBECs, nurses tell stories to each other about ethical dilemmas. The stories provide opportunities for gaining ethical knowledge, managing situations and/or emotions, promoting personal reflection, and yielding insight. Moral reasoning may also be strengthened. UBECs may improve communication and reasoning skills for participants. Over time, nurses may better comprehend ethical principles and concepts (Wocial et al., 2010).

Helft, Bledsoe, Hancock, and Wocial (2009) provided many guidelines for conducting UBECs. Because oncology nurses may struggle to identify the specific issue, facilitators should consider asking targeted questions. Specific answers identify key issues that are likely causing moral distress. Details may be clarified, consensus may be measured, and best practice may be discussed.

Through their experiences with UBECs, the authors identified three important concepts. First, direct care nurses want to understand their unique ethical issues and appreciate the ethical components to their work. Second, easy answers are likely impossible. However, nurses appreciate sharing with and learning from each other. Finally, the facilitator's ability to identify ethical issues is important for UBECs to be perceived as successful. UBEC facilitators should be selected because they have received ethics training (Helft et al., 2009).

Ethics Education for Students and Oncology Nurses

In the *Essentials of Baccalaureate Education for Professional Nursing Practice,* the American Association of Colleges of Nursing (2008) delineated competencies required for new nurses to enter the profession. The call for integrated educational activities related to ethics is evident in several of the essentials. For example, in order to learn professional values, students should be given opportunities to develop ethical reasoning through community-based activities that promote advocacy and social justice as part of their liberal education. Students should also be able to identify and articulate ethical implications of healthcare and economic policies, as well as participate in scenarios that illustrate ethical dilemmas in clinical practice and research.

When students first encounter ethical issues in clinical situations, they often use their personal experiences and environmental resources as the foundations (Numminen & Leino-Kilpi, 2007). Students and novice nurses will develop higher levels of reasoning as they encounter additional moral situations and advance their educations. The undergraduate nursing curriculum should include content about ethical codes and principles. Undergraduate students should also learn how to apply these resources to their clinical experiences. When students complete ethics courses and have ethical content integrated into their curriculum, they are better prepared to address and resolve ethical dilemmas in their practice. Such knowledge will reduce their moral distress (Range & Rotterham, 2010).

Following graduation, novice oncology nurses may experience moral uncertainty and distress because of differences between academic concepts and clinical realities (Cantrell, Browne, & Lupinacci, 2005). Novice nurses may lack confidence with their clinical performance and skills, as well as struggle with critical thinking. Novice nurses may also worry about their integration into healthcare teams and struggle to gain independence. Preceptors and seasoned clinicians are encouraged to support novice nurses by exploring troubling ethical situations with them. Also, preceptors and seasoned clinicians should offer support by encouraging novice nurses to acknowledge their feelings and demonstrating how to handle such situations.

In order to gain confidence in their moral reasoning, judgments, and actions, experienced oncology nurses should complete ethics-related continuing education (Grady et al., 2008). Ethics-related continuing education and in-services help to develop key ethics skills. Attendees will learn how to frame ethical components of complex situations, define their personal ethical values, and build skill sets for addressing future ethical dilemmas. Currently, no specific recommendations related to this topic are available to guide oncology nurses. However, oncology nurses should seek assistance from advanced practice nurses and ethics committees.

Optimal ethics education should incorporate interprofessional and intraprofessional components. Because interprofessional collaborative practice strengthens healthcare delivery and improves health outcomes, interprofessional education (IPE) is necessary for future nurses. IPE should also be offered to practicing nurses (World Health Organization, 2010). Collaborative practice extends beyond daily interactions in clinical settings. Collaborative practice calls for partnerships, mutual responsibility, and shared goals (Alberto & Hearth, 2009; D'Amour, Ferrada-Videla, San Martin-Rodriguez, & Beaulieu, 2005). In order to prevent and alleviate future moral distress originating from nurse-physician conflicts, collaborative-ready healthcare providers should be developed.

Conclusion

Developing and maintaining an ethical nursing practice is a unique journey for each oncology nurse. Student and novice oncology nurses may not easily recognize or articulate ethical dilemmas in patient care situations. Rather, they may be focused on learning psychomotor skills and integrating into organizational cultures. However, oncology nurses should act on their feelings of uncertainty, frustration, and dissatisfaction.

As oncology nurses gain experience and clinical proficiency in caring for complex patients, they will gradually adopt more holistic views of patient situations. These nurses will derive meaning and consider long-term outcomes (Benner, 1984). Ideally, oncology nurses will develop increased ethical sensitivity and confidence. Such traits will enable oncology nurses to communicate with members of interdisciplinary teams. By using correct ethical terminology to communicate, oncology nurses will gain credibility to address ethical issues in everyday practice. Ultimately, every oncology nurse within a healthcare organization is responsible for creating and maintaining their ethical environments. Advanced practice nurses and nurse leaders have additional responsibilities to create and maintain ethical environments.

All oncology nurses are responsible for seeking ethics education. Oncology nurses are encouraged to learn about ethics through various means, such as engaging in ethical dialogue, attending rounds and lectures, participating in ethics committees, and utilizing their professional organizations. ANA and the Oncology Nursing Society (ONS) offer tremendous resources for oncology nurses. The ANA Code of Ethics and the ONS Ethics Special Interest Group are invaluable. Without ethical education and commitment, moral distress will continue to threaten oncology nursing.

References

Alberto, J., & Hearth, K. (2009). Interprofessional collaboration within faculty roles: Teaching, service, and research. *Online Journal of Issues in Nursing, 14*(2). Retrieved from http://nursingworld.org/MainMenuCategories/ANAMarketplace/ANAPeriodicals/OJIN/TableofContents/Vol142009/No2May09/Articles-Previous-Topics/Interprofessional-Collaboration-.aspx

American Association of Colleges of Nursing. (2008). The essentials of baccalaureate education for professional nursing practice. Retrieved from http://www.aacn.nche.edu/Education/pdf/BaccEssentials08.pdf

American Association of Critical-Care Nurses. (n.d.). The 4A's to rise above moral distress. Retrieved from http://www.aacn.org/WD/Practice/Docs/4As_to_Rise_Above_Moral_Distress.pdf

American Association of Critical-Care Nurses. (2005). AACN standards for establishing and sustaining healthy work environments: A journey to excellence. Retrieved from http://www.aacn.org/WD/HWE/Docs/HWEStandards.pdf

American Nurses Association. (2001). Code of ethics for nurses with interpretive statements. Retrieved from http://www.nursingworld.org/MainMenuCategories/EthicsStandards/CodeofEthicsforNurses/Code-of-Ethics.aspx

Aulisio, M.P., & Arnold, R.M. (2008). Role of the ethics committee: Helping to address value conflicts or uncertainties. *Chest, 134*, 417–424. doi:10.1378/chest.08-0136

Austin, W.A. (2007). The ethics of everyday practice: Healthcare environments as moral communities. *Advances in Nursing Science, 20*(1), 81–88.

Baily, M.A., Bottrell, M., Lynn, J., & Jennings, B. (2006). The ethics of using QI methods to improve health care quality and safety. *Hastings Center Report, 36*(4), S1–S40.

Beauchamp, T.L., & Childress, J.F. (2009). *Principles of biomedical ethics* (6th ed.). New York, NY: Oxford University Press.

Benner, P. (1984). *From novice to expert: Excellence and power in clinical nursing practice.* Menlo Park, CA: Addison-Wesley.

Bressler, T. (2010). Professional boundaries: A legal, ethical, and administrative perspective. *APHON Counts, 24*(3), 4–5.

Brown, C.E., Wickline, M.A., Ecoff, L., & Glaser, D. (2009). Nursing practice, knowledge, attitudes and perceived barriers to evidence-based practice at an academic medical center. *Journal of Advanced Nursing, 65*, 371–381. doi:10.1111/j.1365-2648.2008.04878.x

Cantrell, M.A., Browne, A.M., & Lupinacci, P. (2005). The impact of a nurse externship program on the transition process from graduate to registered nurse: Part I quantitative findings. *Journal for Nurses in Staff Development, 21*, 187–195.

Centers for Medicare and Medicaid Services. (2011, September 21). Medicare hospice benefits. Retrieved from http://www.medicare.gov/publications/pubs/pdf/02154.pdf

Cohen, J.S., & Erickson, J.M. (2006). Ethical dilemmas and moral distress in oncology nursing practice. *Clinical Journal of Oncology Nursing, 10*, 775–780. doi:10.1188/06.CJON.775-780

Cohn, E., & Larson, E. (2007). Improving participant comprehension in the informed consent process. *Journal of Nursing Scholarship, 39*, 273–280. doi:10.1111/j.1547-5069.2007.00180.x

D'Amour, D., Ferrada-Videla, M., San Martin-Rodriguez, L., & Beaulieu, M.D. (2005). The conceptual basis for interprofessional collaboration: Core concepts and theoretical frameworks. *Journal of Interprofessional Care, 9*(Suppl. 1), 116–131. doi:10.1080/13561820500082354

de Casterlé, B.D., Izumi, S., Godfrey, N.S., & Denhaerynck, K. (2008). Nurses' responses to ethical dilemmas in nursing practice: Meta-analysis. *Journal of Advanced Nursing, 63*, 540–549. doi:10.1111/j.1365-2648.2008.04702.x

Deshpande, S.P. (2009). A study of ethical decision making by physicians and nurses in hospitals. *Journal of Business Ethics, 90*, 387–397. doi:10.1007/s10551-009-0049-5

Dunlop, B.W. (2010). Should sensitive information from clinical trials be included in electronic medical records? *JAMA, 304*, 685–686. doi:10.1001/jama/2010.1117

Edmonson, C. (2010, September 30). Moral courage and the nurse leader. *Online Journal of Issues in Nursing, 15*(3), Manuscript 5. doi:10.3912/OJIN.Vol15No3Man05

Elkin, E.B., & Bach, P.B. (2010). Cancer's next frontier: Addressing high and increasing costs. *JAMA, 303*, 1086–1087. doi:10.1001/jama.2010.283

Emanuel, L.L. (2008). Advance directives. *Annual Review of Medicine, 59*, 187–198. doi:10.1146/annurev.med.58.072905.062804

Epstein, E.G., & Delgado, S. (2010, September 30). Understanding and addressing moral distress. *Online Journal of Issues in Nursing, 15*(3), Manuscript 1. doi:10.3912/OJIN.Vol15No3Man01

Epstein, E.G., & Hamric, A.B. (2009). Moral distress, moral residue, and the crescendo effect. *Journal of Clinical Ethics, 20*, 330–342.

Freeman, J.M. (2010). Rights, respect for dignity, and end-of-life care: Time for a change in the concept of informed consent. *Journal of Medical Ethics, 36*, 61–62. doi:10.1136/jme.2009.031773

Fry, S.T., & Duffy, M.E. (2001). The development and psychometric evaluation of the ethical issues scale. *Journal of Nursing Scholarship, 33*, 273–277. doi:10.1111/j.1547-5069.2001.00273.x

Gordon, E.J., & Hamric, A.B. (2006). The courage to stand up: The cultural politics of nurses' access to ethics consultation. *Journal of Clinical Ethics, 17*, 231–254.

Grady, C., Danis, M., Soeken, K.L., O'Donnell, P., Taylor, C., Farrar, A., & Ulrich, C.M. (2008). Does ethics education influence the moral action of practicing nurses and social workers? *American Journal of Bioethics, 8*, 4–11. doi:10.1080/15265160802166017

Ham, K. (2004). Principled thinking: A comparison of nursing students and experienced nurses. *Journal of Continuing Education in Nursing, 35*, 66–73.

Hamric, A.B. (1999). The nurse as a moral agent in modern health care. *Nursing Outlook, 47*, 106. doi:10.1016/S0029-6554(99)90001-5

Hamric, A.B., & Blackhall, L.J. (2007). Nurse-physician perspectives on the care of dying patients in intensive care units: Collaboration, moral distress, and ethical climate. *Critical Care Medicine, 35*, 422–429. doi:10.1097/01.CCM.0000254722.50608.2D

Hamric, A.B., Davis, W.S., & Childress, M.D. (2006). Moral distress in health care professionals: What is it and what can we do about it? *Pharos, 69*(1), 16–23.

Hanchate, A., Kronman, A.C., Young-Xu, Y., Ash, A.S., & Emanuel, E. (2009). Racial and ethnic differences in end-of-life costs: Why do minorities cost more than whites? *Archives of Internal Medicine, 169*, 493–501. doi:10.1001/archinternmed.2008.616

Helft, P.R., Bledsoe, P.D., Hancock, M., & Wocial, L.D. (2009). Facilitated ethics conversations: A novel program for managing moral distress in bedside nursing staff. *Journal of Nursing Administration's Healthcare, Law, Ethics, and Regulation, 11*, 27–33. doi:10.1097/NHL.0b013e31819a787e

Hewitt, M., Greenfield, S., & Stovall, E. (Eds.). (2006). *From cancer patient to cancer survivor: Lost in transition*. Retrieved from http://www.iom.edu/Reports/2005/From-Cancer-Patient-to-Cancer-Survivor-Lost-in-Transition.aspx

Howard, D.S., & Pawlik, T.M. (2009). Withdrawing medically futile treatment. *Journal of Oncology Practice, 5*, 193–195. doi:10.1200/JOP.0948501

Hughes, A., Gudmundsdottir, M., & Davies, B. (2007). Everyday struggling to survive: Experiences of the urban poor living with advanced cancer. *Oncology Nursing Forum, 34*, 1113–1118. doi:10.1188/07.ONF.1113-1118.

International Council of Nurses. (2006). The ICN code of ethics for nurses. Retrieved from http://www.icn.ch/about-icn/code-of-ethics-for-nurses

Jameton, A. (1984). *Nursing practice: The ethical issues*. Englewood Cliffs, NJ: Prentice-Hall.

Jukkala, A. (2009). Breast cancer survivors and fertility preservation: Ethical and religious considerations. *Seminars in Oncology Nursing, 25*, 278–283. doi:10.1016/j.soncn.2009.08.005

King, D.A., & Quill, T. (2006). Working with families in palliative care: One size does not fit all. *Journal of Palliative Medicine, 9*, 704–715. doi:10.1089/jpm.2006.9.704

King, L., Quinn, G.P., Vadaparampil, S.T., Gwede, C.K., Miree, C.A., Wilson, C., … Perrin, K. (2008). Oncology nurses' perceptions of barriers to discussion of fertility preservation with patients with cancer. *Clinical Journal of Oncology Nursing, 12*, 467–476. doi:10.1188/08.CJON.467-476

Kohara, I., & Inoue, T. (2010). Searching for a way to live to the end: Decision-making process in patients considering participation in cancer phase I clinical trials. *Oncology Nursing Forum, 37*, E124–E132. doi:10.1188/10.ONF.E124-132

Lachman, V.D. (2007). Moral courage: A virtue in need of development? *MEDSURG Nursing, 16*, 131–133.

Lachman, V.D. (2010, September 30). Strategies necessary for moral courage. *Online Journal of Issues in Nursing, 15*(3), Manuscript 3. doi:10.3912/OJIN.Vol15No03Man03

LaSala, C., & Bjarnason, D. (2010, September 30). Creating workplace environments that support moral courage. *Online Journal of Issues in Nursing, 15*(3), Manuscript 4. doi:10.3912/OJIN.Vol15No03Man04

Lea, D.H. (2008, April 30). Genetic and genomic healthcare: Ethical issues of importance to nurses. *Online Journal of Issues in Nursing, 13*(1), Manuscript 4. doi:10.3912/OJIN.Vol13No01Man04

Lidz, C.W., Appelbaum, P.S., Joffe, S., Albert, K., Rosenbaum, J., & Simon, L. (2009). Competing commitments in clinical trials. *IRB: Ethics and Human Research, 31*(5), 1–6. Retrieved from http://www.medscape.com

Lowrey, K.M. (2004). Legal and ethical issues in cancer genetic nursing. *Seminars in Oncology Nursing, 20,* 203–208. doi:10.1053/j.soncn.2004.04.007

Lynn, J., Baily, M.A., Bottrell, M., Jennings, B., Levine, R.J., Davidoff, F., … James, B. (2007). The ethics of using quality improvement methods in health care. *Annals of Internal Medicine, 146,* 666–673. Retrieved from http://www.annals.org/content/146/9/666.full.pdf

Marik, P.E. (2007). Management of patients with metastatic malignancy in the intensive care unit. *American Journal of Hospice and Palliative Care, 23,* 479–482. doi:10.1177/104/9909106294921

Mayer, D.K. (2011). Evidence-based practice: Challenging what we think we know. *Clinical Journal of Oncology Nursing, 15,* 237. doi:10.1188/11.CJON.237

McBride, D., & Cohen, E. (2009, July). Misuse of social networking may have ethical implications for nurses. *ONS Connect, 24*(7), 17. Retrieved from http://onsconnect.org/wp-content/issues/2009/07.pdf

McCabe, M.S., & Storm, C. (2008). When doctors and patients disagree about medical futility. *Journal of Oncology Practice, 4,* 207–209. doi:10.1200/JOP.0848503

Miller, F.G., & Joffe, S. (2011). Equipoise and the dilemma of randomized clinical trials. *New England Journal of Medicine, 364,* 476–480. doi:10.1056/NEJMsb1011301

Moratti, S. (2009). The development of "medical futility": Towards a procedural approach based on the role of the medical profession. *Journal of Medical Ethics, 35,* 369–372. doi:10.1136/jme.2008.027755

Murray, J.S. (2010, September 30). Moral courage in healthcare: Acting ethically even in the presence of risk. *Online Journal of Issues in Nursing, 15*(3), Manuscript 2. doi:10.3912/OJIN.Vol15no03Man02

Myser, C., Donehower, P., & Frank, C. (1999). Making the most of disequilibrium: Bridging the gap between clinical and organizational ethics in a newly merged healthcare organization. *Journal of Clinical Ethics, 10,* 194–201.

National Database of Nursing Quality Indicators. (n.d.). Frequently asked questions. Retrieved from https://www.nursingquality.org/FAQPage.aspx#1

Nishimura, A., Mueller, P.S., Evenson, L.K., Downer, L.L., Bowron, C.T., Thieke, M.P., … Crowley, M.E. (2007). Patients who complete advance directives and what they prefer. *Mayo Clinic Proceedings, 82,* 1480–1486. doi:10.4065/82.12.1480

Numminen, O.H., & Leino-Kilpi, H. (2007). Nursing students' ethical-decision making: A review of the literature. *Nurse Education Today, 27,* 796–807. doi:10.1016/j.nedt.2006.10.013

Park, M. (2009). Ethical issues in nursing practice. *Journal of Nursing Law, 13,* 68–77. doi:10.1891/1073-7472.13.3.68

Quill, T.E., Arnold, R., & Back, A.L. (2009). Discussing treatment preferences with patients who want "everything." *Annals of Internal Medicine, 151,* 345–349.

Range, L.M., & Rotterham, A.L. (2010). Moral distress among nursing and non-nursing students. *Nursing Ethics, 17,* 225–232. doi:10.1177/0969733009352071

Rice, R.M., Rady, M.Y., Hamrick, A., Verheijde, J.L., & Pendergast, D.K. (2008). Determinants of moral distress in medical and surgical nurses at an adult acute care tertiary hospital. *Journal of Nursing Management, 16,* 260–373. doi:10.111/j.1365-2834.2007.00798.x

Richards, M.M. (2009). Electronic medical records: Confidentiality issues in the time of HIPAA. *Professional Psychology: Research and Practice, 4,* 550–556. doi:10.1037/a0016853

Rodney, P., Doane, G.H., Storch, J., & Varcoe, C. (2006). Toward a safer moral climate. *Canadian Nurse, 102*(8), 24–27.

Rodriguez, K.L., & Young, A.J. (2006). Perceptions of patients on the utility or futility of end-of-life treatment. *Journal of Medical Ethics, 32,* 444–449. doi:10.1136/jme.2005.014118

Rousseau, P. (2002). Aggressive treatment in the terminally ill: Right or wrong? *Journal of Palliative Medicine, 5,* 657–658. doi:10.1089/109662102320880444

Shepard, A. (2010). Moral distress: A consequence of caring. *Clinical Journal of Oncology Nursing, 14,* 25–27. doi:10.1188/10.CJON.25-27

Shirey, M.R. (2005). Ethical climate in nursing practice: The leader's role. *Journal of Nursing Administration's Healthcare Law, Ethics, and Regulation, 7*(2), 59–67. doi:10.1097/00128488-200504000-00006

Sittig, D.F., & Singh, H. (2011). Legal, ethical, and financial dilemmas in electronic health record adoption and use. *Pediatrics, 127,* e1042–e1047. doi:10.1542/peds.2010-2184

Ulrich, C., O'Donnell, P., Taylor, C., Farrar, A., Danis, M., & Grady, C. (2007). Ethical climate, ethics stress, and the job satisfaction of nurses and social workers in the United States. *Social Science and Medicine, 65,* 1708–1719. doi:10.1016/j.socscimed.2007.05.050

Vig, E.K., Starks, H., Taylor, J.S., Hopley, E.K., & Fryer-Edwards, K. (2007). Surviving surrogate decision-making: What helps and hampers the experience of making medical decisions for others. *Society of General Internal Medicine, 22,* 1274–1279. doi:10.1007/s11606-007-0252-y

von Gruenigen, V.E., & Daly, B.J. (2005a). Futility: Clinical decisions at the end-of-life in women with ovarian cancer. *Gynecologic Oncology, 97,* 638–644. doi:10.1016/j.ygyno.2005.01.031

von Gruenigen, V.E., & Daly, B.J. (2005b). Treating ovarian cancer patients at the end of life: When should we stop? *Gynecologic Oncology, 99,* 255–256. doi:10.1016/j.ygyno.2005.09.005

Weissman, D. (2003). Medical oncology and palliative care: The intersection of end-of-life care. *Journal of Palliative Medicine, 6,* 859–861. doi:10.1089/109662103322654721

Wocial, L.D., Hancock, M., Bledsoe, P.D., Chamness, A.R., & Helft, P.R. (2010). An evaluation of unit-based ethics conversations. *Journal of Nursing Administration's Healthcare Law, Ethics, and Regulation, 12*(2), 48–54. doi:10.1097/NHL.0b013e3181de18a2

World Health Organization. (2010). Framework for action on interprofessional education and collaborative practice. Retrieved from http://whqlibdoc.who.int/hq/2010/WHO_HRH_HPN_10.3_eng.pdf

Wynia, M., & Dunn, K. (2009). Dreams and nightmares: Practical and ethical issues for patients and physicians using personal health records. *Journal of Law, Medicine, and Ethics, 38,* 64–73. doi:10.1111/j.1748-720X.2010.00467.x

Zafar, Y., Goetzinger, A.M., Fowler, R., Gblokpor, A., Warhadpande, D., Taylor, D.H., … Abernethy, A.P. (2011). Impact of out-of-pocket expenses on cancer care. *Journal of Clinical Oncology, 29*(Suppl. 18), Abstract 6006.

CHAPTER 10

The Reality of Gero-Oncology for Nursing in an Aging Society

Sarah H. Kagan, PhD, RN, AOCN®

Introduction

Cancer—from detection and diagnosis through periodic and chronic treatment to survivorship and end-of-life care—represents the future illness and caregiving burden of aging societies like the United States, as well as many developed and developing nations around the world (Jemal et al., 2011; Smith, Smith, Hurria, Hortobagyi, & Buchholz, 2009; Thun, DeLancey, Center, Jemal, & Ward, 2010). In our society, where longevity and cancer survivorship are increasing, aging demographics and cancer epidemiology delineate commensurate increases in specific aspects of the human burden of the cancer experience. Symptom profiles and functional decline resulting from cancer and its treatment interact with underlying frailty and comorbid disease.

This complex interplay of disease, symptom, and function generate escalating needs for nursing care. Oncology nurses are the vanguards of health care. Nurses are experts in mitigating individual and family burden of cancer as well as helping to contain familial and social costs of caregiving demands. As a result, oncology nurses possess the necessary skills, perspective, and scope to generate and implement innovative solutions that can improve cancer care in an aging society. Nevertheless, oncology nurses face prospects of astonishing educational, scientific, and clinical challenges as they formulate necessary solutions.

This chapter aims to describe the future of oncology nursing with respect to practice, education, research, and policy. The chapter begins by casting a new light on demographics and epidemiology, reflecting relationships that create impact in cancer care and nursing. Discussion of practice emphasizes advances in cancer treatment and the ways in which sociocultural forces combine with changes in treatment to alter care delivery and settings for care. An agenda to meet the challenges presented by cancer care in an aging society and transform challenge into opportunity concludes the chapter.

Implications of an Aging Society

Demographics and Disease

Gains in life expectancy along with declining birth rates beget an aging society. An aging society determined by rates of birth and death generates consequences through patterns of function and dependency. *Dependency ratios*—the ratios of dependent adults and children to able adults who support and care for them—in aging societies are of great concern to nurses. Although overall dependency ratios may remain stable or decline in light of declining birth rates, current projections predict higher than expected elder dependency ratios in developed nations where mortality is already low (Tuljapurkar, Li, & Boe, 2000). Specific disease-related mortality and morbidity rates for cancer in both developed and developing nations outline improving survival and imply extended periods of possible morbidity (Jemal et al., 2011; Thun et al., 2010). Whether that morbidity is from a cancer diagnosis or its treatment, greater dependency results at a societal level. Greater dependency increases burdens and costs of cancer in aging societies.

Dependency in late life emerges most often as a consequence of more than one chronic condition and multiple functional losses (Fried, Ferrucci, Darer, Williamson, & Anderson, 2004; Fulop et al., 2010; Weiss, 2011). *Underlying frailty*—a physiologic phenomenon mediated by senescence—is compounded by comorbid conditions and syndromes in what is almost certainly a causal cascade resulting in escalating informal care needs and use of healthcare services (Fried et al., 2004). Despite the impetus of an aging population, most biomedical science and health care isolates chronic conditions for investigation and treatment (Bayliss, Edwards, Steiner, & Main, 2008; Institute of Medicine [IOM], 2008). An isolated approach to disease management fragments care and risks triggering polypharmacy and other geriatric syndromes. Importantly, older patients also find it frustrating and confusing (Bayliss et al., 2008; Boyd et al., 2007).

Cancer, long considered an acute and life-threatening condition, is more accurately a chronic disease with sustained physical, emotional, psychosocial, and spiritual dimensions (Adler & Page, 2008; Avis & Deimling, 2008; Holland & Weiss, 2008; Thun et al., 2010). As a chronic disease, cancer increasingly results in long-term survivorship. Importantly, cancer is an age-related disease, disproportionately affecting older adults and those who live to late life after diagnoses earlier in life (Avis & Deimling, 2008; Bellury et al., 2011; Malek & Silliman, 2007; Rao & Demark-Wahnefried, 2006). Disease cure or control both result in long-term survivorship and predominantly exist in the context of comorbid conditions. The commensurate risk of frailty with geriatric syndromes and functional limitations further complicate cancer survivorship in late life.

Aging, Generations, and the Societal Burden of Cancer

Expectations and use of health and social care mediate the social burdens and costs of cancer in an aging society. The current generational shift from the Mature and Silent generations to the sheer magnitude of the Baby Boom generation receives much attention in popular and scientific press (Keehan et al., 2008; Martin, Freedman, Schoeni, & Andreski, 2009; Ricketts, 2011). Some evidence suggests and authors commonly predict that members of the much vaunted Baby Boom generation will demand more and different healthcare services while others attempt to predict the health of this generation (IOM, 2008; Keehan et al., 2008; Martin et al., 2009; O'Neil, 2009; Ricketts, 2011). Only time may reveal true patterns of healthcare use and outcomes. Contemporary epidemiologic trends in age-related diseases such as cancer, combined with clear population projections, however, do point toward manifest healthcare need, clinician and caregiver shortages, and increased expenditures to compensate for both (IOM, 2008; Keehan et al., 2008; O'Neil, 2009).

Older adults may expect and value different elements in health care. Health care, particularly cancer care, may represent different investments, decisions, and potential outcomes for older adults. While much has been made of the "Me" generational character of Baby Boomers, little substantive evidence outlines the ramifications of generationally specific behavior as opposed to developmentally mediated behaviors in health care. Nonetheless, healthcare users—whether they are referred to as *patients* or as *consumers*—are less likely, regardless of age, to agree to curative therapies for cancer without adequate supportive care. As a result, use of supportive care, integrative therapies, and efforts to market these aspects of cancer care will only increase as the older adult population grows in size (Cheung, Wyman, & Halcon, 2007; Lawsin et al., 2007). Oncology nurses, with strengths in symptom management and patient experience, are ideally placed to lead service integration and delivery no matter what generational shifts the Mature, Silent, and Baby Boom generations demand of cancer care.

Perceptions of aging in the culture of cancer care potentially limit capacity to meet the demands of an aging society (Crawford, 2011; Delamothe, 2008; IOM, 2007, 2008; Kagan, 2008a). Persistent ageism shapes responsiveness to challenge and openness to solutions in oncology care delivery systems, education, practice, and policy (Kagan, 2008a, 2009). Issues of ageism require scrutiny as oncology nurses address generational needs and education required to change practice and meet care delivery demands (Bellury et al., 2011; Kagan, 2008a, 2008b; Rao & Demark-Wahnefried, 2006). The many needs of burgeoning patient numbers as well as rapidly evolving treatment paradigms suggest that integrating analysis of possibly ageist assumptions must parallel efforts to advance education and practice (Kagan, 2009). Although ageism is commonly acknowledged as a barrier in the adequacy and effectiveness of clinical trials, the role of benign neglect in regard to unique aspects of caring for older patients and the impact of positively intended parentalism on the part of clinicians is not as well understood (Kagan, 2009). Sensitivity, similar to the proponents of cultural sensitivity, provides integral support to assessment, analysis, and correction of ageist assumptions in cancer care. Effective communication becomes essential with increasingly complex care, multiple options, and critical treatment and goals of care decisions that older people and their families make. Underscoring that ageism is ever more unacceptable as societies and populations age emphasizes a different sensibility in the culture of cancer care and a changing expectation about aging and caring for older adults and their families (Kagan, 2008a; O'Connor, 2011).

Healthcare Policy and Reform

Expectations of cancer care on the part of older patients pair with economic forces shaping current healthcare delivery and reform. Patients with cancer and their families expect both comfort and compassion as elements of effective cancer care, critically evaluating treatment process and outcomes (Bayliss et al., 2008; Repetto,

Piselli, Raffaele, & Locatelli, 2009). Similarly, concerns about the population-based healthcare needs of aging societies drive intense debate and rapidly issued policy directives aimed at cost containment and outcomes improvement (Beverly, Burger, Maas, & Specht, 2010; Bhalla & Kalkut, 2010; Iglehart, 2009; Kizer & Dudley, 2009; Murray & McElwee, 2010; Oberlander, 2010; O'Neil, 2009; Stanley, Werner, & Apple, 2009). Increasingly, contemporary discourse on healthcare reform explicitly considers implications of aging populations and nursing need (Beverly et al., 2010; Bhalla & Kalkut, 2010; O'Neil, 2009). Conversely, more recent conversations about patient and family–centered care remain less clearly connected to aging families and preferences of older people as well as generational concerns (Luxford, Safran, & Delbanco, 2011; Reid Ponte & Peterson, 2008). Discussions of older patient and family preferences for care emphasize communication, goals of care, and advance directives (Bomba & Vermilyea, 2006; Epstein, Fiscella, Lesser, & Stange, 2010; Rose, O'Toole, Koroukian, & Berger, 2009). Bayliss and colleagues suggested that older patients with comorbid conditions express preferences for individualized approaches, care coordination, and a single contact person (Bayliss et al., 2008). Their findings echo precepts of patient and family–centered care mandated at a regulatory level while underscoring well-established markers of quality care for older people (Boyd et al., 2007; Epstein et al., 2010; Happ, Williams, Strumpf, & Burger, 1996; Kizer & Dudley, 2009). Success in future cancer care requires integration of expectations and reforms to achieve effective older patient–centered care that moves beyond the cancer and provider–focused model common today (Epstein et al., 2010; Luxford et al., 2011).

Shifts in the Paradigm of Cancer Care

Three prominent trends in cancer treatment promise to shape care for all patients and imply markedly important consequences for care of older adults. Most obviously, the emergence of targeted therapies presents possibilities for improving responses to therapy, suggesting potential shifts in survivorship and alterations in expected treatment toxicity and side effect profiles, necessitating differential supportive care (Bellury et al., 2011; Rao & Demark-Wahnefried, 2006). The promise of combining targeted therapies with understandings of genomic markers of malignant cell and senescent cell behavior makes personalized cancer therapy a reality. Finally, dual forces of patient expectations and healthcare economics continually drive delivery of the expanding catalog of cancer treatment options into outpatient, ambulatory settings.

Emerging science in targeted therapies creates an ever-faster treadmill of change in oncology nursing education and practice. As biomedical researchers and physician scientists introduce new agents, regimens, and combined modalities into cancer care, oncology nurses and nurse researchers are compelled to keep pace with modifications in practice and timely investigations. Targeted therapies diverge from long-held expectations of anticancer therapy toxicity and side effects. This divergence generates an array of new and altered symptoms with which oncology nurses must contend on behalf of their patients. Combinations of targeted therapies in ever-changing regimens pose the multiplicative effect of drug-drug and drug-therapy interactions. Patient experience of protocols that combine targeted therapies with traditional antineoplastic agents, radiotherapeutic modalities, and minimally invasive surgical and interventional procedures is often poorly delimited by extant evidence.

Limited evidence then places burdens for assessment and management on generalist and advanced practice oncology nurses as they create standards of care ad hoc.

Personalized cancer therapy, the oncologic variant of personalized medicine, connotes futuristic technologies used to individualize diagnosis, treatment, and evaluation (Toyota et al., 2009). The dawn of truly personalized medicine is not a distant possibility but an almost immediate reality in leading academic centers. Anticancer medicine already possesses the science for fundamental elements of personalized cancer therapy, including identified epigenetic biomarkers, cellular targets, and innovative delivery systems (Gal-Yam, Saito, Egger, & Jones, 2008; Rodriguez-Paredes & Esteller, 2011; Toyota et al., 2009; Tsai & Baylin, 2011). The advent of personalized cancer therapy then poses a dualistic challenge to oncology nurses. First, nurses must prepare to deliver these therapies, readying the nursing and interdisciplinary research communities to study the human experience of understanding these therapies, identifying side effects and toxicities, and developing and evaluating management strategies. Ageism presents further threat as nurses and interdisciplinary colleagues ensure that older adults have equal access to emerging therapies and personalized medicine.

Changing Cancer Care Delivery

Cancer care delivery systems are changing almost as quickly as therapeutic options evolve. Oral therapies and other ambulatory treatments are increasingly standard for most cancer diagnoses and most patients (Ma & Adjei, 2009; Maloney & Kagan, 2011). Drug and other technologies are quickly advancing, and care delivery systems and clinicians are more sophisticated than ever in managing the needs of patients receiving complex regimens (Maloney & Kagan, 2011). As a result, care settings for cancer therapies are shifting noticeably from a balance of care delivered in inpatient and select outpatient environments to a continuum that emphasizes home and clinic delivery. This shift in settings for delivery of care results in downstream reliance on high-acuity inpatient care for management of unexpected emergent toxicities and complications as well as aggressive care in advanced disease (Earle et al., 2008). Changes in care delivery create commensurate demands for documentation and communication of that care (Cutler & Everett, 2010; Shortell & Casalino, 2008). Electronic health records that transcend commonplace fragmentation in current healthcare delivery are at a premium, the Holy Grail of delivery systems. Although patients may respect and understand the need for effective electronic records, evidence suggests they and their families desire effective communication and care coordination (Bayliss et al., 2008; Repetto et al., 2009). Similarly, clinicians also prioritize communication, especially in delivering cancer care for older adults, whose needs are more complex (Luxford et al., 2011; Owusu & Studenski, 2009; Rose et al., 2009).

An Agenda for the Future of Oncology Nursing

An agenda that addresses the future of oncology nursing in an aging society must shape professional culture while directing practical initiatives to achieve necessary change. Meeting the demands of an aging society with workforce shortfalls, professional knowledge gaps, limited resources, and mismatched evidence is a pressing yet daunting task. Experts serving on the IOM panel commissioned to deliver a report on health care for our aging society acknowledged significant lack of action despite well-known population demographics and epidemiologic projections (IOM, 2008). Many voices are raised, and yet change is slow and even absent in some domains. Calls for more and different education and for increased research to improve clinical care generally lack explicit analysis of disciplinary, organizational, and institutional culture as foundational to argued change. The agenda presented here then begins with culture before moving forward to recommend changes in education and practice to address cancer care needs for our aging society. This combination of cultural change and recommendations in education and research, although specific to American oncology nursing, may offer resonance for demographically similar societies.

Changing the Culture of Oncology Nursing

The culture of oncology nursing in America is strong and well established, relying on the central organizing function of the Oncology Nursing Society (ONS). A well-respected nursing specialty, oncology nursing holds professional stature and cachet. Through ONS and its leadership in practice and policy, oncology nursing has acknowledged the importance of care of older people for more than a decade (Kagan, 2004). National leadership stemming from ONS actions includes policy statements and educational initiatives. Nevertheless, the frontline culture of oncology nursing is apparently slow to change. Care of older people remains a specialty by individual choice, warranting particular interest and an independent pursuit of knowledge and skills. Although many oncology nurses admit to caring for mostly older patients, still only small numbers claim this population as a primary focus. Research similarly often addresses age as a variable. However, despite this advance in research focus, too few investigators are prepared for and declare primary focus on the older adult population and cancer. Furthermore, chronologic age remains the most evident operational variable, representing unsophisticated interpretations of understanding cancer in late life as well as advancing age in survivorship. Such lags in identifying nurses in research and practice are emblematically a cultural phenomenon within the nursing discipline and the oncology nursing specialty. Overdue improvements in education, research, and practice are likely only achievable with concerted attention and bold activism on the part of nurses to address latent ageism in oncology nursing. Political activism, rather than mere leadership, offers advantages in effecting change in oncology nursing and other nursing specialties in institutions where nurses practice, teach, and investigate and in the professional and lay communities that have a stake in the quality of care for our aging society (Mahlin, 2010).

Educating for Competence and Expertise

Momentum for changing education becomes feasible with the foundation of aging-focused multidisciplinary culture. Many expert voices coalesce in calling for education with two aims (IOM, 2008; Kagan, 2008a, 2008b). Geriatric competence is necessary to ensure adequate care for all patients as they age and receive care in late life (Mezey, Boltz, Esterson, & Mitty, 2005; Mezey, Stierle, Huba, & Esterson, 2007; "Nurse Competence in Aging (NCA) Partners: Association Activities and Resources," 2007; Resnick, 2007; Scholder, Kagan, & Schumann, 2004; Stierle et al., 2006). Although education broadly has been the focus of prominent competency programs, specific relevance is obvious for nursing students, currently practicing nurses in need of continuing education, and research trainees. Importantly, education must move past chronologic age as defining the topic to the many implications of function, generation, culture, and family as they play out in health and social care. The burden of a burgeoning aged population suggests stronger emphasis on contemporary concerns about topics such as care coordination and effective transitions, and patient and family education for self-care and family care holds significant merit.

Education for practice, more broadly, requires specific plans for generalist and advanced practice nurses. Generalist clinical nurses require education to meet the exactingly specialized care needs of older adults diagnosed with and treated for cancer throughout their often long survivorship trajectories across different care settings. Advanced practice nurses must be prepared for oncologic treatment models that combine modalities, center on patient and family goals and needs, and maintain a focus on function, self-care, and care coordination. In addition, artificial distinctions between geriatric and oncologic care are outdated and require new vision to achieve adequate preparation for practice (Rose et al., 2009). Undergraduate nursing and proposed advanced practice nursing regulations offer little guidance in developing visionary curricula to meet this challenge (Benner, Sutphen, Leonard, Day, & Shulman, 2009; Stanley, 2009). Thus, an agenda for nursing education to meet the demands of cancer care in aging requires accommodation as innovative curricula are proposed and tested.

Embracing Gero-Oncology Research

Similar to education, oncology nursing research lacks dedicated focus commensurate with the magnitude of cancer in our aging society. Simply put, if cancer is a disease of aging and the great majority of people diagnosed with and treated for cancer are aged and many of those people experience complex care needs, then a significant proportion of cancer nursing research should reflect these realities (Jemal et al., 2011; Jemal, Siegel, Xu, & Ward, 2010). Research conducted by nurses and their interdisciplinary teams must achieve a pervasive orientation to issues of aging and aging changes at biologic, psychological, social, emotional, and spiritual levels in combination with parallel aspects of cancer and oncology care. Current research is particularly limited by two factors. First, chronologic age remains the default variable to define gero-oncology nursing research. Such use of age results in potentially erroneous and often inconclusive findings, as evidence strongly suggests little exclusive relationship between age and other variables of interest in cancer research. Second, patient populations easily accessed and eager to participate in clinical research, such as women with breast cancer, are almost overstudied, creating imbalance in the reflection of clinical realities in current research. Overly simplistic and convenient sampling limits scientific quality and may divert resources from more needful groups and unexplored phenomena in gero-oncology.

Conclusion

Shifting the culture of oncology nursing to recognize the full import of an aging society and transforming education and research as the new culture takes shape form the foundation of a new oncology nursing practice. In this new practice, care of older people is the core of oncology nursing. Both generalist and advanced practice oncology nurses must be fundamentally competent in this tangibly altered practice. Additionally, some in each group of nurse clinicians must specialize in various aspects of meeting the unique needs of older patients across a variety of diagnostic groups and settings of care. Most significantly, oncology nurses of the future—as they become gero-oncology nurses—must discard isolated approaches to disease and therapeutic modalities to become perceptive and able communicators and coordinators of care for older people contending with comorbid conditions, complex treatment options, and varied functional needs. Masters of transitions in care, gero-oncology nurses anchor individualized cancer care for older people and their families in an age of personalized cancer care.

References

Adler, N.E., & Page, A.E. (Eds.). (2008). *Cancer care for the whole patient: Meeting psychosocial health needs.* Retreived from http://books.nap.edu/openbook.php?record_id=11993&page=R2

Avis, N.E., & Deimling, G.T. (2008). Cancer survivorship and aging. *Cancer, 113*(Suppl. 12), 3519–3529. doi:10.1002/cncr.23941

Bayliss, E.A., Edwards, A.E., Steiner, J.F., & Main, D.S. (2008). Processes of care desired by elderly patients with multimorbidities. *Family Practice, 25,* 287–293. doi:10.1093/fampra/cmn040

Bellury, L.M., Ellington, L., Beck, S.L., Stein, K., Pett, M., & Clark, J. (2011). Elderly cancer survivorship: An integrative review and conceptual framework. *European Journal of Oncology Nursing, 15,* 233–242. doi:10.1016/j.ejon.2011.03.008

Benner, P., Sutphen, M., Leonard, V., Day, L., & Shulman, L.S. (2009). *Educating nurses: A call for radical transformation.* New York, NY: Jossey-Bass.

Beverly, C., Burger, S.G., Maas, M.L., & Specht, J.K.P. (2010). Aging issues: Nursing imperatives for healthcare reform. *Nursing Administration Quarterly, 34,* 95–109. doi:110.1097/NAQ.1090b1013e3181d91718

Bhalla, R., & Kalkut, G. (2010). Could Medicare readmission policy exacerbate health care system inequity? *Annals of Internal Medicine, 152,* 114–117. doi:10.1059/0003-4819-152-2-201001190-00185

Bomba, P.A., & Vermilyea, D. (2006). Integrating POLST into palliative care guidelines: A paradigm shift in advance care planning in oncology. *Journal of the National Comprehensive Cancer Network, 4,* 819–829.

Boyd, C.M., Boult, C., Shadmi, E., Leff, B., Brager, R., Dunbar, L., ... Wegener, S. (2007). Guided care for multimorbid older adults. *Gerontologist, 47,* 697–704. doi:10.1093/geront/47.5.697

Cheung, C.K., Wyman, J.F., & Halcon, L.L. (2007). Use of complementary and alternative therapies in community-dwelling older adults. *Journal of Alternative and Complementary Medicine, 13,* 997–1006. doi:10.1089/acm.2007.0527

Crawford, S.M. (2011). Cancer care in the UK: Updating the professional culture. *Postgraduate Medical Journal, 87,* 243–244. doi:10.1136/pgmj.2010.099085

Cutler, D.M., & Everett, W. (2010). Thinking outside the pillbox—Medication adherence as a priority for health care reform. *New England Journal of Medicine, 362,* 1553–1555. doi:10.1056/NEJMp1002305

Delamothe, T. (2008). Universality, equity, and quality of care. *BMJ, 336,* 1278–1281. doi:10.1136/bmj.a169

Earle, C.C., Landrum, M.B., Souza, J.M., Neville, B.A., Weeks, J.C., & Ayanian, J.Z. (2008). Aggressiveness of cancer care near the end of life: Is it a quality-of-care issue? *Journal of Clinical Oncology, 26,* 3860–3866. doi:10.1200/JCO.2007.15.8253

Epstein, R.M., Fiscella, K., Lesser, C.S., & Stange, K.C. (2010). Why the nation needs a policy push on patient-centered health care. *Health Affairs, 29,* 1489–1495. doi:10.1377/hlthaff.2009.0888

Fried, L.P., Ferrucci, L., Darer, J., Williamson, J.D., & Anderson, G. (2004). Untangling the concepts of disability, frailty, and comorbidity: Implications for improved targeting and care. *Journals of Gerontology Series A: Biological Sciences and Medical Sciences, 59,* M255–M263. doi:10.1093/gerona/59.3.M255

Fulop, T., Larbi, A., Witkowski, J., McElhaney, J., Loeb, M., Mitnitski, A., & Pawelec, G. (2010). Aging, frailty and age-related diseases. *Biogerontology, 11,* 547–563. doi:10.1007/s10522-010-9287-2

Gal-Yam, E.N., Saito, Y., Egger, G., & Jones, P.A. (2008). Cancer epigenetics: Modifications, screening, and therapy. *Annual Review of Medicine, 59,* 267–280. doi:10.1146/annurev.med.59.061606.095816

Happ, M.B., Williams, C.C., Strumpf, N.E., & Burger, S.G. (1996). Individualized care for frail elders: Theory and practice. *Journal of Gerontological Nursing, 22*(3), 6–14.

Holland, J., & Weiss, T. (2008). The new standard of quality cancer care: Integrating the psychosocial aspects in routine cancer from diagnosis through survivorship. *Cancer Journal, 14,* 425–428. doi:10.1097/PPO.1090b1013e31818d38934

Iglehart, J.K. (2009). The struggle for reform—Challenges and hopes for comprehensive health care legislation. *New England Journal of Medicine, 360,* 1693–1695. doi:10.1056/NEJMp0902651

Institute of Medicine. (2007). *Cancer in elderly people: Workshop proceedings.* Retrieved from http://www.nap.edu/openbook.php?record_id=11869&page=R1

Institute of Medicine. (2008). *Retooling for an aging America: Building the health care workforce.* Retrieved from http://books.nap.edu/openbook.php?record_id=12089&page=R2

Jemal, A., Bray, F., Center, M.M., Ferlay, J., Ward, E., & Forman, D. (2011). Global cancer statistics. *CA: A Cancer Journal for Clinicians, 61,* 69–90. doi:10.3322/caac.20107

Jemal, A., Siegel, R., Xu, J., & Ward, E. (2010). Cancer statistics, 2010. *CA: A Cancer Journal for Clinicians, 60,* 277–300. doi:10.3322/caac.20073

Kagan, S.H. (2004). Gero-oncology nursing research. *Oncology Nursing Forum, 31,* 293–299. doi:10.1188/04.ONF.293-299

Kagan, S.H. (2008a). Ageism in cancer care. *Seminars in Oncology Nursing, 24,* 246–253. doi:10.1016/j.soncn.2008.08.004

Kagan, S.H. (2008b). Moving from achievement to transformation. *Geriatric Nursing, 29,* 102–104. doi:10.1016/j.gerinurse.2008.01.005

Kagan, S.H. (2009). The plateau of recognition in specialty acute care. *Geriatric Nursing, 30,* 130–131. doi:10.1016/j.gerinurse.2009.01.005

Keehan, S., Sisko, A., Truffer, C., Smith, S., Cowan, C., Poisal, J., & Clemens, M.K. (2008). Health spending projections through 2017: The baby-boom generation is coming to Medicare. *Health Affairs, 27,* w145–w155. doi:10.1377/hlthaff.27.2.w145

Kizer, K.W., & Dudley, R.A. (2009). Extreme makeover: Transformation of the veterans health care system. *Annual Review of Public Health, 30,* 313–339. doi:10.1146/annurev.publhealth.29.020907.090940

Lawsin, C., DuHamel, K., Itzkowitz, S., Brown, K., Lim, H., Thelemaque, L., & Jandorf, L. (2007). Demographic, medical, and psychosocial correlates to CAM use among survivors of colorectal cancer. *Supportive Care in Cancer, 15,* 557–564. doi:10.1007/s00520-006-0198-3

Luxford, K., Safran, D.G., & Delbanco, T. (2011). Promoting patient-centered care: A qualitative study of facilitators and barriers in healthcare organizations with a reputation for improving the patient experience. *International Journal for Quality in Health Care, 23,* 510–515. doi:10.1093/intqhc/mzr024

Ma, W.W., & Adjei, A.A. (2009). Novel agents on the horizon for cancer therapy. *CA: A Cancer Journal for Clinicians, 59,* 111–137. doi:10.3322/caac.20003

Mahlin, M. (2010). Individual patient advocacy, collective responsibility and activism within professional nursing associations. *Nursing Ethics, 17,* 247–254. doi:10.1177/0969733009351949

Malek, K., & Silliman, R. (2007). Cancer survivorship issues in older adults. In P.A. Ganz (Ed.), *Cancer survivorship* (pp. 215–224). New York, NY: Springer.

Maloney, K.W., & Kagan, S.H. (2011). Adherence and oral agents with older patients. *Seminars in Oncology Nursing, 27,* 154–160. doi:10.1016/j.soncn.2011.02.007

Martin, L.G., Freedman, V.A., Schoeni, R.F., & Andreski, P.M. (2009). Health and functioning among baby boomers approaching 60. *Journals of Gerontology Series B: Psychological Sciences and Social Sciences, 64B,* 369–377. doi:10.1093/geronb/gbn040

Mezey, M., Boltz, M., Esterson, J., & Mitty, E. (2005). Evolving models of geriatric nursing care. *Geriatric Nursing, 26,* 11–15. doi:10.1016/j.gerinurse.2004.11.012

Mezey, M., Stierle, L.J., Huba, G.J., & Esterson, J. (2007). Ensuring competence of specialty nurses in care of older adults. *Geriatric Nursing, 28,* 9–14. doi:10.1016/j.gerinurse.2007.10.013

Murray, R.K., & McElwee, N.E. (2010). Comparative effectiveness research: Critically intertwined with health care reform and the future of biomedical innovation. *Archives of Internal Medicine, 170,* 596–599. doi:10.1001/archinternmed.2010.50

Nurse Competence in Aging (NCA) Partners: Association activities and resources. (2007). *Geriatric Nursing, 28*(Suppl. 6), 34–39. doi:10.1016/j.gerinurse.2007.10.011

Oberlander, J. (2010). Perspective: A vote for health care reform. *New England Journal of Medicine, 362,* e44. doi:10.1056/NEJMp1002878

O'Connor, S.J. (2011). Prevention is better than cure and collaboration better than insularity: Reasons why oncologists should embrace the international, public health and care of the elderly agendas in their research activities. *European Journal of Cancer Care, 20,* 283–285. doi:10.1111/j.1365 -2354.2011.01252.x

O'Neil, E. (2009). Four factors that guarantee health care change. *Journal of Professional Nursing, 25,* 317–321. doi:10.1016/j.profnurs.2009.10.004

Owusu, C., & Studenski, S.A. (2009). Shared care in geriatric oncology: Primary care providers' and medical/oncologist's perspectives. *Journal of the American Geriatrics Society, 57,* S239–S242. doi:10.1111/j.1532-5415.2009.02501.x

Rao, A.V., & Demark-Wahnefried, W. (2006). The older cancer survivor. *Critical Reviews in Oncology/ Hematology, 60,* 131–143. doi:10.1016/j.critrevonc.2006.06.003

Reid Ponte, P., & Peterson, K. (2008). A patient- and family-centered care model paves the way for a culture of quality and safety. *Critical Care Nursing Clinics of North America, 20,* 451–464. doi:10.1016/j.ccell.2008.08.001

Repetto, L., Piselli, P., Raffaele, M., & Locatelli, C. (2009). Communicating cancer diagnosis and prognosis: When the target is the elderly patient—A GIOGer study. *European Journal of Cancer, 45,* 374–383. doi:10.1016/j.ejca.2008.08.020

Resnick, B. (2007). Nurse competence in aging: From dream to reality. *Geriatric Nursing, 28*(Suppl. 6), 7–8. doi:10.1016/j.gerinurse.2007.10.014

Ricketts, T.C. (2011). The health care workforce: Will it be ready as the boomers age? A review of how we can know (or not know) the answer. *Annual Review of Public Health, 32,* 417–430. doi:10.1146/ annurev-publhealth-031210-101227

Rodriguez-Paredes, M., & Esteller, M. (2011). Cancer epigenetics reaches mainstream oncology. *Nature: Medicine, 17,* 330–339. doi:10.1038/nm.2305

Rose, J.H., O'Toole, E.E., Koroukian, S., & Berger, N.A. (2009). Geriatric oncology and primary care: Promoting partnerships in practice and research. *Journal of the American Geriatrics Society, 57,* S235–S238. doi:10.1111/j.1532-5415.2009.02500.x

Scholder, J., Kagan, S., & Schumann, M.J. (2004). Nurse competence in aging overview. *Nursing Clinics of North America, 39,* 429–442. doi:10.1016/j.cnur.2004.02.006

Shortell, S.M., & Casalino, L.P. (2008). Health care reform requires accountable care systems. *JAMA, 300,* 95–97. doi:10.1001/jama.300.1.95

Smith, B.D., Smith, G.L., Hurria, A., Hortobagyi, G.N., & Buchholz, T.A. (2009). Future of cancer incidence in the United States: Burdens upon an aging, changing nation. *Journal of Clinical Oncology, 27,* 2758–2765. doi:10.1200/JCO.2008.20.8983

Stanley, J. (2009). Reaching consensus on a regulatory model: What does this mean for APRNs? *Journal for Nurse Practitioners, 5,* 99–104. doi:10.1016/j.nurpra.2008.11.005

Stanley, J.M., Werner, K.E., & Apple, K. (2009). Positioning advanced practice registered nurses for health care reform: Consensus on APRN regulation. *Journal of Professional Nursing, 25,* 340–348. doi:10.1016/j.profnurs.2009.10.001

Stierle, L.J., Mezey, M., Schumann, M.J., Esterson, J., Smolenski, M.C., Horsley, K.D., ... Gould, E. (2006). Professional development. The Nurse Competence in Aging initiative: Encouraging expertise in the care of older adults. *American Journal of Nursing, 106*(9), 93–94. doi:10.1097/00000446 -200609000-00040

Thun, M.J., DeLancey, J.O., Center, M.M., Jemal, A., & Ward, E.M. (2010). The global burden of cancer: Priorities for prevention. *Carcinogenesis, 31,* 100–110. doi:10.1093/carcin/bgp263

Toyota, M., Suzuki, H., Yamashita, T., Hirata, K., Imai, K., Tokino, T., & Shinomura, Y. (2009). Cancer epigenomics: Implications of DNA methylation in personalized cancer therapy. *Cancer Science, 100,* 787–791. doi:10.1111/j.1349-7006.2009.01095.x

Tsai, H.-C., & Baylin, S.B. (2011). Cancer epigenetics: Linking basic biology to clinical medicine. *Cell Research, 21,* 502–517. doi:10.1038/cr.2011.24

Tuljapurkar, S., Li, N., & Boe, C. (2000). A universal pattern of mortality decline in the G7 countries. *Nature, 405,* 789–792. doi:10.1038/35015561

Weiss, C.O. (2011). Frailty and chronic diseases in older adults. *Clinics in Geriatric Medicine, 27,* 39–52. doi:10.1016/j.cger.2010.08.003

CHAPTER 11

Oncology Community Health

Mary Pat Johnston, RN, MS, AOCN®

Introduction

Several trends will present challenges to the delivery of care for people living with cancer, including (a) the aging population, (b) cancer as a chronic disease, (c) older cancer survivors, and (d) workforce shortages among physicians and nurses. The purpose of this chapter is to describe these challenges and identify the opportunities in the community, exploring palliative care and other supportive care services where care is delivered close to home.

The population of the United States is aging as the first of the baby boomers approach 65 years old. Men and women older than 65 comprise 12% of the U.S. population, which is expected to double between 2000 and 2030 (Bellizi, Mustain, Balesh, & Diefenbach, 2008). Cancer has become a chronic disease demonstrating an increased incidence with age. As such, the number of cancer survivors older than age 65 in the United States is estimated at 6.5 million and rising (Bellizi et al., 2008; Griffith, McGuire, & Russo, 2010). Healthcare systems focused on an acute care model are unlikely to meet the needs of cancer survivors who are now living with a chronic disease and their families because neither the system nor the culture are oriented to the person's own role in self-management, consistent disease follow-up, and secondary prevention (Phillips & Currow, 2010). According to Wagner (1998), who developed a model for improvement of chronic illness care, people with chronic disease and their families "require planned, regular interactions with their caregivers, with a focus on function and prevention of exacerbations and complications" (p. 2). The keys to success of this model are patient-provider interactions that develop essential relationships and yield improved patient care outcomes, including self-management support to increase patient confidence and self-care skills and regular communication among clinicians about the care of a defined patient group. The members of the patient care team extend beyond the usual scope of services and providers of a single practice or institution, combining specialists and generalists as well as community agencies (Wagner, 1998, 2000). Frequently, older cancer survivors have coexisting and multifaceted medical conditions that can affect cancer prognosis and lead to poor quality-of-life outcomes (Bellizi et al., 2008). Often, these survivors cope with late effects of cancer and its treatment, which may include secondary malignancies such as chemotherapy-induced leukemia, peripheral neuropathy, osteopenia potentially leading to bone fractures, and cardiomyopathy. In addition, they may have other comorbid diseases, such as hypertension, stroke, myocardial infarction, diabetes, and osteoarthritis (Griffith et al., 2010). Higher morbidity and mortality may occur with older cancer survivors because they are disparately affected by more post-treatment healthcare needs (Bellizi et al., 2008).

In the community, cancer care services are offered in outpatient clinics or infusion centers (either hospital-based or freestanding clinics), home care (both private and county services), and community clinics, including free medical clinics, to serve people who would not otherwise receive care. The services may include cancer prevention and early detection through cancer screening, of which breast, cervical, prostate, and colon cancers are more common, and health promotion and intervention, such as tobacco cessation. Genetic services for patients with familial cancers are emerging in community settings. Nurse-managed clinics expand access, provide quality, deliver evidence-based care, and improve outcomes (Institute of Medicine [IOM], 2010). Outpatient clinics, infusion centers, and home care provide symptom management, such as pain management and IV antibiotics, to avoid post-course hospitalization. To further explore palliative care services offered in communities, the four basic clinical models for palliative care services include hospice care, palliative care programs, outpatient palliative care, and community palliative care (National Consensus Project [NCP], 2009).

Hospice Care

Hospice care is a specific programmatic model for delivering palliative and end-of-life care to patients with life-limiting, advanced disease and a prognosis of less than six months (Ferris et al., 2009). "Hospice emphasizes that accepting death is a natural part of life and seeks neither to prolong nor hasten death" (Quest, Marco, & Derse, 2009, p. 94). It is widely available and a longstanding model for managing end-of-life care that pioneered the interdisciplinary model. However, it has been plagued with underutilization as patients are enrolled days to weeks prior to death rather than benefit from the services for weeks to months (Ferris et al., 2009). Hospice care is delineated within the Medicare Hospice Benefit with services provided in the patient's own home, a nursing home, a residential facility, or an inpatient unit (NCP, 2009). Several reasons have been cited for the delay in accessing hospice care, including patient, family, and/or physician reluctance, indicating that it is not yet time (Ferrell, 2005). Medicare requires physicians to certify that patients have less than six months to live, which limits access as hospices struggle to accept people with conditions where estimation of prognosis is difficult, especially with diseases other than cancer (Ferris et al., 2009). More often, people in extended care facilities die from other diseases or conditions, such as myocardial infarction, congestive heart failure, or stroke. Another reason for poor utilization of these services is that patient and families feel forced to choose between treatment and comfort care because of the lack of integration of hospice and palliative care (IOM, 2001).

Palliative Care

The World Health Organization (2008) defined *palliative care* as an approach that "improves the quality of life of patients and their families who face life-threatening illness, by providing pain and symptom relief, spiritual and psychosocial support from diagnosis to the end of life and bereavement." With this approach, life-prolonging therapies are balanced with interventions, maximizing quality of life, symptom management through the prevention and relief by astute assessments and early interventions, and good communication between the healthcare providers and the patient and family, understanding prognosis and clarifying goals of care and patient wishes (NCP, 2009; Quest et al., 2009). Palliative care is optimally achieved through close coordination and partnership along the continuum of care and living situations (NCP, 2009). "The goal of palliative care is to prevent and relieve suffering and to support the best possible quality of life for patients and their families regardless of the stage of the disease or the need for other therapies" (NCP, 2004, p. 3). It allows for people living with an advanced disease, like cancer, to choose to receive disease-modifying treatments at any stage of their chronic illness (Quest et al., 2009).

The NCP (2004) *Clinical Practice Guidelines for Quality Palliative Care* described several palliative care models that are partially defined by care setting. Palliative Care Programs provide services in institutional-based hospitals, meaning academic, community, rehabilitation, or skilled care facilities. In contrast, Outpatient Palliative Care provides services in ambulatory care settings, supporting the continuum of care. Finally, Community Palliative Care Programs have consultative teams to support patients with life-limiting disease and their families at home who have not yet accessed hospices services. The consultative team works in collaboration with hospice and home healthcare agencies. The core elements of palliative care are further described in the second edition of the NCP (2009) *Clinical Practice Guidelines for Quality Palliative Care* and serve as the foundation for some of the later demonstration projects in palliative care.

Demonstration Projects

In 1997, the Robert Wood Johnson Foundation funded a national program, Promoting Excellence in End-of-Life Care, for 22 demonstration projects to develop innovative models for delivering palliative care for people living with advanced disease and to create institutional change to improve palliative care for these individuals and their families (Byock, Twohig, Merriman, & Collins, 2006). Project Safe Conduct, Simultaneous Care, and Project ENABLE (Educate, Nurture, Advise Before Life Ends) are examples of the demonstration projects involving comprehensive cancer centers that expanded palliative care services. First, Project Safe Conduct developed a palliative care team to provide support for patients with lung cancer while they were concurrently receiving life-prolonging treatment through clinical trials at a comprehensive cancer center (Byock et al., 2006; Pitorak, Beckham, & Sivec, 2003). Over time, the program has been sustained and expanded to include other cancer diagnoses. Secondly, Simultaneous Care is a model in which patients with cancer receive supportive care through an educational model while patients were receiving life-prolonging treatment by participating in clinical trials. Through satellite telecommunication, academic physicians at a university were connected to physicians in rural settings, reducing the conflict for patients of choosing between treatment and supportive care, offering earlier access to palliative services (Byock et al., 2006; Meyers et al., 2004). Finally, Project ENABLE was conducted in a regional cancer center, community-based oncology practice, and rural community. The goal was to increase utilization of palliative care services by people with cancer and their families through education and empowerment (Bakitas, Bishop, Caron, & Stephens, 2010; Bakitas et al., 2004; Byock et al., 2006). Key functions included (a) a palliative care nurse or nurse practitioner to coordinate the care of patients and families, (b) offer a workshop series for patients and families with life-limiting cancer, and (c) integrate palliative care and hospice services into routine oncology care (Bakitas et al., 2004). The participants of the program had poor prognoses, such as advanced lung, late-stage gastrointestinal, and metastatic or recurrent breast cancer. Over 18 months, the palliative care nurse and nurse practitioner identified patients and families for this program by telephone, at a clinic appointment, or in the hospital. On the initial clinic visit, the palliative care nurse described the program and invited the patient and family to participate. Subsequently, the palliative care nurse met with the patient and families with the scheduled oncology clinic visit and regularly communicated by telephone for symptom management. A four-session series of psychoeducational workshops was offered to promote self-management of symptoms of cancer and its treatment as well as acquire new skills for communicating and navigating the healthcare system. Although 240 patients and families enrolled in the program, only 107 of them attended the workshops because patients were too ill to attend or lived a distance from the site of the workshop, making it difficult to travel for workshop sessions and clinic appointments. Those who attended the workshops evaluated them positively. The model, utilizing concepts of prevention and early detection through assessment of symptoms and intervention with patients with cancer at the time of diagnosis, was a reasonable, effective approach for the regional cancer center and community-based oncology practice; however, the rural community presented several challenges related to the economy and commitment of leadership within the rural community. Outcomes were (a) increased referrals to hospice, (b) integrated outpatient palliative care with oncology care, (c) establishment of educational workshops, "Charting Your Course: A Whole-Person Approach to Living With Cancer," that provided support and education in a new way, (d) availability of palliative care concurrently with clinical trials, and (e) improved symptom management. Project ENABLE set the stage for a clinical trial to further evaluate this model (Bakitas et al., 2004, 2010; Byock et al., 2006).

From November 2003 to May 2008, Project ENABLE II was a randomized controlled trial to determine if nurse-led palliative care interventions have an effect on quality of life, symptom intensity, mood, and resource utilization in 322 patients with advanced cancer receiving cancer care services in a rural National Cancer Institute–designated comprehensive cancer center in New Hampshire and its affiliated clinics and a Veterans Administration medical center in Vermont (Bakitas et al., 2009). The NCP *Clinical Practice Guidelines for Quality Palliative Care* (2004) were utilized for the palliative care interventions. With a chronic care model case management approach, an advanced practice registered nurse (APRN) led the palliative care interventions. The interventions included education to encourage self-management and empowerment, ongoing assessment of symptoms, coaching in problem-solving, advance care planning, strategies for communication with family and healthcare team, crises prevention, and timely referrals to services through a telephone-based format to improve access to palliative care in a rural area (Bakitas et al., 2009, 2010). Similar to the previous project, the participants were newly diagnosed with advanced cancer that involved solid tumors, such as lung, breast, and gastrointestinal; patients with advanced genitourinary cancers; and patients with a prognosis of less than one year to live. The study demonstrated that the participants in the intervention arm (n = 161) reported higher quality of life and lower depressed mood states with APRN palliative care interventions with concurrent cancer therapies than those participants who received usual care (n = 161). However, these palliative care interventions had limited effect on symptom intensity scores and use of resources when comparing intervention participants to usual care participants.

The demonstration projects described identify opportunities for the future, emphasizing the APRN role in palliative care services, innovation through technology, such as telephone or satellite telecommunication, and outreach to community as well as more rural settings. In addition, these projects conveyed the importance of care coordination through an interdisciplinary team or led by a nurse, psychoeducational strategies, and a follow-up plan for monitoring or surveillance of symptoms from late effects of cancer and its treatment. ENABLE II utilized concepts in the chronic care model to more effectively deliver palliative care to people living with advanced disease, incorporating self-management and empowerment interventions for patients and families to acquire new skills in managing a chronic disease and navigating the healthcare system.

Other Models

Griffith et al. (2010) described survivorship care and palliative care as "natural partners" and offered an integrated framework for survivorship and palliative care. The IOM report *From Cancer Patient to Cancer Survivor: Lost in Transition* (Hewitt, Greenfield, & Stovall, 2006) advocated for changes to ensure that survivors are supported in these key areas: prevention to reduce the risk of recurrence, development of new cancers, and late effects of cancer treatment; surveillance for cancer progression, recurrence, and late effects; interventions for late effects of cancer and its treatment; and coordination between specialist and generalist providers, including physicians, nurses, and other healthcare providers. The definitions of both *palliative* and *survivorship care* refer to beginning at the time of diagnosis. The challenge for clinicians who are developing palliative care and survivorship programs is to define the patient population for these programs and services. Griffith and colleagues (2010) offered an integrated framework, identifying a critical intersection between survivorship and palliative care as physical function, psychosocial strain, quality of life, assistance with legal issues, and advance directives. The proposed framework consists of the Domains of Palliative Care (National Quality Forum, 2006) and the Essential Components of Survivorship Care (Hewitt et al., 2006). The eight domains are structure and process, physical, psychological, social, spiritual, cultural, dying, and ethical/legal, and the essential components are coordination of care, prevention and surveillance of new/recurrent cancers and late effects, and interventions for cancer or its treatment (Griffith et al., 2010; National Quality Forum, 2006). It is an evolving structure for comprehensive clinical care and may lead to the identification of new opportunities to meet the needs of patients and families, especially older cancer survivors living with this chronic disease and their families, through program evaluation and further research.

Further research in the population of patients receiving palliative care and cancer survivors greater than 65 years old is another challenge. Although 61% of new cancer cases occur among older adults, they comprise only 25% of the participants in clinical trials (Lewis et al., 2003). In addition, study design eligibility criteria may restrict older adults related to their disease burden and comorbidities. However, more recently researchers are challenged as to how to identify and recruit patients for clinical trials. The paradigm is changing about what being over age 65 even looks like because this population is living a more active lifestyle with a continuation of work, parenting or grandparenting responsibilities, exercise, hobbies, church, volunteerism, and other self-fulfillment activities. The opportunity is to explore how to access older adults in the community, meeting potential participants where they live in community groups, churches, and volunteer organizations. There is a growing trend toward partnerships between community-based healthcare institutions and academic centers for accrual of participants to clinical trials and the opportunity for more collaboration between nurse researchers and APRNs in the community settings.

Workforce Shortages

Finally, workforce shortages of both physician and nurse specialists will affect the community with a greater impact on rural settings. Emergency department physicians and primary care physicians will struggle with the complex care needs of people living with the chronic disease of cancer (Ferris et al., 2009; Quest et al., 2009). With an insufficient number of specialists, not enough skilled clinicians with knowledge, skills, and experience to manage people with cancer in community settings are available. Emergency department and primary care physicians will struggle to manage the complex care needs of people living with cancer and the changing paradigms, especially in rural communities (Ferris et al., 2009; Quest et al., 2009). According to Rieger (2009), "One of our greatest challenges is to address the future workforce shortage with prepared professionals who are representative of the populations that they serve, embrace diversity, and keep pace with new developments in cancer care" (p. S22). Ferris et al. (2009) described the American Society of Clinical Oncology's vision for 2020 that national cancer control plans have palliative care as a routine part of cancer care for all patients that is "consistently delivered to prevent and relieve the suffering of patients and families from the day of diagnosis" (p. 3056). To live this vision, access to skilled physicians and specialists with an increased number and expansion of roles for nonphysicians will be necessary for delivery of cancer care and palliative care.

Nurses play a key role in educating and assisting patients with this new paradigm (Rieger, 2009). Oncology nurses will have many opportunities to bridge the challenges in the community, some of which have been described by demonstration models for palliative care, emphasizing the chronic care model, and supported by the core components of palliative care demonstration projects and survivorship models of care. Other new opportunities are emerging with the institution of oncology nurse navigator and APRN programs. Oncology nurse navigation programs are oncology nurse–led programs designed to support patients by reducing barriers to timely access to care, increase patient satisfaction, and facilitate best possible patient outcomes; these programs continue to evolve as they are evaluated with the goal of improving cancer care to all patients (Koh, Nelson, & Cook, 2011). Second, oncology nurse practitioners (NPs) are expanding their traditional practice sites from primary, acute, and tertiary settings to practice in nontraditional healthcare sites, including survivorship and symptom management clinics. The oncology NPs' objectives are to improve quality care outcomes, increase patient satisfaction through establishing a relationship with patients and families, and promote cost-effective interventions (Nevidjon et al., 2010). Third, clinical nurse specialists (CNSs) are uniquely prepared as change agents to address the gap of evidence-based practice in palliative care services regardless of the setting. CNSs ensure competency and training of staff on new developments and evidence-based practice changes, supporting staff through coaching to not only integrate change but thrive in it. For example, hospice and palliative care programs have been slow to embrace evidence-based practice guideline recommendations related to barriers such as staff support for new practices, values, and perception of the community culture on implementation of evidence-based practice, including patient, physician, and organizational factors that may affect the ability of the agency to implement evidence-based practice (Sanders et al., 2010). In addition, the CNS is well prepared and integral to the development of new programs, monitoring outcomes, and facilitating research at the point of care. Another opportunity for oncology nurses and APRNs is to explore and address the needs of family caregivers. O'Hara et al. (2010) found that high levels of caregiver objective burden and stress were associated with lower patient quality of life, higher symptom intensity, and higher depressed mood. Further research on palliative care interventions is warranted for both patients and caregivers with attention to caregivers' perceptions of patient care. These are just a few of the opportunities for oncology nurses and APRNs that are emerging to address the needs of people with cancer and their families in the oncology community.

However, none of it will be embraced for our future if we do not develop action plans utilizing recommendations from IOM's (2011) *Future of Nursing: Leading the Change, Advancing Health.* Community-based hospitals and hospital systems have been leaders in the bachelor of science in nursing (BSN) entry into practice, demonstrating a preference toward BSN-prepared nurses as new hires and supporting currently employed RNs to pursue BSN completion programs. Some employers have partnered with schools of nursing to offer BSN completion programs on-site. In southeastern Wisconsin, ProHealth Care at Waukesha Memorial Hospital partnered with the School of Nursing at Concordia University to provide the courses at the hospital and support their RNs with tuition reimbursement. Nursing curricula for both entry into practice and advanced practice should include more content on community health. In the transition from acute to chronic care models, nursing students will need increased exposure to principles of community care and provision of direct patient care in community settings (IOM, 2010). With the statistics for a growing number of cancer survivors, the community health content should incorporate oncology. Anderson and Mercer (2004) evaluated the impact of community health content on primary NPs' and nurse midwives' practice, comparing classroom and Web-based training. The findings indicated that the concepts of community were incorporated into the advanced practice roles; however, no difference was noted between the classroom and Web-based methods. Clearly, the opportunity is in exploring innovative options for inclusion of oncology community health content.

Conclusion

So, where do we go from here? Given that the oncology community setting is broad, comprising a variety of living situations and spaces that people call home, the opportunities to be harvested from the challenges are vast. Although some of the changes are in process or under exploration through evaluation and research, many of the opportunities are yet to be created. Innovative oncology nurses and APRNs are poised to seize these opportunities if they stretch themselves to envision them. Key aspects from the chronic care model described by Wagner (1998) and evaluated in the demonstration projects may serve as a guide to innovation, including the following.

- Establish a relationship between a person living with cancer, family caregivers, and the healthcare team.
- Coordinate care by a skilled oncology nurse or APRN, promoting early access to care.
- Support the person with cancer with an interdisciplinary team with members who are knowledgeable about their own scope of practice, and facilitate good communication beyond the boundaries of institution, setting, and traditional care providers.
- Communicate among interdisciplinary team members, especially regarding prognosis and goals of care with respect to the person's wishes.
- Teach self-management and empowerment skills to people with cancer and their families, and coach them on navigation of the health care.

Traditional silos, such as institution, community, and disciplines, are broken down to avoid fragmented care so that people with cancer and their families receive proactive, streamlined, and coordinated care regardless of where the patient calls home in the community, such as home, hospice, extended care facilities, rehabilitation centers, and nontraditional living sites. Imagine a day when people with cancer and their families do not have to choose between treatment and comfort and survivorship resources or palliative care because they understand the prognosis and care goals and feel empowered to manage their chronic condition. Support from healthcare providers with the skill and expertise to guide patients with cancer can make this happen.

References

Anderson, E.T., & Mercer, Z.B. (2004). Impact of community health content on nurse practitioner practice: A comparison of classroom and web-based training. *Nursing Education Perspectives, 25,* 171–175.

Bakitas, M., Bishop, M.F., Caron, P., & Stephens, L. (2010). Developing successful models of palliative care services. *Seminars in Oncology Nursing, 26,* 266–284. doi:10.1016j.soncn.2010.08.006

Bakitas, M., Lyons, K.D., Hegel, M.T., Balan, S., Brokaw, F.C., Seville, J., ... Ahles, T.A. (2009). Effects of a palliative care intervention on clinical outcomes in patients with advanced cancer: The project ENABLE II randomized controlled trial. *JAMA, 302,* 741–749. doi:10.1001/jama.2009.1198

Bakitas, M., Stevens, M., Ahles, T., Kirn, M., Skalla, K., Kane, N., & Greenberg, E.R. (2004). Project ENABLE: A palliative care demonstration project for advanced cancer patients in three settings. *Journal of Palliative Medicine, 7,* 363–372. doi:10.1089/109662104773709530

Bellizzi, K.M., Mustian, K.M., Palesh, O.G., & Diffenbach, M. (2008). Cancer survivorship and aging: Moving the science forward. *Cancer, 113*(Suppl.), 3530–3539. doi:10.1002/cncr.23942

Byock, I., Twohig, J.S., Merriman, M., & Collins, K. (2006). Promoting excellence in end-of-life care: A report on innovative models of palliative care. *Journal of Palliative Medicine, 9,* 137–146.

Ferrell, B.R. (2005). Late referrals to palliative care. *Journal of Clinical Oncology, 23,* 908–909. doi:10.1200/JCO.2005.11.908

Ferris, F.D., Bruera, E., Cherny, N., Cummings, C., Currow, D., Dudgeon, D., … Von Roenn, J.H. (2009). Palliative cancer care a decade later: Accomplishments, the need, the next steps—From the American Society of Clinical Oncology. *Journal of Clinical Oncology, 27*, 3052–3058. doi:10.1200/JCO.2008.20.1558

Griffith, K.A., McGuire, D.B., & Russo, M. (2010). Meeting survivors' unmet needs: An integrated framework for survivor and palliative care. *Seminars in Oncology Nursing, 26*, 231–242. doi:10.1016/j.soncn.2010.08.004

Hewitt, M., Greenfield, S., & Stovall, E. (Eds.). (2006). *From cancer patient to cancer survivor: Lost in transition.* Washington, DC: National Academies Press. Retrieved from http://www.nap.edu

Institute of Medicine. (2001). *Improving palliative care for cancer: Summary and recommendations.* Retrieved from http://books.nap.edu/catalog.php?record_id=10147#toc

Institute of Medicine. (2010). *A summary of the December 2009 forum on the future of nursing: Care in the community—Workshop summary.* Washington, DC: National Academies Press. Retrieved from http://www.iom.edu/Reports/2010/A-Summary-of-the-December-2009-Forum-on-the-Future-of-Nursing-Care-in-the-Community.aspx

Institute of Medicine. (2011). *The future of nursing: Leading change, advancing health.* Retrieved from http://www.nap.edu/catalog.php?record_id=12956

Koh, C., Nelson, J.M., & Cook, P.F. (2011). Evaluation of a patient navigation program. *Clinical Journal of Oncology Nursing, 15,* 41–48. doi:10.1188/11.CJON.41-48

Lewis, J.H., Kilgore, M.L., Goldman, D.P., Trimble, E.L., Kaplan, R., Montello, M.J., … Escarce, J.J. (2003). Participation of patients 65 years of age or older in cancer clinical trials. *Journal of Clinical Oncology, 21,* 1383–1389. doi:10.1200/JCO.2003.08.010

Meyers, F.J., Linder, J., Beckett, L., Christensen, S., Blais, J., & Gandara, D.R. (2004). Simultaneous care: A model approach to perceived conflict between investigational therapy and palliative care. *Journal of Pain and Symptom Management, 28,* 548–556. doi:10.1016/j.jpainsymman.2004.03.002

National Consensus Project. (2004). *Clinical practice guidelines for quality palliative care.* Brooklyn, NY: National Consensus Project for Quality Care.

National Consensus Project. (2009). *Clinical practice guidelines for quality palliative care* (2nd ed.). Brooklyn, NY: National Consensus Project for Quality Care.

National Quality Forum. (2006). *A national framework and preferred practices for palliative and hospice care quality: A consensus report.* Washington, DC: Author.

Nevidjon, B., Rieger, P., Murphy, C.M., Rosenzweig, M.Q., McCorkle, M., & Baileys, K. (2010). Filling the gap: Development of the oncology nurse practitioner workforce. *Journal of Oncology Practice, 6,* 2–6. Retrieved from http://www.ncbi.nlm.nih.gov/pmc/articles/PMC2805339/?tool=pubmed

O'Hara, R.E., Hull, J.G., Lyons, K.D., Bakitas, M., Hegel, M.T., Zhongze, L., & Ahles, T.A. (2010). Impact of caregiver burden of patient-focused palliative care intervention for patients with advanced cancer. *Palliative and Supportive Care, 8,* 395–404. doi:10.1017/S1478951510000258

Phillips, J.L., & Currow, D.C. (2010). Cancer as a chronic disease. *Collegian, 17,* 43–45. doi:10.1016/j.colegn.2010.04.007

Pitorak, E.F., Beckham, A.M., & Sivec, H.D. (2003). Project Safe Conduct integrates palliative care goals into comprehensive cancer care. *Journal of Pain and Symptom Management, 6,* 645–655. doi:10.1089/109662103768253812

Quest, T.E., Marco, C.A., & Derse, A.R. (2009). Hospice and palliative medicine: New subspecialty, new opportunities. *Annals of Emergency Medicine, 54,* 94–102. doi:10.1016/j.annemergmed.2008.11.019

Rieger, P.T. (2009). Shaping oncology care for the future: An oncology nursing perspective. *Journal of Cancer Education, 24,* S22–S23. doi:10.1080/08858190903400427

Sanders, S., Mackin, M.L., Reyes, J., Herr, K., Titler, M., Fine, P., & Forcucci, C. (2010). Implementing evidence-based practices: Considerations for the hospice setting. *American Journal of Hospice and Palliative Medicine, 27,* 369–376. doi:10.1177/1049909109358695

Wagner, E.H. (1998). Chronic disease management: What will it take to improve care for chronic illness? *Effective Clinical Practice, 1,* 2–4.

Wagner, E.H. (2000). The role of patient care teams in chronic disease management. *BMJ, 320,* 569–572. doi:10.1136/bmj.320.7234.569

World Health Organization. (2008). WHO definition of palliative care. Retrieved from http://www.who.int/cancer/palliative/definition/en

CHAPTER 12

Mental Health Issues in Cancer

Kathleen Murphy-Ende, RN, PsyD, PhD, AOCNP®

Introduction

Oncology clinicians encounter numerous challenges in trying to meet the biopsychosocial needs of each individual patient. Symptoms of psychological distress and existential concerns are more prevalent than pain and other physical symptoms in patients with cancer (Portenoy et al., 1994). Based upon theories of adjustment and coping, professionals are beginning to understand how psychological problems develop in those with cancer. An awareness and better understanding of the mental health issues that impact people living with cancer is necessary so that professionals can address these psychological healthcare needs. The Institute of Medicine (IOM) recommended providing cancer care for the whole patient, including mental health services (Adler & Page, 2008). The IOM report recommended provision of care for patients with cancer by properly trained mental healthcare providers who have expertise and experience in an effort to address the psychological complexities that arise. The National Comprehensive Cancer Network's (NCCN, 1999) original guideline, which is updated annually, was based on the recognition of the importance of managing emotional distress and recommended procedures for evaluating patients with cancer with the use of psychological, psychiatric, social work, and pastoral care services. The NCCN (2012) guideline recommends that all patients be routinely screened to identify the level and source of their distress so that further evaluation and resources can be implemented. Commonly, clinicians recognize that identifying and treating psychological issues is complex and beyond the scope of their practice. Psychological needs vary depending upon the individual, the available resources, and the phase of disease trajectory.

Much is written about psychological needs at the time of diagnosis and recurrence. In the past decade, more information has been published in the palliative and supportive care literature on the topics of anxiety, depression, and existential suffering. Regardless of the scientific data documenting the prevalence and seriousness of mental health issues in cancer, according to Hewitt, Greenfield, and Stovall (2006) and the President's Cancer Panel (2004), we know that the psychological needs of cancer survivors are not being met. The disconnect between the research that identifies the mental health needs of patients with cancer and clinical practice is tragic, causing much unnecessary suffering.

The purpose of this chapter is to discuss contemporary psycho-oncology issues frequently experienced along the cancer continuum by patients with cancer. Having this information will encourage clinicians to consider the unique emotional challenges and transitions that these patients face. It is important for healthcare providers to be aware of the complex psychological issues that their patients may face in order to be alert to those who are experiencing or are at risk for psychological distress and initiate referral to a cancer psychologist.

The first section of this chapter highlights the importance of clinical screening, initial assessment, the challenges of measuring psychological distress, and tracking outcomes. The mental health issues that occur during the cancer experience covered in this chapter include depression, anxiety, cognitive changes, post-traumatic stress disorder (PTSD), hope during cancer, and common psychological interventions. The chapter concludes with a discussion of the phenomena of compassion fatigue in professional staff.

Clinical Screening and Outcome Measures

The evaluation and treatment of psychological distress in patients with cancer should ideally be based on research or best practice whenever possible. Clinical screening and diagnostic instruments used to detect psychological distress should be practical and accurately measure the specific subjective state. Knowing what to look for in scales as well as the limitations of measuring subjective states is important. Numerous scales are designed to measure psychological distress and the domains that contribute to quality of life (QOL).

Reliability of an instrument, which is the extent to which the characteristic of interest is measured, should be taken into account. Likewise, when ascertaining the degree of validity of an instrument, it is important to consider if the studies were done with a similar population. Other issues to consider about clinical scales include the length of time it takes to administer and complete the scale, practicality of physically completing the scale, reading level, native language, culture, and amount of time needed to score the instrument.

Clinicians and researchers should think about the goals of treatment and how to objectively evaluate the treatment's effectiveness by measuring specific outcomes. In the cancer population, health-related QOL is an important outcome to track. Many well-established instruments for patients with cancer as well as disease-specific scales are available, and these should be used in the context for which they were originally intended. In the global context of measuring QOL, the generic instruments assess all domains of QOL. Disease-specific instruments focus on concerns that tend to occur with a specific illness or treatment. Although the general instruments cover a broad arena, they can be used across different treatment groups and types of cancer in order to evaluate the effects of disease and treatment on QOL. The generic instruments tend to be superficial, yet the advantage is that they can be used for making comparisons with the general population. Disease-specific instruments are more sensitive in detecting changes in symptoms and treatment effects, providing more statistical power (Ferrans & Hacker, 2011). The other key element to consider in QOL measurement is the extent to which individuals' personal values are summarized. The importance patients place upon each indicator of QOL or being free of distress symptoms should be incorporated into the measurement scores by a weighting process. The Quality of Life Inventory and Quality of Life Index both measure the magnitude of worth that patients place on each item.

Another major instrumentation consideration pertains to the studying of patients at the end of life. Practitioners need to be sensitive to the difficulty in determining the risks and benefits of trials in those with limited life span. Typical outcome measures in palliative care consist of patient and family satisfaction, relief of symptoms, provider continuity, life closure, and grieving.

Psychological treatment interventions should be individualized and based on evidence-based practice or best practice to date whenever possible. The oncology literature has empirical support for psychological interventions based on randomized clinical trials; however, fewer empirical studies are available on the palliative care population than other phases of the cancer continuum because this type of research is challenging to conduct at the end of life. Healthcare providers and researchers must consider that the focus of care needs to be on the areas that interfere with the current problems that are negatively affecting well-being and the issues that the patient and family value the most.

The outcomes of psychological treatment should be measureable and congruent with the treatment goal. Ideally, the outcomes should be based on the individual's goals of care, accurately measure the subjective phenomena of interest, and collect objective data including pertinent and specific functional status when applicable. These outcomes serve to assist the psychologist in evaluating the effectiveness of the intervention and for positive feedback for the patient.

Anxiety and Depression

Anxiety and depression, which commonly occur in those with cancer, are closely related concepts sharing an element of emotional distress or "negative affect." The symptoms of negative affect include altered mood, difficulty concentrating, altered sleep, and irritability. Anxiety is characterized by high negative affect with symptoms of feeling distressed, fearful, hostile, jittery, nervous, and scornful. Depression is characterized by low positive affect with symptoms of anhedonia and cognitive and motor slowing. It is critical that a qualified mental health practitioner such as a psychologist or psychiatrist properly evaluate the patient using diagnostic criteria so that the correct diagnosis and treatment can be offered. Although these two common symptoms tend to occur concurrently, they will be discussed separately in this section.

The exact prevalence of anxiety in patients with cancer is uncertain due to the variability in measurement methods and diagnostic criteria used and differences in age, gender, time from diagnosis, stage and extent of disease, presence of comorbid conditions, history of anxiety disorder, current medications, and type and phase of treatment. When standardized psychiatric interviews and diagnostic criteria are used, the range of anxiety in patients with cancer is 10%–30% (Stark et al., 2002).

Several types of anxiety disorders can occur as a maladaptive response and can impair functioning in those with cancer. Adjustment disorder with anxious mood is the most common anxiety disorder requiring psychological or psychiatric referral in the cancer population (Noyes, Holt, & Massie, 1998). The features of adjustment disorder occur within three months of the stressor; cause significant distress or so-

cial impairment; exclude other psychiatric diagnoses, personality disorders, or bereavement; and resolve within six months of the trigger. Adjustment disorder may be
subtyped by predominant anxiety or mixed anxiety and depressed mood. It is classi-
fied as acute if symptoms last for less than six months and chronic if symptoms last
more than six months (American Psychiatric Association [APA], 2000). The degree
of impairment and duration of anxiety is not predictable, and its effects can greatly
impinge upon QOL. Professionals tend to expect that patients will experience anxiety, and validating their emotional response is important; however, additional attention needs to be given to assessing this symptom. Professionals are responsible for ap-
praising the level of distress and functional impairment caused by the anxiety symptoms so that early diagnosis and treatment can be implemented to minimize the severity and interval of symptoms.

Anxiety disorder associated with a general medical condition is caused by the direct physiologic consequence of a medical disorder or its treatment. This can occur in patients with cancer experiencing uncontrolled pain. Medications associated
with symptoms of anxiety (e.g., emotional lability, insomnia, agitation, restlessness)
include steroids, interferon, bronchodilators, antipsychotics, stimulants, and anti-
emetics. Patients undergoing withdrawal from alcohol, nicotine, opioids, or anxio-
lytics are at risk for developing sudden agitation. Metabolic abnormalities that can
lead to symptoms of anxiety include hypoxemia, sepsis, hypoglycemia, hyperkale-
mia, hypo- or hypercalcemia, hyperthermia, hyponatremia, hypovolemia, and bleeding. Hormonal changes that occur in hyper- or hypothyroidism, hyperparathyroid-
ism, carcinoid syndrome, and adrenocorticotropic-producing tumors can similarly
cause anxiety. Cardiovascular and pulmonary abnormalities often produce physical
and emotional symptoms of anxiety. If anxiety is the consequence of a medical condition, the underlying condition should be corrected whenever possible concurrently with symptom management of the anxiety.

Preexisting anxiety disorders, genetics, age, and gender influence the expression/
manifestation of anxiety. PTSD can reemerge during the cancer experience, or the
trauma associated with the cancer experience can cause PTSD. The PTSD diagnosis should be considered in those exhibiting anxiety symptoms, and this is discussed
in detail in the section on PTSD that follows. Generalized anxiety disorder (GAD) is
difficult to differentiate from adjustment disorders when looking at symptoms alone;
however, those with GAD have experienced excessive anxiety and worry for at least
six months or frequently for many years preceding the cancer diagnosis. Obtaining
a history directly from the patient may reveal an undiagnosed or underreported anxiety subtype such as GAD. Panic disorder, which causes acute sudden symptoms of
fear, palpitations, shortness of breath, chest pain, fear of losing control, going crazy,
or dying (APA, 2000), may be reactivated during any time of the disease trajectory
but may be more apparent during treatment or procedures or upon receiving unexpected or unpleasant news. It is important to be aware of the history of a specific
phobia, which can have a negative effect on treatment and care. Agoraphobia, claus-
trophobia, and blood/injection/injury–type phobias can be extremely distressing
to patients undergoing cancer treatment or surveillance. Avoidance of imaging, radiation, injections, and procedures may be the first indication that a phobia exists,
and in these situations healthcare workers should investigate by asking questions in
a nonjudgmental and nonthreatening way.

Epidemiologic studies suggest that genetic factors contribute to the development
of anxiety disorders in generalized anxiety, panic, agoraphobia, and specific phobias

(Hettema, Prescott, Myers, Neale, & Kendler, 2005). Inquiring about the family history of anxiety may help to identify those at higher risk.

Although all patients should be screened for anxiety, it is important to consider risk factors that have been associated with a higher prevalence rate of anxiety. Female gender, younger age, marital separation, divorce, being widowed, and lower socioeconomic status are factors associated with more anxiety in the oncology population (Brintzenhofe-Szoc, Lenin, Li, Kissane, & Zahora, 2009). In working with this population, it is important to consider the commonalities in people with certain risk factors that contribute to anxiety. Those who are younger may have less experience and social resources than the older cohort. Some older adults may have cumulative losses that contribute to social isolation and fear of future loss. Those of lower socioeconomic status may not have insurance coverage for medical and psychological treatment. Specific individual differences related to risk factors that affect coping with anxiety can be identified after establishing trust and rapport.

Anxiety frequently occurs in the later phases of cancer and end of life. Medical complications such as pain and dyspnea, physical symptoms, changes in role function, financial concerns, fear of dependence, spiritual concerns, fear of isolation, fear of being a burden, and existential issues surface at this time. Patients face many complex issues at the end of life, and special consideration should be given to the individual's needs based upon his or her value system, goals of care, and priorities.

Treatment for anxiety should be aimed at the exact cause while incorporating psychotherapeutic, pharmacologic, and supportive interventions. Psychoeducational interventions with a focus on providing information about the medical system and treatment process, with anticipatory guidance, are likely to help reduce anxiety. In a randomized clinical trial, patients who received an orientation at the clinic, information about available coping resources (support groups), and time for questions and answers with a counselor had reduced anxiety at follow-up (McQuellon et al., 1998). Psychotherapy in the form of cognitive therapy has been efficacious in numerous studies of patients with anxiety, but results are difficult to interpret in the oncology population because of individual variables. Brief supportive psychotherapy by trained professionals is useful in crisis-related situations including end-of-life issues (Massie, 1989). Support groups can be used to dissipate fears and anxieties. Support groups for women with stage IV breast cancer have been effective in alleviating anxiety (Spiegel, Bloom, & Yalom, 1981). Many different support groups are available, and for some patients, this option is effective in reducing emotional distress.

It is helpful for all healthcare providers who offer psychological support to recognize typical phases of anxiety during the cancer trajectory. At the time of diagnosis, shock, irritability, disrupted sleep, impaired concentration, and fear of treatment may occur and last several days to weeks. Those undergoing treatment may be fearful of side effects and have concern about their ability to remain fully functional. At the end of treatment, patients may fear abandonment and be uncomfortable about not being surveyed as closely as they were during treatment. During the posttreatment phase, isolation and fear of recurrence as well as a sense of survival guilt may occur. Disease recurrence is a difficult time and can be accompanied by fear of death, existential distress, worry of becoming a burden, and anxiety regarding the future of children or a significant other.

Nurses contribute to psychological care by providing support and evaluating the effectiveness of the treatment for anxiety and depression. When working with anxious patients, it is helpful to validate their feelings and assist them to find a balanced perspective of their emotional reactions. Anxiety and depression are natural responses. Apprehension and anxiety are essential emotions required for creative adaptability and protection from danger. Anxiety can serve as a motivating factor to make positive changes. Nurses can assist patients by listening to the patients' concerns, endorsing their feelings, promoting self-reflection, and providing referral to available resources such as support groups and individual psychotherapy. Referral to psychology services is indicated in those with preexisting anxiety disorders, presence of intolerable symptoms, severe physical symptoms from the anxiety, and anxiety that interferes with treatment.

Depression is an important problem to identify because it negatively affects all domains of QOL, can result in suicide, and often can be effectively treated. Depression increases morbidity and hospital stays and is correlated with decreased patient compliance (Pasquini & Biondi, 2007). Unfortunately, professionals and patients may mistakenly believe that depression is normal or expected for those who have cancer, and this misconception may be one barrier to accurate evaluation and effective treatment. Cultural and ethnic groups vary in their interpretations regarding the meaning of depressive symptoms or beliefs about the appropriateness of expressing symptoms and may use different terms to describe their symptoms. These differences may cause an underdiagnosis of depression.

Data on the prevalence of depression vary because of the lack of standardization of methodology and diagnostic criteria used, but the prevalence rates of major depressive disorder are documented to be between 10% and 25% (Pirl, 2004), and up to 58% for depression spectrum syndromes (Massie, 2004). The occurrence of depression may be correlated with certain types of cancer. Depression is two to three times greater in patients with pancreatic cancer than in patients with other intra-abdominal cancers and has been noted to predate the pancreatic cancer diagnosis by up to 43 months before physical symptoms (Makrila, Indeck, Syrigos, & Saif, 2009). The prevalence of suicide in patients with cancer is twice that of the general population (Misono, Weiss, Fann, Redman, & Yueh, 2008). In a large cohort study examining the period immediately after a cancer diagnosis, the immediate risk of suicide was 12.6 during the first week and 3.1 during the first year, as compared with people without cancer (Fang et al., 2012).

One can never predict who will develop depression; therefore, all patients should periodically be screened for it. Certain factors were identified in a review of the literature as well as observed in practice that may place patients with cancer at risk for developing depression. Severe active disease may lead to feelings of uncertainty about the future and may be accompanied by pain, nausea, dyspnea, or physical limitations. Older adult patients may be dealing with other comorbidities, a spouse's illness, family, and numerous cumulative losses of friends and family members. Social support tends to act as a buffer to the ill effects of stress, and social isolation may contribute to depression. Other unexpected life events and stressors can decrease one's coping reserves. A family history of depression and personal history of major depression are known risk factors for developing depression. Certain medications can cause depression, and patients exhibiting symptoms of depression should have their medication list reviewed.

Diagnosing whether a patient has clinical depression is challenging. Because many patients with cancer have physical symptoms and anxiety, psychologists and psychiatrists need to use clinical judgment and other criteria besides those of the APA (2000) *Diagnostic and Statistical Manual of Mental Disorders* (DSM-IV TR). As in the clinical situation of evaluating anxiety, the skills needed to detect major depression require special training by mental health workers such as psychologists or psychiatrists, who also perform diagnostic interviews, and these services may not be readily available. A review of the literature found that nurses underestimated the level of depressive symptoms in patients who were depressed (McDonald et al., 1999), and physicians only identified one-third of psychiatric morbidity in patients with cancer (Fallowfield, Ratcliffe, Jenkins, & Saul, 2001). Nurses and physicians are responsible for monitoring and addressing multiple aspects of the patient. The physiologic, pharmacologic, educational, and emotional needs of patients with cancer are complex, and it is not realistic for a clinician to be able to address all of the patient's needs. Therefore, a multidisciplinary team that includes psychological services will provide comprehensive care to meet all of the needs of the patient and family.

The classic symptoms of depression include depressed mood, increased or decreased appetite, insomnia or hypersomnia, psychomotor agitation or retardation, fatigue or loss of energy, guilt or a sense of worthlessness, diminished concentration, thoughts of death or suicide, or anhedonia. The cognitive symptoms of depression are noteworthy in patients with cancer because somatic symptoms may be related to the disease or treatment. It is apparent that the presence of the aforementioned symptoms does not necessarily equivocate with depression. Several quick screening tools are available to identify patients with depression and measure subjective distress. The advantage of using depression screening tools is that they are an efficient way to identify individuals with depressive symptoms so that further evaluation can be implemented. Commonly used scales for screening for depression are the Beck Depression Inventory, the Hamilton Rating Scale, the Hospital Anxiety and Depression Scale, the Zung Self-Rating Depression Scale, and the Patient Health Questionnaire.

Other distinct conditions that are similar to depression that occur in the cancer trajectory should be considered as part of the evaluation process. Demoralization syndrome is accompanied by existential despair, hopelessness, and helplessness with loss of meaning and purpose for life, but unlike depression, one does not experience anhedonia (Clarke & Kissane, 2002). Adjustment disorder consists of symptoms in response to an identifiable stressor (other than bereavement) occurring within three months of the onset of the stressor, with marked distress or impairment in social or occupational functioning. Mood disorder associated with a general medical condition is easily misdiagnosed as major depression and is discussed previously with anxiety. The hallmark of dysthymic disorder is depressed mood for two or more years. Hypoactive delirium may start with the patient being easily distracted, withdrawn, or irritable, or demonstrating an altered level of consciousness. Noogenic neurosis consists of frustration of the will to find meaning, with despair over the worthlessness of life. Those who are in an existential vacuum have no meaning in life or no awareness of values, a sense of boredom, and a tendency to conform to what others do or to do what others want them to do. Consideration of these conditions is necessary so that psychological and spiritual issues can be appropriately addressed.

The ideal treatment intervention for an individual should be based on both the evidence of efficacy and the individual preference, with the goal of improving mood and, when possible, increasing the functional status. The amount of evidence from research-based interventions is limited; therefore, any psychological treatment plan should include objective and subjective measurements to evaluate the effectiveness of treatment. Interventions should be chosen based upon the individual patient's needs, evidence from a similar oncology population, if available, and evidence extrapolated from the general population. Psychotherapy in the form of individual, family, or group is a commonly used intervention. Counseling, psychotherapy, guided relaxation, psychoeducation, problem solving, and coordination of oncologic and psychiatric care are effective interventions for depression in patients with cancer (Rodin et al., 2007). Cognitive-behavioral therapy, supportive psychotherapy, and problem solving reduce depressive symptoms in patients with incurable cancer, according to a meta-analysis of six studies (Akechi, Okuyama, Onishi, Morita, & Furukawa, 2008). Logotherapy, which is existential in nature, can be used at any time during the disease trajectory and may be the most appropriate form of therapy for those who are nearing death.

It is critical for nurses to know when to go beyond validation and reassurance and initiate a referral for psychological services. Patients who express thoughts of suicide or the desire to hasten death need immediate psychological evaluation. Early referral for those with preexisting anxiety or depressive disorders should be offered. Patients who are experiencing intolerable and severe psychological symptoms deserve to be further evaluated. Any patient who meets the diagnostic criteria for major depression should be further evaluated and treated. When the physical symptoms from anxiety or depression are severe, consultation is advised. Patients whom staff report as having "behavioral problems" should undergo psychological evaluation. A psychology/psychiatry consultation should be offered anytime anxiety or depressive symptoms interfere with the patient's treatment or ability to function to the fullest capacity given the current situation.

Cognitive Function

Cognitive functioning is a multidimensional concept that describes the domains of healthy brain performance, consisting of attention and concentration, executive function, information processing speed, language, visuospatial skill, psychomotor ability, learning, and memory (Jansen, Miaskowski, Dodd, Dowling, & Kramer, 2005). Cognitive impairment may reflect a specific decline or deficit in one or multiple domains of cognitive functioning. Numerous cognitive changes may occur as a direct effect of cancer or its treatment or indirectly from concurrent problems associated with cancer. Direct effects of cancer include tumor type and location and treatment modalities of radiation, chemotherapy, and biologic response modifiers. Indirect factors that may impair cognition include secondary organ toxicity, vascular injury to small vessels in the central nervous system (CNS), infection, alterations in hormones, release of tumor necrosis factor and cytokines, anemia, electrolyte imbalance, comorbid psychiatric diagnoses, depression, anxiety, pain, poor nutrition, and sleep deprivation. Cerebral impairments are beginning to be documented more frequently than in the past. The interest in this problem has escalated over the past 15 years, and randomized trials examining the effects of cancer treatment on cognition are growing. Clinical reports and research have examined the impact on cognition from the specific location of tumors on brain structures, type of cancer, effects of treatment such as radiation and chemotherapy, hormone effects, and variation of genetic polymorphisms.

An estimated 22,910 new cases of primary brain and other nervous system tumors will be diagnosed in the United States in 2012 (Siegel, Naishadham, & Jemal, 2012). Primary brain tumors can impair cognition as a result of increased intracranial pressure, with symptoms ranging from short-term memory loss and forgetfulness to impaired judgment or difficulty concentrating. Intracranial tumors can also cause cognitive changes from direct pressure, and the abnormal symptoms vary depending upon the function of the involved brain anatomy. Frontal lobe tumors can impair intellect, judgment, abstract thinking, or long-term memory. Parietal lobe tumors can impair ability to write or calculate. Temporal lobe tumors can cause memory loss and intellectual impairment. Occipital lobe tumors can cause the inability to identify objects or symbols or understand the meaning of written words (Hannay, Howieson, Loring, Fischer, & Lezak, 2005).

An estimated 20%–40% of patients with cancer develop brain metastasis (Armstrong, 2011). Melanoma and lung and breast cancers have the tendency to metastasize to the brain. Metastatic brain lesions may present with symptoms similar to primary glioblastoma multiforme brain tumors, with cognitive changes that progress over weeks to months (Victor & Ropper, 2001). By the time neurologic symptoms of brain metastases present, the disease is usually widespread. The incidence of cognitive dysfunction in both metastatic lesions and primary brain tumors is likely underestimated because past studies have focused on mental status examination, which has a low sensitivity for detecting cognitive impairment. Providentially, the National Cancer Institute Brain Tumor Progress Review Group (2005) report recommended that routine cognitive assessment become the standard care for all patients with primary brain tumors. This will provide further information on the effects of brain tumors and treatments on cognition.

One of the most frequently reported complications among long-term cancer survivors is cognitive dysfunction from brain radiation (Behin & Delattre, 2003). Radiation to the brain can cause irreversible and progressive damage to the CNS. Vascular injury causes ischemia to the surrounding tissue and demyelination of the white matter and necrosis (Sheline, Wara, & Smith, 1980). Radiation can disrupt hippocampal neurogenesis (Dietrich, Han, Yang, Mayer-Proschel, & Nobel, 2006), which may account for problems in memory. The function of retrieval from verbal memory may be vulnerable to adverse effects from radiation (Armstrong, Stern, & Corn, 2001). Whole-brain radiation can initially cause transient confusion caused by cerebral edema, diminution of cognitive and functional status attributed to transient cerebral demyelination, and late effects from severe demyelination and necrosis seen months to years after treatment (Filley, 2001). The effects of whole-brain radiation are consistent with frontal-subcortical dysfunction, affecting the domains of attention, executive functions, learning retrieval of new information, and psychomotor speed (Wefel, Kayl, & Meyers, 2004). Radiation may affect myelin-producing cells, interrupting the myelin synthesis process and causing a subacute somnolence syndrome consisting of sleepiness, drowsiness, and lethargy; this tends to be noted more in children and those undergoing whole-brain radiation (Haas, 2011). Risk factors for developing cognitive changes associated with brain radiation include high total dose radiation, young or old age, individuals with vascular risk factors, and patients receiving concomitant chemotherapy (Armstrong et al., 2001). The precise frequency and specificity of cognitive problems are not well documented and likely vary because of the insensitivity of assessment measures, variability in duration of follow-up studies, location of tumor, site and dose of radiation, and the amount of cerebral edema or increased intracranial pressure. Because the effects of radiation can be delayed up to two years after treatment, the effects on patients with shorter survival rates are not obtainable. Referral for neuropsychology consultation is indispensable for obtaining baseline neuropsychological evaluation, identifying cognitive defects, managing behavioral issues, making recommendations for pharmacologic agents and suggestions for rehabilitation and compensatory coping strategies, and managing specific cognitive problems.

Chemotherapy-induced cognitive impairment is distressing and greatly affects patients' QOL, can diminish one's role at work, and may change relationships. Cognitive impairment affects approximately 25%–33% of patients undergoing chemotherapy (Coyne & Leslie, 2004). The cognitive functions noted to be impaired in research studies are information processing speed, memory, executive function, spatial abilities, and simple attention span. Most of the studies exploring the effects of chemotherapy on cognition have been done on women with breast cancer. In women with breast cancer, the physical effects of chemotherapy on brain structure showed a decrease in the density of brain gray matter on magnetic resonance imaging scans (McDonald, Conroy, Ahles, West, & Saykin, 2010). Demyelination of white matter fibers is also associated with chemotherapy (Saykin, Ahles, & McDonald, 2003). Neuropathologic evidence documents a change in glial cells that support the alignment of neurons (Inagaki et al., 2007). These alterations are consistent with the type of cognitive symptoms and impairment found in neurocognitive studies. Certain chemotherapeutic agents pass through the blood-brain barrier, thus allowing a direct toxic effect on brain structure. Other agents may alter the permeability of the blood-brain barrier, allowing the agents to have contact with the brain tissue. High-dose chemotherapy may pose a greater risk of developing cognitive difficulties. Some evidence suggests that variation in genetic polymorphisms may play a role in causing some patients to be at higher risk for chemotherapy-induced cognitive changes. Those with lower cognitive reserve may be more vulnerable to cognitive decline from chemotherapy. The cognitive changes from chemotherapy can last for months to years after treatment.

Interventions used to improve cognitive function include medication, nutrition, cognitive rehabilitation, stress reduction, exercise, and patient education. Stimulants such as dexmethylphenidate and methylphenidate have been used in clinical practice in an attempt to improve cognitive function in patients receiving opioids and in the palliative care population, but the benefits for chemotherapy-induced cognitive impairment are not documented. Donepezil, a cholinesterase inhibitor used for Alzheimer disease, has been studied, but it is difficult to ascertain if the benefits are directly from the medication or from other anticancer treatments. Modafinil, a CNS stimulant, has been tried with some improvement in speed of processing, psychomotor speed, depression, and drowsiness (Lundorff, Jonsson, & Sjogren, 2009). Erythropoiesis-stimulating agents, which stimulate the production of red blood cells, have been tried with little if any benefit on cognition reported.

Nutritional interventions include diets high in antioxidants found in certain fruits and vegetables for the purpose of reduction of oxidative stress. Anemia treated with iron, folic acid, or vitamin B complex may help counter the effects of anemia on cognition. Vitamin E is thought to stop production of reactive oxygen species and showed improvement in global cognition, verbal and visual memory, and cognitive flexibility (Chan, Cheung, Law, & Chan, 2004), but it should be used with caution because of the risk of bleeding.

Cognitive rehabilitation may be the most promising intervention, and much research is being conducted in this area. Positive results were found in Poppelreuter, Weis, and Bartsch's (2009) randomized controlled trial, which offered occupational therapy for memory and attention or computer-based training. Both treatment arms obtained benefit in cognitive function. The Memory/Attention Adaptation Training intervention, which focused on arousal reduction through relaxation training and use of compensatory strategies, resulted in improved verbal memory, executive function, psychomotor function, and cognition (Ferguson et al., 2007). Patients can use many simple measures to organize their routine and daily habits that may assist in attention, concentration, and memory. Examples of strategies that can aid cognition include setting priories, using a day planner and notebook for lists, developing daily routines, preparing ahead of time, rehearsing before interactions, cueing the senses, breaking numbers into chunks, posting checklists, labeling items with respective and commonly used numbers or names, assigning a specific place for items, using timers, and working the mind with puzzles, reading, or memory games.

Stress reduction through meditation may repair brain tissue and strengthen the immune system. Researchers have linked many types of meditation practices with changes in brain electrical patterns and structure. During meditation, gamma brain waves are more synchronized, suggesting that meditation changed the brain's electrical pattern and improved blood flow in the area responsible for positive thoughts and emotions (Lutz, Greisch, Rawlings, Ricard, & Davidson, 2004). Brain regions associated with sensory processing and attention were thicker in those who meditated, and older subjects who meditated had cortical thickening instead of the expected thinning that occurs with aging as noted in Lazar and colleague's (2005) study. The documented positive benefits of meditation, along with the fairly easy accessibility of teaching this technique, make it a practical approach worth offering to patients.

Exercise is recommended to promote general well-being. Blood flow and oxygenation to the brain is improved with exercise (Nelson, Nandy, & Roth, 2007). Exercise may promote relaxation and improve sleep patterns, causing positive effects on alertness and concentration. Proinflammatory hormone-like proteins such as cytokines are associated with decreased learning and inability to concentrate (Jansen et al., 2005), and these levels are reduced with improvement in cognition in long-term exercise programs (Wilson, Finch, & Cohen, 2002).

Patient education needs to be initiated prior to starting chemotherapy or radiation. Patients have a right to know the potential side effects and risks associated with treatment. Education should be integrated into the care regarding which cognitive changes may be expected with brain involvement. In primary brain tumors and brain metastases, practitioners should offer anticipatory guidance on possible changes in cognitive functioning. With the patient's permission, family and friends should be included in the educational process with the goal of obtaining understanding, assistance, and emotional support. The education needs to be delivered in a nonthreatening way with ample time for the patient and significant others to reflect on and express their concerns and questions. Abundant mention of "chemobrain" is in the general public domain, and providing factual information may alleviate fears and clarify misconceptions about the potential cognitive difficulties associated with chemotherapy.

The cognitive changes associated with cancer and its treatment can greatly affect patients' QOL. Over the past decade, more attention has been given to understanding the etiology of the neuropsychological effects in order to develop effective psychological treatment, patient education, and medication interventions to help compensate for these effects. We are in the early stages of understanding the numerous variables in the process of cognitive impairment. An accurate account of cognitive defects from cancer and its treatment do not exist for multiple reasons. The inconsistencies of research findings, the low sensitivity of measurement tools used in the past, the limited number of longitudinal studies, the often long duration between treatment and the development of cognitive changes, and the short survival in some populations are challenges that researchers and clinicians face.

A lack of pretreatment neurologic functioning prohibits us from documenting the extent of the changes within individuals and participants undergoing the same treatment. Performing pretreatment cognitive testing, however, can result in practice effects seen in cognitive retesting, which may minimize or mask changes, and this needs to be accounted for and factored into research designs. Referral for neuropsychology consultation is indispensable for obtaining baseline neuropsychological evaluation; identifying cognitive defects; managing behavioral issues; recommending pharmacologic agents, rehabilitation, and compensatory coping strategies; and managing specific cognitive problems. Cancer psychologists can identify the patient's specific concerns and provide advice and guidance on finding routines, writing lists, color-coding items, using notes, and teaching new skills that serve to reinforce the retention of information. Additionally, psychologists can offer cognitive-behavioral therapy, acceptance and commitment therapy, or psychodynamic therapeutic approaches to assist patients to adjust to the numerous challenges of living with cancer. Providing patient education with anticipatory guidance on the possibility of cognitive changes is an important role of the oncology nurse. Nurses should inquire about cognitive changes so that further evaluation can occur. Validating the existence and the impact that cognitive impairment has on patients' QOL is critical.

Post-Traumatic Stress Disorder

The traumatic events that might cause PTSD include military combat, violent personal assault, and being diagnosed with a life-threatening illness. Psychological trauma is caused by sudden and unexpected events in which the person perceives a dramatic loss of personal control and safety (Ehlers & Steil, 1995). The unexpected diagnosis and often aggressive treatment for cancer can lead to thoughts of loss of control and threats to safety. After a traumatic event, the brain is not able to reconcile the thoughts, memories, and images of the trauma with one's core beliefs (Brewin, Dalgleish, & Joseph, 1996). Avoidance and denial are temporary defenses in response to a trauma, but eventually, the individual usually is able to integrate the event into his or her existing worldview (Horowitz, 1986). The process of integrating new information from the distressing event with one's current worldview is manifested by re-experiencing the event or in the form of intrusive thoughts. Avoidance is the process used to defend the mind from the emotional distress and will prevent emotional processing from occurring. Adaptation occurs when traumatic information is gradually integrated into one's core beliefs through the process of mentally oscillating between intrusive thoughts and avoidance (Dalgleish, 2004).

Typically the traumatic event is persistently re-experienced, and any stimuli associated with the trauma are avoided. Persistent symptoms of increased arousal include difficulty falling or staying asleep, irritability, outbursts of anger, difficulty concentrating, hypervigilance, or exaggerated startle response. PTSD is considered acute PTSD if the duration of symptoms is less than three months, chronic PTSD if the symptoms are three months or more, and PTSD with delayed onset if the symptoms are at least six months or more after the stressor.

Historically, PTSD was thought to occur mainly in combat veterans. PTSD was not considered a formal diagnosis until 1980. Prior to this, combat veterans may have been told that they had shell shock, combat fatigue, war neurosis, transient situational disturbance, or survivor syndrome (Averill & Beck, 2000). Since the nosology used to describe PTSD in the DSM-IV TR (APA, 2000) was developed according to responses from younger individuals, the diagnostic features may present differently in older adults. Currently the DSM-IV TR delineates the specific diagnostic criteria for the diagnosis of PTSD, which includes facing a life-threatening illness as a possible traumatic stressor. Cancer as the traumatic stressor is triggered at numerous points of time such as the time of diagnosis, active treatment, post-treatment, recurrence, and the terminal phase. The term *direct traumatization* applies to individuals diagnosed with cancer, whereas *indirect traumatization* applies to those who are informed that their child or significant other has cancer.

It is difficult to obtain accurate prevalence rates of PTSD in patients with cancer because it may go undetected or underreported. In the general adult population in the United States, the prevalence rate is approximately 8% (APA, 2000). Rates of cancer-related PTSD assessed by structured clinical diagnostic interview ranged widely across studies up to 35%; however, Kangas, Henry, and Bryant's (2002) empirical review found that most studies confirmed a rate of 4%–6%, and Andrykowski and Kangas's (2010) review found a prevalence rate range of 0%–36%. The diagnosis of cancer can cause PTSD or symptom reactivation in those with a previous history of PTSD.

Why some cancer survivors develop PTSD is not clear. Potential risk factors for developing PTSD after a cancer diagnosis include high level of perceived threat, prior trauma history, younger age, lower income, less education, less social support, and difficult interactions with medical staff (Jim & Jacobsen, 2008). These risk factors should be considered when screening for PTSD.

Living with cancer may lead to a persistence of PTSD symptoms without necessarily leading to the full syndrome of PTSD (Smith, Redd, Peyser, & Vogl, 1999). The trauma associated with cancer is different from other types of traumatic events. Specifically, the intrusive thoughts in cancer frequently consist of fears of future threats such as pain, physical changes, or death rather than a specific past memory. Therefore, the patient's concept and core belief about the prognosis may reflect the intensity of the threat and degree of emotional trauma. A review of the literature shows that other types of intrusive thoughts that cancer survivors experience consist of recurrent or distressing thoughts or dreams about the cancer, thinking about the cancer when they do not want to, and high levels of distress when reminded of the cancer. It is important to note that many of these studies have been on women with breast cancer and that many of the studies were cross-sectional with a wide range of time from diagnosis. Nonetheless, the literature supports the importance that PTSD symptoms have on QOL in patients with cancer, and this issue needs to be addressed.

Conceptually, PTSD in people with cancer is different than PTSD from other traumatic events such as combat. Most of the perceived threats associated with cancer are preoccupation with somatic symptoms (somatic distress) and fear of recurrence (Somerfield, Stefanek, Smith, & Padberg, 1999). Fifty-one percent of an ethnically diverse cancer population indicated wanting help with overcoming their fears (Moadel et al., 1999). Another key difference is the intense and immediate psychosocial support that people newly diagnosed with cancer or those undergoing treatment often receive. Support in the form of time with family and friends, attention from medical and nursing staff, support groups, and individual counseling or psychotherapy provides an opportunity for individuals to give a narrative of their experience. The disorganization of trauma memories is known to interfere with processing of information (Foa & Cahill, 2001).

It is important for patients who have symptoms of PTSD to be evaluated by a psychologist or psychiatrist for proper diagnosis and to initiate a treatment plan. Differentiating between PTSD and other mental conditions in the oncology population is complex. The differential diagnosis should include adjustment disorder, acute stress disorder, major depressive episode, and a mental disorder (e.g., mood disorder, anxiety disorder, sleep disorder) associated with a general medical condition. One major difference between PTSD and acute stress disorder is that the disturbance in the latter lasts for a minimum of two days and a maximum of four weeks after the traumatic event. If the symptoms of acute stress disorder persist, the diagnosis of PTSD may be given.

Treatment of PTSD with psychotherapeutic interventions is effective in alleviating the symptoms. Trauma-focused cognitive-behavioral and exposure therapy and desensitization therapy are the most effective (Jim & Jacobsen, 2008). Stress reduction approaches with guided imagery and progressive muscle relaxation may be less threatening to some patients. Supportive-expressive group therapy has shown symptom improvement in one randomized clinical trial (Classen et al., 2001). Fifty-one percent of patients with cancer endorsed the need to overcome fears (Moadel et al., 1999), supporting the importance of assessing for and treating PTSD. Numerous approaches have documented effective treatment of PTSD; therefore, assessing for this problem and early referral are likely to result in a positive outcome.

Hope

The emotion of hope is central to mental well-being. Hope is an everyday emotion that adds or detracts from QOL. QOL is reduced with loss of hope (Rusteon, 1995). Hopelessness is associated with poorer survival rates in women with breast cancer (Watson, Haviland, Greer, Davidson, & Bliss, 1999) and higher rates of suicide, suicidal ideation, and desires for hastened death (Breitbart et al., 2010). Psychological distress was related to hopelessness in 37% of inpatient hospice patients (Moadel et al., 1999). Forty-two percent of ethnically diverse patients with cancer in the clinic setting indicated wanting help with finding hope (Moadel et al., 1999). Healthcare providers play a pivotal role in assisting the patient to find, maintain, or enhance a sense of hope.

The nursing literature includes several working definitions, concept analyses, and research that describes the nature of hope and its impact of hope on suffering and well-being and supports the importance of maintaining and restoring hope during the cancer trajectory. Merriam-Webster ("Hope," 2011) defines *hope* as the "desire accompanied by expectation of or belief in fulfillment" and "someone or something on which hopes are centered." Tulsky (2002) points out the competing interpretations of this definition of hope with the first being a sense of trust that implies faith and does not depend on the outcome. The other interpretation is the expectation of fulfillment of a specific outcome. When hope consists of expectation that something will or will not happen, the risk for despair exists. Unfortunately, all too often the hope for cure is not possible, leading to profound disappointment. The goal of the psychologist is to assist the patient who may expect cure to also find realistic expectations that are focused upon the present and near future and provide a sense of peace and comfort.

Based on my clinical observations, I have concluded that some patients with cancer have a common misconception that hope is necessary for cure or remission. Taken to the extreme, some patients may hold the belief that hope is the essential ingredient necessary to make the cure occur. If the cure or improvement does not occur, a patient can potentially self-blame. The patient's beliefs may be based on magical thinking or be influenced by the current societal constructs that focus on unrealistic expectations of medical technology and an unrealistic belief in cure, miracles, and spontaneous remissions. These expectations may be unrealistic in certain diagnoses or in later stages of cancer and should be differentiated from denial. In addition, healthcare providers may unknowingly contribute to unrealistic hope by trying to instill hope as a sincere way of improving mental well-being. Unrealistic hope sometimes presents as the belief that one's frame of mind is able to completely control one's physiology.

Hope is a multidimensional and dynamic concept that is a complex blend of thoughts that are constantly changing. This point is dissected by the work of Dufault and Martocchio (1985), who developed a conceptualization of hope based on clinical data collected on patients with cancer ages 14 years and older and on older adult patients. These authors found that hope is "characterized by a *confident* yet *uncertain* expectation of achieving a *future* good which, to the hoping person, is *realistically* possible and *personally significant*" (p. 380). This definition includes interpersonal relatedness. Based on their empirical data Dufault and Martocchio (1985) found two spheres of hope: generalized and particularized hope. *Generalized hope* is a sense of some future benefit, and this protects against despair. *Particularized hope* is concerned with a specific valued outcome or state of being. Both generalized hope and particularized hope encompass six dimensions: affective, cognitive, behavioral, affiliative, temporal, and contextual.

Groopman (2004) described the practical concept of hope as "the elevating feeling we experience when we see—in the mind's eye—a path to a better future. Hope acknowledges the significant obstacles and deep pitfalls along that path. True hope has not room for delusion" (p. xiv). This definition incorporates the essential ingredient of truthfulness and trust. Numerous studies have documented that patients value honest information from healthcare providers as very important; therefore, honesty should be considered when planning interventions to enhance hopefulness. Patients tend to trust nurses and often inquire about their status. These are teachable moments, when nurses can help patients identify the realistic future events, goals, or accomplishments that they can hope for.

A related concept to hope and depression is demoralization syndrome. Hopelessness, loss of meaning, and desire for death form the triad of the demoralization syndrome (Kissane et al., 1997), causing spiritual and existential suffering. Demoralization syndrome is a prominent form of existential distress in which meaninglessness, hopelessness, purposelessness, and helplessness predominate and which may lead to the desire to die. Demoralization can be differentiated from depression, anhedonia, and grief. It is different from depression in that in spite of feeling demoralized, one can find pleasure because the lack of hope is restricted to the future. Anhedonia is characterized by the inability to experience pleasure. Interventions for demoralization syndrome include implementing cognitive-behavioral therapy to counter the pessimistic beliefs, promoting goal setting, exploring the patient's role and purpose, and reducing feelings of isolation and dependence.

Hope has been studied extensively in the oncology and mentally ill populations, and numerous instruments are available to measure hope. A complete listing and discussion of these instruments is beyond the scope of this chapter; suffice it to say that careful selection should occur before using a particular instrument in clinical practice or research. The Herth Hope Scale is a 30-item, 0–3-point summated rating scale that captures the multidimensionality of hope. It has three subscales: the cognitive-temporal dimension, affective-behavioral dimensions, and the affiliative-contextual dimension. This scale was tested in both healthy adults and in patients with cancer and has a Cronbach reliability coefficient range from 0.75–0.94 (Herth, 1991). Another commonly used hope scale is the Beck Hopelessness Scale. This is a 20-item, true-false test based on the definition of hopelessness and measures negative expectancies concerning oneself and one's future (Beck, Weissman, Lester, & Trexler, 1974). The Miller Hope Scale (Miller & Powers, 1988) is a 40-item, five-point Likert scale questionnaire specifically designed to measure the degree of the patient's anticipation for a continued good state, an improved state, or a release from a perceived entrapment. It has been tested in medically ill adults and adults with psychiatric illness. In addition, other useful clinical scales are available to measure hope, including the Hopefulness Scale for Adolescents, a 24-item visual analog scale tested in both healthy adolescents and those with cancer. The Snyder Hope Scale, which has been tested in healthy adults, adults with psychiatric illness, and children, is a 12-item, four-point Likert scale that focuses on goal identification and achievements. Practitioners can use these instruments as an efficient way to assess patients' level of hope at baseline and throughout the disease trajectory.

Interventions aimed at maintaining and building hope should be part of the psychological support plan. Moadel and colleagues' (1999) survey reported that 41% of patients with cancer needed help to find hope. Herth (2000) found that participants with recurrence who were randomized to a hope intervention had higher scores on hope than did those randomized to the informational group or control group at two weeks and three, six, and nine months after the intervention.

Psychological support programs grounded on the research of the constructs and dimensions of hope have successfully assisted those living with cancer to gain hope. The Hope Process Framework (Farran, Wilken, & Popovich, 1992) is based on four attributes of hope: the experiential process, the spiritual or transcendent process, the rational process, and the relational process. An eight-session hope intervention program based on the Hope Process Framework, which focused on the four attributes of hope, helped patients increase, rebuild, and maintain hope (Herth, 2001). The Living With Hope Program, a brief intervention program for older adults with cancer, provided greater hope and existential QOL (Duggleby et al., 2007). Other similar successful findings have been documented, supporting the effectiveness of structured programs on enhancing hope.

Many approaches and actions are available that practitioners can take to foster hope on an individual basis. First, when listening to patients describe their sense of hope, it is important to identify which dimension (affective, cognitive, behavioral, affiliative, temporal, or contextual) applies in order to support and facilitate the individual's hope. Comprehensive interviews that assess each domain of hope will identify other desires that patients may have or areas in which they have not yet identified hope. Because hope is a dynamic process, attention should be given to it at each visit. For this reason, it is necessary to develop stage-specific hope that is realistic to the patient at that time during the disease trajectory.

What one hopes for will change over time. Consideration of the central attributes of hope is only part of the story. Attention must be given to how the stage of one's illness influences hope. The place along the cancer trajectory affects the priority level for the specific events for which a patient expresses hope. Those newly diagnosed or cured have different concerns than those near the end of life. Hope, honesty, information, emotional expression, and discussion of issues related to death and dying were the five major needs critically ill patients identified in Young-Brockopp's (1982) study. Indeed, healthcare professionals increase hospice patients' sense of hope by being present, giving accurate information, and showing that they care (Koopmeiners et al., 1997). It may be necessary to clarify patients' hope and assist them in moving perception to a realistic one by providing information and correcting misinformation or misrepresentations.

Interventions

Patients experiencing psychological distress deserve to be treated. Psychotherapeutic interventions, such as individual psychotherapy, logotherapy, group psychotherapy, and narrative work, are a few examples of approaches found to be extremely useful in alleviating psychological symptoms and restoring emotional well-being.

Individual therapy provided by a trained licensed mental health provider offers patients a safe and confidential environment in which to communicate concerns, process feelings, reframe the meaning of the situation, learn coping skills, and identify personal values. Whether individuals are receptive to individual therapy depends upon how the treatment is presented, their cultural belief on the acceptability of therapy, their level of distress, available support systems, and access to a professional therapist. Different types of psychotherapy exist, and individuals' backgrounds and preferences should be evaluated in order to determine the best fit. Commonly used therapeutic approaches that are appropriate but not restrictive to the oncology population include logotherapy, cognitive-behavioral therapy, supportive-expressive therapy, emotion-focused therapy, brief psychodynamic psychotherapy, dream analysis, hypnotherapy, and acceptance and commitment therapy. Providing the details of these complex approaches is beyond the scope of this chapter; however, logotherapy and narrative therapies will be discussed briefly as examples.

Logotherapy, also known as *meaning-centered psychotherapy*, is based on the work of Victor E. Frankl, a professor of neurology and psychiatry at the University of Vienna who was a Holocaust Auschwitz survivor (Frankl, 1967). The basic concepts of meaning-centered psychotherapy include
- Meaning of life (life has meaning and never ceases to have meaning)
- Will to meaning (the desire to find meaning in human existence is a third primary and basic motivation for human behavior)
- Freedom of will (freedom to find meaning in existence and to choose one's attitude toward suffering).

The focus of this therapy is to assist the patient to identify the sources of meaning and achieve transcendence through experience, creativity, attitude, and legacy. The treatment goals are to find spiritual well-being and a sense of purpose and meaning in life. In a randomized controlled trial, Breibart et al. (2010) document-

ed significantly greater improvements in spiritual well-being and anxiety with an enhanced sense of meaning. The comparison group did not show any significant improvement in these domains. Although this was a small pilot study (N = 90), it documents the potential benefits of meaning-centered group psychotherapy as an intervention for psychologists to consider.

Narrative therapy is an approach that assists those with serious illness or grief to
begin to develop a new perspective on their situation and life. Narrative therapy can
be implemented in several ways, including writing and storytelling. The written narrative has shown to improve immune response (Pennebaker, Kiecolt-Glaser, & Glaser, 1988). The oral narrative approach is thought to help patients think differently by hearing themselves tell their stories, absorb others' reactions, and experience
their stories being shared. Frank (1995) described three different narrative ways to
frame illness and loss: restitution, chaos, and quest. The restitution narrative enhances concrete hope, which may be realistic or unfortunately may only serve to lock the
individual into his or her past body-self relationships and way of being in the world
with the false belief that he or she can return to this former state of being. The chaos narrative describes the person whose story has no sense of distance from what is
happening because he or she is in the story and not reflecting on it. This often is
seen in bereavement work and includes strong emotions of anger, fear, depression,
and overwhelming emotion. Often the chaos story is told as events as they happened
without clear causality with the theme of loss of control and frustration. Listening
to chaos narratives is difficult because they are threatening and anxiety provoking.
The lack of coherence can be confusing. The focus of therapy during chaotic stories
should be on listening and steering the patient toward his or her feelings. In listening, it can be helpful to challenge, redirect, and reframe. The quest narrative is the
belief that something is to be gained from the illness and the storyteller has a voice
in what the illness means to him or her.

Group psychotherapy for patients with cancer is effective in improving QOL by
reducing psychological distress and increasing coping skills (Spiegel, Stein, Earhart,
& Diamond, 2000). The three basic types of groups are education, support, and psychotherapy. These approaches are efficient and offer an opportunity for patients to
give and receive support and find alternative ways of coping through the lived experience of other cancer survivors. As in all interventions, the patients' preferences
must be considered when making recommendations, and staff can assist patients by
explaining what the available options entail and encouraging them to try different
approaches because the exact fit or effectiveness is not predictable. It may be helpful for patients to gather information from other cancer survivors about what was
particularly useful for their individual needs.

Workplace Stress: Compassion Fatigue and Burnout

Nurses working with the oncology population face numerous challenges and need
to understand and recognize their own stress, grief, anxiety, depression, and PTSD.
Understanding one's emotional reactions to the clinical situation is necessary in order to recognize how these feelings influence response to the patient and family.
It is imperative to honor the reality that oncology clinical practice affects staff on a
deep personal level. Those who bear witness to their patients' suffering are likely at
risk for compassion fatigue or burnout. Bearing witness means being present with

the suffering person and accepting the risk of suffering alongside the patient (Cody, 2007), and this makes the caregiver open and vulnerable to experiencing suffering with the patient (Arman, 2007). Compassion fatigue, also referred to as *secondary traumatic stress disorder* or *vicarious traumatization*, occurs as a result of professionals putting out more energy and compassion than they receive and manifests as physical, emotional, psychological, and spiritual exhaustion. Burnout occurs in response to chronic interpersonal stressors on the job (Maslach, Schaufeli, & Leiter, 2001).

In providing compassionate care, the professional may be traumatized. The symptoms of compassion fatigue are closely related to PTSD, which Figley (2002) defined as "a state of tension and preoccupation with the individual or cumulative trauma of clients as manifested in one or more ways" (p. 127). Compassion fatigue can emerge suddenly, resulting in a sense of helplessness and confusion. Burnout, a similar concept, is the result of cumulative and prolonged stress accompanied by physical, emotional, occupational, and social symptoms. Burnout is a form of mental distress manifested in "normal" people who did not suffer from prior psychopathology who experience decreased work performance resulting from negative attitudes and behaviors (Maslach & Leiter, 2008). The negative attitude characterizing burnout was described by Edelwich and Brodsky (1980) as "the progressive loss of idealism, energy, and purpose experienced by people in the helping professions as a result of the conditions of their work" (p. 12). The overwhelming exhaustion, feelings of cynicism and detachment from the job, and sense of ineffectiveness or incompetence reflect the impact that prolonged stress has on the personal, interpersonal, and self-evaluative dimensions of the individual. The main difference between compassion fatigue and burnout is that in the former, one can still care and be involved, whereas in burnout, the individual may have cynicism or a detached response.

Recognizing and managing symptoms of stress is necessary in order to function at one's highest potential. Sources of work-related stress may be personal, interpersonal, or organizational in nature. Feelings of stress and chronic loss can cause a sense of helplessness or hopelessness. Symptoms of burnout reported in the literature include fatigue, physical and emotional exhaustion, headaches, gastrointestinal disturbances, weight loss, sleeplessness, depression, anxiety, irritability, depersonalization, boredom, frustration, low morale, job turnover, and impaired job performance including decreased empathy and increased absenteeism.

The literature on oncology staff mental well-being identifies potential risks for compassion fatigue. Factors that may place a healthcare provider at risk for compassion fatigue are numerous. Sherman's (2000) findings noted that nurses who experienced reverberations from the past and unresolved personal issues found it difficult to provide appropriate care for certain types of patients. Holding high or unrealistic expectations of one's emotional strength may lead to disappointment when emotional exhaustion occurs. Providing care or treatment that induces pain or suffering is a threat that causes distress to nurses (Rowe, 2003). Other risk factors that are likely to put staff at risk for compassion fatigue are situations that block a supportive environment. The culture of a professional healthcare community that promotes silence versus the sharing of stressful experiences may put staff at risk for compassion fatigue. Working in an environment that does not validate the legitimacy of the caregiver's distress may lead to withdrawal, apathy, and depression.

The effects of burnout and compassion fatigue negatively impact patient care in terms of patient safety and satisfaction. Emotional stability was identified as a predictor of patient safety in a study of nurses, and the authors concluded that managers should strive to create a climate that promotes the emotional stability of staff to prevent adverse events (Teng, Chang, & Hsu, 2009).

Patient satisfaction is influenced by numerous factors, including staff's level of mental well-being. In oncology practice, the relationship between the patient and staff is an essential tool of service provision necessary to provide quality comprehensive care to a complex patient population. Factors that interfere with the patient-staff relationship would predictably diminish patient satisfaction. Staff burnout and compassion fatigue lead to psychological distress. The professional staff's mental well-being directly affects patient care as documented in numerous studies. Patient care satisfaction scores were significantly low in patients cared for by staff who reported higher levels of emotional exhaustion in a tertiary care hospital study (Leiter, Harvie, & Frizzell, 1998). Poor patient satisfaction rates correlated with group-level staff burnout scores in Garman, Corrigan, and Morris's (2002) study on behavioral health teams. These findings indicate that staff burnout at both the individual and team levels strongly influences patients' appraisal of care received.

Healthcare providers respond when they are exhausted or psychologically overwhelmed in a number of ways that may or may not be helpful. Defenses against the stress of witnessing suffering may include distancing behaviors. The act of distancing themselves from patients may depersonalize and dehumanize care, leading to undignified care. Professional techniques are often used to remain somewhat detached and objective. Two examples are therapeutic empathy, consisting of a learned empathetic response, and informative reassurance, which consists of providing information and explanations of the suffering. It is necessary for professionals to find a realistic balance of bearing witness to suffering with the recognition that it is not possible to connect deeply with all patients. Patients' emotional and psychological needs should never be ignored, and the most appropriate healthcare team member should be matched to meet the specific needs of the patient. Utilizing mental health professionals such as cancer psychologists may serve to alleviate the staff's emotional burden while addressing the needs of the patient.

The six domains of the work environment that may influence the level of occupational stress as listed by Maslach et al. (2001) include workload, control, reward, community, fairness, and values. The work environment and emotion-work variables (expectation) influence one's response to stress. The emotion-work variables consist of the normative expectations of the employment community as to whether professionals should display or suppress emotions. Not fitting into the expected emotion-work requirements can lead to additional emotional stress. Those planning interventions to prevent compassion fatigue and burnout should consider how the work environment may be contributing to the individual's stress. It is important to consider the congruency between professionals' and employers' value systems because the amount of synchronization influences engagement versus burnout. Assisting staff in identifying which domains of the work environment are most valued and how that causes or prevents stress may be helpful in beginning to understand and validate the current level of compassion fatigue or burnout. Conceptualizing the match or mismatch between the employee and the domains of the work environment would allow astute administrators to identify areas that need to be changed and programs to assist staff with the reality of stressful job requirements.

Lamentably, healthcare providers' ability to alleviate patients' pain and suffering is sometimes less than ideal. Recognizing the limitations of how much one is able to impact patients' well-being is necessary to avoid a sense of guilt, grief, depression, self-blame, or incompetence. Numerous interventions and programs have been studied or suggested to reduce or avoid compassion fatigue and burnout. Sherman (2000) found that nurses learned to alleviate their emotional stress by acknowledging unresolved losses, sharing with a colleague or a counselor, obtaining assistance and emotional support from professionals, finding time for laughter, and taking time to take care of themselves. Oncology nurses who participated in a qualitative study suggested interventions aimed at providing support for managing grief and loss with focus on improving interpersonal functioning and resiliency (Wenzel, Shaha, Klimmek, & Krumm, 2011). Staff bereavement programs provide an opportunity for staff to address their grief. Psychoeducational programs offering topics on effective communication strategies and self-care strategies could be offered informally or incorporated into other continuing education programs. Creating moments of connection with patients was found to prevent compassion fatigue in oncology nurses (Perry, 2008). Encouraging staff to reflect on these positive work experiences may serve to sustain professional well-being. Narrative reflection provides an avenue for staff to document meaningful and pivotal experiences, as well as a method to debrief, resolve their loss, and safely express their feelings.

Assisting caregivers to be mindfully present to their experience without judgment has been documented as an effective intervention. An eight-week mindfulness-based stress reduction program decreased burnout scores with decreased emotional exhaustion and depersonalization and increased personal accomplishment; these changes lasted three months (Cohen-Katz et al., 2004). Programs that increase self-awareness by assisting staff members to identify their emotions and responses will contribute to personal wellness and can be offered in a variety of venues.

Other interventions to consider are those that promote self-awareness, search for meaning of the experience, and value clarification. Fillion et al. (2009) developed and tested a meaning-centered psychoeducational group intervention based on Frankl's logotherapy. The purpose of this study was to assess and address existential and emotional demands. Licensed psychologists provided the intervention that applied didactic and process-oriented strategies, including guided reflections, experiential exercises, and education. The nurses in the experimental group reported more perceived benefits of working in palliative care after the intervention and at follow-up than the control group.

The importance of self-care is often suggested and offered in staff support programs. Oncologists who used self-care and wellness strategies had greater work satisfaction than those who did not (Shanafelt et al., 2005). Based on what is known about the nature of staff stress, those preparing intervention content and design aimed at preventing or reducing staff stress should consider the type of oncology setting, length of work experience, personality factors, and educational level. Consultation from a mental health professional should be obtained if symptoms of burnout and compassion fatigue are severe.

Clearly, healthcare providers must establish a balance between their personal and professional lives by routinely taking care of themselves. The personality variables such as optimism, self-efficacy, resilience, hardiness, sense of coherence, and emotional sensitivity, as well as the sense of spirituality, social support, and history of significant life events, influences how individuals conceptualize and respond to occupational stress. Self-acknowledgment of one's tendencies to respond, react, and behave in specific situations is the first step toward a mindfulness-based practice. Being in tune with one's personality traits allows for attaining self-acceptance, transforming emotional pain, and avoiding negative self-judgment. Clarifying values and finding meaning in one's work enhances the commitment to work that is inspiring, fulfilling, and promotes professional growth.

Conclusion

The numerous psychological symptoms that are frequently associated with cancer often impose a significant negative impact on quality of life, and in some cases, the magnitude of emotional distress results in patients' desire to hasten their death or commit suicide. Psychological problems may not always be obvious to healthcare providers; therefore, screening all patients with cancer for psychological distress is recommended. The screening process is an ideal time to begin to address current or potential mental health issues. During these conversations, patients can be provided with information about available psychological support services. The process of asking patients about their mental well-being may convey the message that distress is a common reaction and a safe topic to discuss with the staff.

By the nature of their professional relationship with patients with cancer, nurses are in a prime position to identify psychological problems. The common types of mental health issues seen in the oncology population include anxiety, depression, acute or chronic adjustment disorder, cognitive dysfunction, PTSD, suicidal ideation, desire to hasten death, and hopelessness. Those with a comorbid psychiatric illness may be at risk for relapse or additional psychological symptoms. Identified psychological symptoms or emotional distress can be further evaluated and treated by cancer psychologists. Numerous psychological interventions have empirically demonstrated an improvement in mental health outcomes in the oncology population.

Oncology nurses are admirably passionate about their work. The responsibilities and challenges that nurses face daily can impact their psychological well-being. Work environments that validate the reality of compassion fatigue and offer support to staff can reduce burnout and promote safe and comprehensive cancer care.

References

Adler, N.E., & Page, A.E. (Eds.). (2008). *Cancer care for the whole patient: Meeting psychosocial health needs*. Retrieved from http://www.iom.edu/Reports/2007/Cancer-Care-for-the-Whole-Patient-Meeting-Psychosocial-Health-Needs.aspx

Akechi, T., Okuyama, T., Onishi, J., Morita, T., & Furukawa, T. (2008). Psychotherapy for depression among incurable cancer patients (review). *Cochrane Database of Systematic Reviews, 2008*(2), Art. No.: CD005537. doi:10.1002/14651858

American Psychiatric Association. (2000). *Diagnostic and statistical manual of mental disorders* (4th ed., text rev.). Washington, DC: Author.

Andrykowski, M., & Kangas, M. (2010). Posttraumatic stress disorder associated with cancer diagnosis and treatment. In J. Holland, W. Breitbart, P. Jackobsen, M. Lederber, J. Loscalzo, & R. McCorkle (Eds.), *Psycho-oncology* (2nd ed., pp. 348–357). New York, NY: Oxford University Press.

Arman, M. (2007). Bearing witness: An existential position in caring. *Contemporary Nurse, 27,* 84–94. doi:10.5172/conu.2007.27.1.84

Armstrong, C., Stern, C.D., & Corn, B. (2001). Memory performance used to detect radiation effects on cognitive functioning. *Applied Neuropsychology, 8,* 129–139. doi:10.1207/S15324826AN0803_1

Armstrong, T. (2011). Central nervous system cancers. In C.H. Yarbro, D. Wujcik, & B.H. Gobel (Eds.), *Cancer nursing: Principles and practice* (7th ed., pp. 1146–1187). Burlington, MA: Jones and Bartlett.

Averill, P., & Beck, J. (2000). Posttraumatic stress disorder in older adults: A conceptual review. *Journal of Anxiety Disorders, 14,* 133–156. doi:10.1016/S0887-6185(99)00045-6

Beck, A., Weissman, A., Lester, D., & Trexler, L. (1974). The measurement of pessimism: The hopelessness scale. *Journal of Consulting and Clinical Psychology, 42,* 861–865. doi:10.1037/h0037562

Behin, A., & Delattre, J.-Y. (2003). Neurologic sequelae of radiotherapy on the nervous system. In D. Schiff & P. Wen (Eds.), *Cancer neurology in clinical practice* (pp. 173–191). Totowa, NJ: Humana Press.

Breitbart, W., Rosenfeld, B., Gibson, C., Pessin, H., Poppito, S., Nelson, C., ... Olden, M. (2010). Meaning-centered group psychotherapy for patients with advanced cancer: A pilot randomized controlled trial. *Psycho-Oncology, 19,* 21–28. doi:10.1002/pon.1556

Brewin, C., Dalgleish, T., & Joseph, S. (1996). A dual representation theory of posttraumatic stress disorder. *Psychological Review, 103,* 670–686. doi:10.1037/0033-295X.103.4.670

Brintzenhofe-Szoc, K., Levin, T., Li, Y., Kissane, D., & Zahora, J. (2009). Mixed anxiety/depression symptoms in a large cancer cohort: Prevalence by cancer type. *Psychosomatics, 50,* 383–391. doi:10.1176/appi.psy.50.4.383

Chan, A., Cheung, M.C., Law, S., & Chan, J. (2004). Phase II study of alpha-tocopherol in improving cognitive function of patients with temporal lobe radionecrosis. *Cancer, 100,* 398–404. doi:10.1002/cncr.11885

Clarke, D., & Kissane, D. (2002). Demoralization: Its phenomenology and importance. *Australian and New Zealand Journal of Psychiatry, 36,* 733–742. doi:10.1046/j.1440-1614.2002.01086.x

Classen, C., Butler, L.D., Koopman, C., Miller, E., DiMiceli, S., Giese-Davis, J., ... Spiegel, D. (2001). Supportive-expressive group therapy and distress in patients with metastatic breast cancer: A randomized clinical intervention trial. *Archives of General Psychiatry, 58,* 494–501. doi:10.1001/archpsyc.58.5.494.

Cody, W. (2007). Bearing witness to suffering: Participating in contrascendence. *International Journal for Human Caring, 11*(2), 17–21.

Cohen-Katz, J., Wiley, S., Capuano, T., Baker, D., Deitrick, L., & Shapiro, S. (2005). The effects of mindfulness-based stress reduction on nurse stress and burnout: A quantitative and qualitative study. *Holistic Nursing Practice, 19,* 78–86.

Coyne, B., & Leslie, M. (2004). Chemo's toll on memory. *RN, 67*(4), 40–43.

Dalgleish, T. (2004). Cognitive approaches to posttraumatic stress disorder: The evolution of multi-representational theorizing. *Psychological Bulletin, 130,* 228–260. doi:10.1037/0033-2909.130.2.228

Dietrich, J., Han, R., Yang, Y., Mayer-Proschel, M., & Nobel, M. (2006). CNS progenitor cells and oligodendrocytes are targets of chemotherapeutic agents in vitro and vivo. *Journal of Biology, 5,* 1–23. doi:10.1186/jbiol50

Dufault, K., & Martocchio, B. (1985). Symposium on compassionate care and the dying experience. Hope: Its spheres and dimensions. *Nursing Clinics of North America, 20,* 379–391.

Duggleby, W., Degner, L., Williams, A., Wright, K., Cooper, D., Popkin, D., & Holtslander, L. (2007). Living with hope: Initial evaluation of a psychosocial hope intervention for older palliative care patients. *Journal of Pain and Symptom Management, 33,* 247–257. doi:10.1016/j.jpainsymman.2006.09.013

Edelwich, J., & Brodsky, A. (1980). *Burn-out: Stages of disillusionment in the helping professions.* New York, NY: Springer.

Ehlers, A., & Steil, R. (1995). Maintenance of intrusive memories in posttraumatic stress disorder: A cognitive approach. *Behavioral and Cognitive Psychotherapy, 23,* 217–249. doi:10.1017/S135246580001585X

Fallowfield, L., Ratcliffe, D., Jenkins, V., & Saul, J. (2001). Psychiatric morbidity and its recognition by doctors in patients with cancer. *British Journal of Cancer, 84,* 1011–1015. doi:10.1054/bjoc.2001.1724

Fang, F., Fall, K., Mittleman, M., Sparén, P., Ye, W., Adami, H., & Valimarsdóttir, U. (2012). Suicide and cardiovascular death after a cancer diagnosis. *New England Journal of Medicine, 366,* 1310–1318. doi:10.1056/NEJMoa1110307

Farran, C., Wilken, C., & Popovich, J. (1992). Clinical assessment of hope. *Issues in Mental Health Nursing, 13,* 129–138. doi:10.3109/01612849209040528

Ferguson, R., Ahles, T., Saykin, A., McDonald, B., Furstenberg, C., Cole, B., & Mott, L. (2007). Cognitive behavioral management of chemotherapy-related cognitive changes. *Psycho-Oncology, 16,* 772–777. doi:10.1002/pon.1133

Ferrans, C.E., & Hacker, E.D. (2011). Quality of life as an outcome of cancer care. In C.H. Yarbro, D. Wujcik, & B.H. Gobel (Eds.), *Cancer nursing* (7th ed., pp. 201–231). Burlington, MA: Jones and Bartlett.

Figley, C.R. (2002). *Treating compassion fatigue.* New York, NY: Brunner-Routledge.

Filley, D. (2001). *Behavioral neurology of white matter.* New York, NY: Oxford University Press.

Fillion, L., Duval, S., Dumont, S., Gagnon, P., Tremblay, I., Bairati, I., & Breitbart, W. (2009). Impact of a meaning-centered intervention on job satisfaction and on quality of life among palliative care nurses. *Psycho-Oncology, 18,* 1300–1310. doi:10.1002/pon.1513

Foa, E., & Cahill, S. (2001). Psychological therapies: Emotional processing. In H.J. Smelser & P.B. Bates (Eds.), *International encyclopedia of the social and behavioral sciences* (pp. 1263–1269). Oxford, England: Elsevier.

Frank, A. (1995). *The wounded storyteller: Body, illness and ethics.* Chicago, IL: University of Chicago Press.

Frankl, V. (1967). *Psychotherapy and existentialism: Selected papers on logotherapy.* New York, NY: Simon and Schuster.

Garman, A., Corrigan, P., & Morris, S. (2002). Staff burnout and patient satisfaction: Evidence of relationships at the care unit level. *Journal of Occupational Health Psychology, 7,* 235–241. doi:10.1037/1076-8998.7.3.235

Groopman, J. (2004). *The anatomy of hope.* New York, NY: Random House.

Haas, M. (2011). Radiation therapy: Toxicities and management. In C.H. Yarbro, D. Wujcik, & B.H. Gobel (Eds.), *Cancer nursing: Principles and practice* (7th ed., pp. 312–351). Burlington, MA: Jones and Bartlett.

Hannay, J., Howieson, D., Loring, D., Fischer, J., & Lezak, M. (2005). Neuropathology for neuropsychologists. In M. Lezak, D. Howieson, & D. Loring (Eds.), *Neuropsychological assessment* (4th ed., pp. 157–285). New York, NY: Oxford University Press.

Herth, K. (1991). Development and refinement of an instrument to measure hope. *Scholarly Inquiry for Nursing Practice, 5,* 39–51.

Herth, K. (2000). Enhancing hope in people with a first recurrence of cancer. *Journal of Advanced Nursing, 32,* 1431–1441. doi:10.1046/j.1365-2648.2000.01619.x

Herth, K. (2001). Development and implementation of a hope intervention program. *Oncology Nursing Forum, 28,* 1009–1017.

Hettema, J., Prescott, C., Myers, J., Neale, M., & Kendler, K. (2005). The structure of genetic and environmental risk factors for anxiety disorders in men and women. *Archives of General Psychiatry, 62,* 182–189. doi:10.1001/archpsyc.62.2.182

Hewitt, M., Greenfield, S., & Stovall, E. (Eds.). (2006). *From cancer patient to cancer survivor: Lost in transition.* Retrieved from http://www.nap.edu/catalog.php?record_id=11468

Hope. (2011). In *Merriam-Webster's online dictionary.* Retrieved from http://www.merriam-webster .com/dictionary/hope

Horowitz, M. (1986). *Stress response syndromes* (2nd ed.). New York, NY: Jason Aronson.

Inagaki, M., Yoshikawa, E., Matsuoka, Y., Sugawara, Y., Nakano, T., Akechi, T., … Uchitomi, Y. (2007). Smaller regional volumes of gray and white matter demonstrated in breast cancer survivors exposed to adjuvant chemotherapy. *Cancer, 109,* 146–156. doi:10.1002/cncr.22368

Jansen, C., Miaskowski, C., Dodd, M., Dowling, G., & Kramer, J. (2005). Potential mechanisms for chemotherapy-induced impairments in cognitive function. *Oncology Nursing Forum, 32,* 1151–1163. doi:10.1188/05.ONF.1151-1163

Jim, H., & Jacobsen, P. (2008). Posttraumatic stress and posttraumatic growth in cancer survivorship: A review. *Cancer Journal, 14,* 414–419. doi:10.1097/PPO.0b013e31818d8963

Kangas, M., Henry, J.L., & Bryant, R. (2002). Posttraumatic stress disorder following cancer: A conceptual and empirical review. *Clinical Psychology Review, 22,* 499–524. doi:10.1016/S0272-7358(01)00118-0

Kissane, D., Bloch, S., Miach, P., Smith, G., Seddon, A., & Keks, N. (1997). Cognitive existential group therapy for patients with primary breast cancer—Techniques and themes. *Psycho-Oncology, 6,* 25–33. doi:10.1002/(SICI)1099-1611(199703)6:1<25::AID-PON240>3.0.CO;2-N

Koopmeiners, L., Post-White, J., Gutknecht, S., Ceronsky, C., Nickelson, K., Drew, D., … Kreitzer, M. (1997). How healthcare professionals contribute to hope in patients with cancer. *Oncology Nursing Forum, 24,* 1507–1513.

Lazar, S., Kerr, C., Wasserman, R., Gray, J., Greve, D., Treadway, M., … Fischl, B. (2005). Meditation experience is associated with increased cortical thickness. *NeuroReport, 16,* 1893–1897. doi:10.1097/01.wnr.0000186598.66243.19

Leiter, M.P., Harvie, P.L., & Frizzell, C. (1998). The correspondence of patient satisfaction and nurse burnout. *Social Science and Medicine, 47,* 1611–1617. doi:10.1016/S0277-9536(98)00207-X

Lundorff, L., Jonsson, B., & Sjogren, P. (2009). Modafinil for attentional and psychomotor dysfunction in advanced cancer: A double-blind, randomized, cross-over trial. *Palliative Medicine, 23,* 731–738. doi:10.1177/0269216309106872

Lutz, A., Greisch, L., Rawlings, N., Ricard, M., & Davidson, R. (2004). Long-term mediators self-induce high amplitude gamma synchrony during mental practice. *Proceedings of the National Academy of Sciences, 101,* 16369–16373. doi:10.1073/pnas.0407401101

Makrila, N., Indeck, B., Syrigos, K., & Saif, M. (2009). Depression and pancreatic cancer: A poorly understood link. *Journal of Pain, 10,* 69–76.

Maslach, C., & Leiter, M. (2008). Early predictors of job burnout and engagement. *Journal of Applied Psychology, 93,* 498–512. doi:10.1037/0021-9010.93.3.498

Maslach, C., Schaufeli, W., & Leiter, M. (2001). Job burnout. *Annual Review of Psychology, 52,* 397–422. doi:10.1146/annurev.psych.52.1.397

Massie, J. (1989). Anxiety, panic, and phobia. In J. Holland & J. Rowland (Eds.), *The handbook of psychooncology: The psychological care of the cancer patient* (pp. 300–309). New York, NY: Oxford University Press.

Massie, M. (2004). Prevalence of depression in patients with cancer. *Journal of the National Cancer Institute Monographs, 2004*(32), 57–71. doi:10.1093/jncimonographs/lgh014

McDonald, B., Conroy, S., Ahles, T., West, J., & Saykin, A. (2010). Gray matter reduction associated with systemic chemotherapy for breast cancer: A prospective MRI study. *Breast Cancer Research and Treatment, 12,* 819–828. doi:10.1007/s10549-010-1088-4

McDonald, M., Passik, S., Dugan, W., Rosenfeld, B., Theobald, D., & Edgerton, S. (1999). Nurses' recognition of depression in their patients with cancer. *Oncology Nursing Forum, 26,* 593–599.

McQuellon, R., Wells, M., Hoffman, S., Craven, B., Russell, G., Cruz, J., ... Savage, P. (1998). Reducing distress in cancer patients with an orientation program. *Psycho-Oncology, 7,* 207–217.

Miller, J., & Powers, M. (1988). Development of an instrument to measure hope. *Nursing Research, 37,* 6–10. doi:10.1097/00006199-198801000-00002

Misono, S., Weiss, N., Fann, J., Redman, M., & Yueh, B. (2008). Incidence of suicide in persons with cancer. *Journal of Clinical Oncology, 26,* 4731–4738. doi:10.1200/JCO.2007.13.8941

Moadel, A., Morgan, C., Fatone, A., Grennan, J., Carter, J., Laruffa, G., ... Dutcher, J. (1999). Seeking meaning and hope: Self-reported spiritual and existential needs among an ethnically diverse cancer patient population. *Psycho-Oncology, 8,* 378–385. doi:10.1002/(SICI)1099-1611(199909/10)8:5<378::AID-PON406>3.0.CO;2-A

National Cancer Institute Primary Brain Tumor Progress Review Group. (2005). *Report of the Brain Tumor Progress Review Group.* Retrieved from http://www.ninds.nih.gov/find_people/groups/brain_tumor_prg/frontpage.htm

National Comprehensive Cancer Network. (1999). NCCN practice guidelines for the management of psychosocial distress. *Oncology, 13,* 113–147.

National Comprehensive Cancer Network. (2012). *NCCN Clinical Practice Guidelines in Oncology: Distress management* [v.1.2012]. Retrieved from http://www.nccn.org/professionals/physician_gls/pdf/distress.pdf

Nelson, C., Nandy, N., & Roth, A. (2007). Chemotherapy and cognitive deficits: Mechanisms, finding, and potential interventions. *Palliative and Supportive Care, 5,* 273–280. doi:10.1017/S1478951507000442

Noyes, R., Holt, D., & Massie, J. (1998). Anxiety disorders. In J. Holland (Ed.), *Psycho-oncology* (pp. 548–563). New York, NY: Oxford University Press.

Pasquini, M., & Biondi, M. (2007). Depression in cancer patients: A critical review. *Clinical Practice and Epidemiology in Mental Health, 3,* 2. doi:10.1186/1745-0179-3-2

Pennebaker, J., Keicolt-Glaser, J., & Glaser, R. (1988). Disclosure of traumas and immune function: Health implications for psychotherapy. *Journal of Consulting and Clinical Psychology, 56,* 239–245. doi:10.1037/0022-006X.56.2.239

Perry, B. (2008). Why exemplary oncology nurses seem to avoid compassion fatigue. *Canadian Oncology Nursing Journal, 18,* 87–99.

Pirl, W. (2004). Evidence report on the occurrence, assessment and treatment of depression in cancer patients. *Journal of the National Cancer Institute Monographs, 2004*(32), 32–39. doi:10.1093/jncimonographs/lgh026

Poppelreuter, M., Weis, J., & Bartsch, H. (2009). Effects of specific neuropsychological training program for breast cancer patients after adjuvant chemotherapy. *Journal of Psychosocial Oncology, 27,* 274–296. doi:10.1080/07347330902776044

Portenoy, R.K., Thaler, H.T., Kornblith, A.B., Lepore, J.M., Friedlander-Klar, H., Kiyasu, E., ... Norton, L. (1994). The Memorial Symptom Assessment Scale: An instrument for evaluation of symptom prevalence, characteristics and distress. *European Journal of Cancer, 30A,* 1326–1336. doi:10.1016/0959-8049(94)90182-1

President's Cancer Panel. (2004). *Living beyond cancer: Finding a new balance.* Bethesda, MD: National Cancer Institute.

Rodin, G., Lloyd, N., Katz, M., Green, E., Mackay, J., & Wong, R. (2007). The treatment of depression in cancer patients: A systematic review. *Supportive Care in Cancer, 15,* 123–136. doi:10.1007/s00520-006-0145-3

Rowe, J. (2003). The suffering of the healer. *Nursing Forum, 38*(4), 16–20. doi:10.1111/j.0029-6473.2003.00016.x

Rusteon, T. (1995). Hope and quality of life, two central issues for cancer patients: A theoretical analysis. *Cancer Nursing, 15,* 355–361.

Saykin, A., Ahles, T., & McDonald, B. (2003). Mechanisms of chemotherapy-induced cognitive disorders: Neuropsychological, pathophysiological and neuroimaging perspectives. *Seminars in Clinical Neuropsychiatry, 8,* 201–216.

Shanafelt, T., Novotny, P., Johnson, M., Zhao, X., Steensma, D., Lacy, M., ... Sloan, J. (2005). The well-being and personal wellness promotion strategies of medical oncologists in the North Central Cancer Treatment Group. *Oncology, 68,* 23–32. doi:10.1159/000084519

Sheline, G., Wara, W., & Smith, V. (1980). Therapeutic irradiation and brain injury. *International Journal of Radiation Oncology, Biology, Physics, 6,* 1215–1228. doi:10.1016/0360-3016(80)90175-3

Sherman, D. (2000). Experiences of AIDS-dedicated nurses in alleviating the stress of AIDS caregiving. *Journal of Advanced Nursing, 31,* 1501–1508. doi:10.1046/j.1365-2648.2000.01439.x

Siegel, R., Naishadham, D., & Jemal, A. (2012). Cancer statistics, 2012. *CA: A Cancer Journal for Clinicians, 62,* 10–29. doi:10.3322/caac.20138

Smith, M., Redd, W., Peyser, C., & Vogl, D. (1999). Post-traumatic stress disorder in cancer: A review. *Psycho-Oncology, 8,* 521–537. doi:10.1002/(SICI)1099-1611(199911/12)8:6<521::AID-PON423>3.0.CO;2-X

Somerfield, M., Stefanek, M., Smith, T., & Padberg, J. (1999). A systems model for adaptation to somatic distress among cancer survivors. *Psycho-Oncology, 8,* 334–343. doi:10.1002/(SICI)1099-1611(199907/08)8:4<334::AID-PON392>3.0.CO;2-E

Spiegel, D., Bloom, J., & Yalom, I. (1981). Group support for patients with metastatic cancer. A randomized outcome study. *Archives of General Psychiatry, 38,* 527–533. doi:10.1001/archpsyc.1980.01780300039004

Spiegel, D., Stein, S., Earhart, Z., & Diamond, S. (2000). Group psychotherapy and the terminally ill. In H. Chochinov & W. Breibart (Eds.), *The handbook of psychiatry in palliative medicine* (pp. 241–251). New York, NY: Oxford University Press.

Stark, D., Kiely, M., Smith, A., Velikova, G., House, A., & Selby, P. (2002). Anxiety disorders in cancer patients: Their nature, associations, and relation to quality of life. *Journal of Clinical Oncology, 20,* 3137–3148. doi:10.1200/JCO.2002.08.549

Teng, C.I., Chang, S.S., & Hsu, K.H. (2009). Emotional stability of nurses: Impact on patient safety. *Journal of Advanced Nursing, 65,* 2088–2096. doi:10.1111/j.1365-2648.2009.05072.x

Tulsky, J. (2002). Hope and hubris. *Journal of Palliative Medicine, 5,* 339–341. doi:10.1089/109662102320135225

Victor, M., & Ropper, A. (2001). *Adams' and Victor's principles of neurology* (7th ed.). New York, NY: McGraw-Hill.

Watson, M., Haviland, J., Greer, S., Davidson, J., & Bliss, M. (1999). Influence of psychological response on survival in breast cancer population-based cohort study. *Lancet, 354,* 1331–1336. doi:10.1016/S0140-6736(98)11392-2

Wefel, J., Kayl, A., & Meyers, C. (2004). Neuropsychological dysfunction associated with cancer and cancer therapies: A conceptual review of an emerging target. *British Journal of Cancer, 90,* 1691–1696. doi:10.1038/sj.bjc.6601772

Wenzel, J., Shaha, M., Klimmek, R., & Krumm, S. (2011). Working through grief and loss: Oncology nurses' perspectives on professional bereavement [Online exclusive]. *Oncology Nursing Forum, 38,* E272–E282. doi:10.1188/11.ONF.E272-E282

Wilson, C., Finch, D., & Cohen, H. (2002). Cytokines and cognition—The case for a head-to-toe inflammatory paradigm. *Journal of the American Geriatrics Society, 50,* 2041–2056. doi:10.1046/j.1532-5415.2002.50619.x

Young-Brockopp, D. (1982). Cancer patients' perceptions of five psychosocial needs. *Oncology Nursing Forum, 9*(4), 31–35.

Primary Care of the Cancer Survivor: A Collaborative Continuum-Based Model for Care

Sandra Kurtin, RN, MS, AOCN®, ANP-C

Introduction

The most recent cancer statistics provide several key messages relevant to the clinical and social challenges we will face as oncology professionals and as human beings. Estimates for the lifetime risk of developing cancer are staggering: one in two individuals when all age groups and all cancer sites are considered (National Cancer Institute, 2011). When age, gender, and ethnicity are considered, the lifetime risk of selected cancers varies greatly. Progress has been made to effectively treat many cancer types, offering hope for cancer survivors. The current estimate for cancer survivors in the United States, defined as any person living with a diagnosis of cancer including those who are cured of their disease and those with active disease, is approximately 12 million (Bober et al., 2009; Siegel, Naishadham, & Jemal, 2012). The estimated number of deaths declined for men (22.2%) and women (13.9%) between 1990 and 2007 with an estimated 898,000 deaths averted during that time period (Bober et al., 2009; Siegel et al., 2012). The number of cancer survivors is expected to double by 2050, and the majority of these patients will be older than 65 years old (Bober et al., 2009; Siegel et al., 2012). Current estimates indicate as many as 65% of cancer survivors will live beyond five years from their diagnosis and will require ongoing care (Schulman et al., 2009). Yet, there is a projected shortage of oncologists and primary care providers (PCPs) to manage this growing population (Ganz, 2011; Shulman et al., 2009).

Cancer survivors require ongoing health and wellness interventions, including routine screening, health promotion, and management of comorbid conditions. The complexity of health needs for cancer survivors together with a shift toward a chronic illness model presents unique challenges in providing these services. Many chronic illnesses are managed by PCPs, gerontologists, and other medical specialists. Patients with multiple health problems and multiple healthcare providers (HCPs), particularly older adults, may be at risk for duplication of services, medication interactions, missed diagnoses, or conflicting recommendations (Kurtin, 2010). Living and feeling well while surviving cancer is a universal goal for cancer survivors. Wellness requires an individualized approach with a focus beyond the cancer diagnosis. The effective management of the cancer survivor's care will require a collaborative continuum-based model of care that incorporates multiple disciplines, familiarity with current health maintenance and wellness strategies, incorporation of consensus guidelines for management of common comorbidities, and promotion of patients and their caregivers adopting self-management strategies.

The Continuum of Care for a Cancer Survivor: Who Is Responsible for Primary Care?

The concept of survivorship care emerged following the release of the Institute of Medicine (IOM) report *From Cancer Patient to Cancer Survivor: Lost in Transition* (Hewitt, Greenfield, & Stovall, 2006). The IOM report identified key elements of cancer survivorship care along with recommendations for practices and programs to support these. Recommendations included development and implementation of interdisciplinary evidence-based clinical practice guidelines, multidisciplinary healthcare teams, and communication strategies that address cancer survivors' healthcare needs throughout the continuum of care (Ganz, 2009; Morgan, 2009; Stricker et al., 2011). Among the healthcare needs for cancer survivors are evaluation and management of treatment toxicities and late effects, continued cancer surveillance, prevention, and health promotion (Shapiro et al., 2009; Sticker et al., 2011).

Primary care typically focuses on health promotion and primary prevention as well as the management of common medical and psychosocial diagnoses (Mao et al., 2009; Potosky et al., 2011). For patients with more complex needs, medical specialists are commonly consulted. PCPs and other medical specialists, such as surgeons and gastroenterologists, are the most common source of referrals to oncologists and often make the initial cancer diagnosis. PCPs include general medicine, family practice, internal medicine, geriatric medicine, and preventive medicine providers (Pollack, Adamanche, Ryerson, Ehemen, & Richardson, 2009). Medical specialists include endocrinologists, nephrologists, pulmonologists, urologists, neurologists, rheumatologists, psychiatrists, and other subspecialties. Cancer survivors may have relationships established with a number of these providers at the time of diagnosis and often require continued collaborative management.

Incorporating the unique needs of cancer survivors into the primary care model presents some challenges. The healthcare needs of cancer survivors will vary throughout the continuum of care. Patients' perceptions of who should take the lead role in managing their healthcare needs may vary throughout their lifetime (Mao et al., 2009). In addition, patients' age, caregiver support, socioeconomic status, and cultural, spiritual, and healthcare beliefs will also affect how and when they utilize HCP services. In addition to the variability in patient preference and utilization of HCP services, there is a general discordance between PCPs' and oncologists' perceptions of who carries the primary responsibility for survivorship care, often confused with primary care (Potosky et al., 2011). A mailed survey of PCPs (n = 1,072) and medical oncologists (n = 1,130) in the United States confirmed the lack of agreement on who should assume the primary role in cancer survivorship care (Potosky et al., 2011). The majority of medical oncologists (60%) favored an oncologist-led model based on continued cancer surveillance, evaluation of treatment effects, and psychosocial support. Almost half of PCPs favored a shared model for cancer survivorship or one led by the PCP. Many of the PCPs (60%) admitted to a lack of knowledge relative to specific guidelines for cancer surveillance in cancer survivors and screening for late effects of treatment. Similar findings were noted in a survey of 299 PCPs in the United States, with 47.9% of the responders noting a level of uncertainty with evaluating and managing the long-term effects of cancer treatment (Bober et al., 2009). A general lack of consensus guidelines for primary care of cancer survivors was identified as a perceived barrier by 82% of the PCPs surveyed (Bober et al., 2009). However, these studies do not address the management of common comorbid conditions or other health-related needs. Thus, the concept of cancer survivorship care must not be confused with general primary care but should incorporate key elements of primary care into the overall plan of care for cancer survivors (see Table 13-1).

Planning and implementation of evidence-based guidelines for primary care requires familiarity with common comorbid conditions with adaptation for the individual cancer survivor. The patient's life expectancy and intensity of cancer treatment must be considered. Patients with extensive disease, limited life expectancy, or those undergoing intensive therapy such as allogeneic hematopoietic cell transplantation will require different monitoring and treatment. These patients are more likely to remain under the direct care of the oncologist with consultation from appropriate specialists or PCPs. In some cases, the cancer diagnosis may not present the greatest risk for morbidity and mortality. Patients with a more favorable prognosis and patients with potentially curable disease are more likely to have a shared care model with PCPs, oncologists, and other medical specialists (O'Toole, Step, Engelhardt, Lewis, & Rose, 2009). Long-term survivors, in particular those more than 10 years out from their diagnosis, are likely to be managed by their PCP (Pollack et al., 2009). For most patients, a model of shared care with oncology providers, PCPs, and other medical specialists will provide the best option for comprehensive medical care that incorporates elements of prevention, health promotion, and cancer surveillance while effectively managing existing illnesses or effects of cancer treatment (Ganz, 2011) (see Figure 13-1). General cancer survivorship care is not within the scope of this chapter. Suggested guidelines for the surveillance and management of common illnesses including cancer, primary prevention, health and wellness recommendations, and promotion of self-management strategies in cancer survivors will be reviewed.

Cancer Surveillance in Cancer Survivors

A history of cancer is a known risk factor for developing a second cancer (American Cancer Society [ACS], 2011). The risk of recurrence is another concern. A review of cancer statistics provides a guide for risk-adapted cancer screening. The cancer diagnoses with the highest incidence in 2012 included prostate (29%), lung, and colorectal for men, and breast (30%), lung, and colorectal for women (Siegel et al., 2012). These same cancer diagnoses represent the highest mortality rates in men and women primarily because of the high incidence, with lung cancer being the

Table 13-1. Key Elements of a Shared Model for Primary Care of the Cancer Survivor

Element	Description
Cancer-focused medical history	Description of the cancer diagnosis including stage, treatment plan, response and duration, any recurrences and subsequent treatment, and any treatment-related adverse events
Three-generation family history	Evaluation of risk for secondary cancers, hereditary risk, or increased risk for other disease states
Lifestyle and health habits	Details of diet, nutrition, exercise habits, and tobacco, alcohol, and illicit drug use
Social and personal history	Marital status, caregiver and social support, employment, hobbies, educational level, depression, self-care capabilities, and learning styles
Emotional history	Assessment of depression, stress response
Financial history	Review of financial resources, insurance
Medication profile	Review of prescription medications including prescriber and rationale and any complementary or alternative therapies, over-the-counter medications, or nutritional supplements. Incorporates mandatory regulatory medication reconciliation.
Detailed cancer treatment–related exposures	Review of all treatments including surgeries, radiation, and systemic therapies (e.g., chemotherapy, targeted therapies, hormonal therapy, transfusions, antibodies) will allow focused assessment for late effects and secondary health problems.
Cancer-focused review of systems	Review of systems to identify potential late effects of cancer treatment as well as areas for health promotion and prevention
Comprehensive review of systems	Standard review of systems questionnaire to identify any changes in symptoms, new symptoms, or improvement after interventions. This review of systems incorporates mandatory regulatory questions for pain and safety. Patient questionnaires completed at the time of the visit provide a useful tool for focused discussion with providers.
American Society of Clinical Oncology and American Cancer Society cancer surveillance guidelines	Health maintenance history that incorporates screening guidelines for breast, colorectal, prostate, lung, cervical, endometrial, and skin cancers—adapted for the individual risk for age at diagnosis, familial risk, and risk of treatment-related or second malignancies
Communication among providers and with the patient	Ongoing written and, when necessary, verbal communication between primary providers relative to the phase of treatment, particularly at key transition points. Written communication may be incorporated into the electronic medical record, faxed to key providers, and shared with the patient to improve self-care management and continuity of care.

Note. Based on information from Ganz, 2009; Hahn & Ganz, 2011; Landier, 2009; McCorkle et al., 2011; Smith et al., 2011.

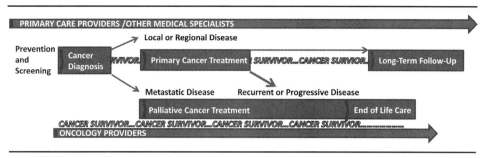

Figure 13-1. Model of Shared Care for Patients With Cancer

leading cause of death in both groups. Cancer screening guidelines proposed by ACS are intended for asymptomatic patients at average risk (Church, 2011; Hollowell et al., 2010; Smith et al., 2011). Cancer survivors represent a unique population when considering the risk of cancer associated with a number of factors, including exposure to antineoplastic agents, exposure to radiation (therapeutic and diagnostic), genetic instability, hereditary predisposition, underlying cancer, and continued at-risk behaviors (Hollowell et al., 2010). Therefore, an individualized risk-adapted model for cancer screening is required for cancer survivors (see Table 13-2). Diagnostic evaluations at the time of initial diagnosis are generally adapted for continued surveillance of the primary cancer and may be adapted further for screening of second cancers. For example, a female patient who is diagnosed in her 30s and found to have stage II *BRCA2*-positive adenocarcinoma of the breast would require modified screening to include increased surveillance for ovarian and colorectal cancers with use of magnetic resonance imaging scans in addition to mammography, and initiation of colonoscopy upon completion of her primary therapy for breast cancer (Holowell et al., 2010). Similarly, a young man with stage III rectosigmoid colorectal cancer (CRC) treated with chemoradiotherapy and resection with a family history of familial polyposis would require adapted screening for CRC recurrence as well as cancers of the testes and prostate because they are in the radiation field (Smith et al., 2011). Potential late effects of treatment for this patient include bowel changes, including pain with bowel movements, bowel incontinence, or tenesmus, which may not only affect quality of life but may also cause fear of local recurrence (Sweed, 2011).

The majority of new cancer diagnoses are found because of patient-reported signs and symptoms, physical examinations, or diagnostic screening during routine HCP visits or urgent visits for more severe symptoms. Similarly, cancer recurrence or the development of second cancers will most often be detected by comprehensive review of systems, physical examination, and selected diagnostic testing. Patients will often seek care for symptoms similar to those experienced at the time of the original diagnosis. The risk of recurrence for most tumor types is greatest in the first two to three years following diagnosis. However, late recurrences are not uncommon, and treatment-related cancers such as leukemia and myelodysplastic syndromes may not be evident for 7–10 years (Kurtin, 2011). For young patients receiving radiation, second cancers may not be evident for up to 20 years (Newhauser & Durante, 2011). Thus, continued risk-adapted surveillance for cancer survivors

Table 13-2. Five-Year Survival Rates (2011) for Common Cancer Sites and Risk-Adapted Cancer Screening for Cancer Survivors

Cancer Site	Five-Year Relative Survival for All Ages and Races (%)	ACS Recommendations for the Early Detection of Cancer in Average-Risk, Asymptomatic Individuals and Risk-Adapted Cancer Screening for Cancer Survivors and High-Risk Individuals
Breast	All stages: 78–90 Localized: 93–99 Distant: 15–23	Average risk/asymptomatic: • BSE: Encouragement of personal awareness and reportable signs and symptoms beginning in the early 20s (BSE is no longer a component of the ACS screening guidelines.) • Clinical breast examination: age 20–30, included in the PE every 3 years; age > 40, included in the PE yearly • Mammography: Annually beginning at age 40 High risk: • *BRCA* mutation carriers or women with a first-degree relative who is *BRCA+*, radiation to the chest for Hodgkin disease, women with overall high-risk disease (20%–25% greater risk of disease) based on risk models, including a personal history of breast cancer. • Annual screening mammography and breast MRI starting at age 30 • Referral to a genetic counselor for *BRCA+* patients, increased surveillance for cervical, ovarian, colorectal, and pancreatic cancers
Cervical	All stages: 61–72 Localized: 91–94 Distant: 12–17	Average risk/asymptomatic: • Pap test beginning at age 21 or within three years of the first sexual activity, repeated every 1–2 years, • Frequency of testing is decreased to every 2–3 years in women age ≥ 30 years with three consecutive negative Pap tests, and may be discontinued in women age ≥ 70 years or those who have had a complete hysterectomy High risk: • Women with a history of cervical cancer, with in utero exposure to diethylstilbestrol, or who are immunocompromised because of organ transplantation or HIV infections should continue the screening annually. • Screening should continue yearly for women with a history of cervical intraepithelial neoplasia type 1 or 2 until testing has been negative for 10 years after diagnosis.
Colorectal	All stages: 56–66 Localized: 86–91 Distant: 8–12	Average risk/asymptomatic: • Screening should begin at age 50 for both men and women with consideration of the sensitivity and limitations of various testing as well as test availability, cost, and patient willingness to obtain testing. • FOBT (sequence of three at home tests), FSIG, CT colonography (repeated every five years if negative), colonoscopy (repeated every 10 years if negative).

(Continued on next page)

Table 13-2. Five-Year Survival Rates (2011) for Common Cancer Sites and Risk-Adapted Cancer Screening for Cancer Survivors *(Continued)*

Cancer Site	Five-Year Relative Survival for All Ages and Races (%)	ACS Recommendations for the Early Detection of Cancer in Average-Risk, Asymptomatic Individuals and Risk-Adapted Cancer Screening for Cancer Survivors and High-Risk Individuals
		High risk: • Personal history of adenomatous polyps, curative intent resection of CRC or inflammatory bowel disease • Family history of first-degree family relative with CRC or colorectal adenomas (recommendations vary based on relative's age at diagnosis), HNPCC, or FAP • Colonoscopy beginning at an earlier age based on symptoms, overall risk, and family history
Lung	All stages: 13–16 Localized: 45–54 Distant: 3–4	Currently no recommendations for early screening of asymptomatic individuals. High risk: • Personal exposure to tobacco or occupational exposure to asbestos and secondary smoke • More recent studies have indicated a potential benefit of early diagnosis in high-risk individuals using spiral CT technology.
Prostate	All stages: 96–100 Localized: 100 Distant: 29–30	Average risk/asymptomatic: • Men age > 50 years, digital rectal examination and prostate-specific antigen monitoring • Men should have open discussion with their healthcare provider regarding the relatively long life expectancy for local or regional disease and cost-benefit ratio of screening frequency. High risk: • African American men and men with a first-degree relative with prostate cancer before age 65, discussions of screening options should begin at age 45.

ACS—American Cancer Society; BSE—breast self-examination; CRC—colorectal cancer; CT—computed tomography; FAP—familial adenomatous polyposis; FOBT—fecal occult blood test; FSIG—flexible sigmoidoscopy; HNPCC—hereditary nonpolyposis colorectal cancer; MRI—magnetic resonance imaging; Pap—Papanicolaou; PE—physical examination

Note. Based on information from Hollowell et al., 2010; Siegel et al., 2012; Smith et al., 2011.

is imperative. However, recent studies have indicated continued challenges and deficits in the healthcare system. The PCPs' and oncology specialists' roles have been the focus of some of these studies.

A retrospective review of medical records for 270 stage I to stage III female patients with breast cancer with a mean follow-up of six years showed that oncology specialists adhered to the American Society of Clinical Oncology (ASCO) recommendations for surveillance and follow-up more often than PCPs (89% versus 63%, $p < 0.01$) (Hollowell et al., 2010). Of particular interest was the lack of documented breast examinations (44% versus 92%), axillary examinations (52% versus 94%), and yearly mammography (48% versus 78%) performed by PCPs compared to specialists. However, at six years of follow-up, many patients fell below the recommended thresholds for surveillance and follow-up. The percentage of patients being screened by PCPs in accordance with the ASCO surveillance criteria declined over time, whereas those continuing to see specialists remained fairly constant. Early detection of recurrent disease or a second cancer provides a more favorable patient outcome. Effective surveillance and screening together with patient involvement and self-awareness provide key tools for early diagnosis as well as opportunities for prevention and health promotion that may reduce risk.

A large study used Surveillance, Epidemiology, and End Results data linked to Medicare data for 104,895 patients with prostate, colorectal, female breast, bladder, and uterine cancers diagnosed more than five years from the time of the study (Pollack et al., 2009). The most common diagnoses had incidence and prevalence rates similar to those reported by ACS for the same year with prostate (47,954), breast (26,972), and colorectal cancers (16,671) being most common. The mean age for the group was 71.7 years, and the majority of patients had local or regional disease as would be expected for long-term cancer survivors (Pollack et al., 2009). Despite the predominantly older population, comorbidities were less common in this patient population (71% with no comorbidities). However, visits to PCPs or specialists were similar for patients with no comorbidities and those with two or more comorbidities. Visits to specialists declined after the sixth year of follow-up, whereas visits to PCPs and non-cancer specialists did not. Thus, PCPs play a critical role in the long-term follow-up of cancer survivors, particularly those who have surpassed the five year milestone often associated with cure. Yet, the risk of late recurrence and late-onset adverse events including second cancers persists beyond five years. Improved communication among providers; refinement of risk-adapted screening and surveillance guidelines for cancer recurrence, second cancers, and late effects of treatment specific to cancer survivors; and empowerment of the patient and caregivers will be necessary to reduce the risk for these patients.

Health Maintenance, Health Promotion, and Prevention Strategies for Cancer Survivors

Health promotion and prevention are key elements of what is considered traditional primary care. Health promotion includes risk avoidance (modifiable risk factors) and integration of elements of a healthy lifestyle including diet and exercise. These same principles apply to cancer survivors regardless of prognosis, yet they require realistic adaptation for each patient.

Nutrition and Physical Activity

ACS proposed guidelines for nutrition and exercise based on the phase of cancer survivorship. The phases identified include active treatment, the immediate post-treatment phase (recovery), the post-recovery phase, and patients living with advanced cancer (Doyle et al., 2006). More than 50% of newly diagnosed patients with cancer exhibit symptoms of nutritional deficits (Doyle et al., 2006). Substantial weight loss prior to diagnosis is considered an unfavorable prognostic finding, implying more aggressive or advanced disease. Thus, patients initiating treatment with existing nutritional deficits will be at particular risk for further decline. Referral to a registered dietitian at the time of diagnosis is advised. The registered dietitian will be able to calculate the caloric needs for the patient—the balance of fat, protein, and carbohydrates—and together with the patient will assess existing eating habits, preferred foods and food intolerances, and any special dietary restrictions. If possible, family members and caregivers should meet with the patient and the dietitian to reinforce the goals and strategies for improved nutrition. Nutritional supplements may be required for patients who are not able to meet their caloric needs. Aggressive management of treatments or disease-related symptoms, such as nausea, vomiting, gastroesophageal reflux disease, constipation, diarrhea, pain, and depression, will improve nutritional intake. In severe cases of malnutrition, enteral or parenteral nutrition may be required. For patients with incurable disease, diet and nutrition remain challenging, particularly toward the end of life. Rapid weight loss and cachexia are frightening to the patient and family and often are a primary focus when meeting with clinicians.

The use of dietary supplements, vitamins, minerals, and herbal compounds should be avoided during active treatment because of unclear effects on treatment outcomes in most instances (Velicer & Ulrich, 2008). Dietary soy in moderate quantities is thought to be safe and potentially beneficial for breast cancer survivors; however, more concentrated sources such as isoflavone supplements or soy powders may increase estrogen levels, thereby increasing the risk of stimulating estrogen-dependent tumors (Shu et al., 2009). Select supplements are safe and have no known interaction with cancer therapies; however, patients should be instructed to discuss this in detail with their providers. Providers must familiarize themselves with the current literature for use of supplements and herbal compounds during treatment.

Cancer survivors in the immediate post-treatment phase and into long-term survivorship often struggle with trying to normalize their diet. Aversion or intolerance to certain foods is common during treatment. These symptoms often resolve; however, patients may continue to avoid these foods because of fear of gastrointestinal symptoms. Patients who have received radiation to the head and neck present a particular challenge because of xerostomia and taste alterations (Kurtin, 2009). Reinforcement of nutrition goals at each provider (oncology or primary care) visit will promote continued patient involvement and identify those patients who may require more focused interventions. For example, patients with gastroesophageal tumors who undergo chemoradiotherapy may develop strictures and progressive dysphagia interfering with nutrition. Endoscopy with possible balloon dilation for these patients is required to detect any evidence of recurrence and allow for opening of any stricture. Patients with pancreatic cancer who undergo Whipple procedures will be prone to pancreatic insufficiency and may require lifelong insulin therapy (Daniel & Kurtin, 2010). Surgical resection of the stomach or gastric bypass procedures for gastroduodenal tumors may render patients vitamin B_{12} and iron deficient along with other metabolic deficiencies. For all of these patients, eating may become a daily struggle. Simplifying the regimen, avoiding unnecessary restrictions, and allowing "forbidden foods" in small quantities now and then will make the diet seem less like work and more natural for the patient.

Maintaining a healthy weight is a primary goal for all cancer survivors. Obesity is a known risk factor for a number of cancers and has been shown to increase the risk of recurrence and decrease survival for several tumors types including breast, colorectal, liver, gallbladder, pancreatic, kidney, uterus, and advanced prostate (Chalasani, Downey, & Stopeck, 2010; Doyle et al., 2006; Eheman et al., 2012; Smith et al., 2011). Patients who are obese at the time of diagnosis may be overwhelmed with the cancer diagnosis, and adequate nutrition during treatment is important for tolerance. However, the introduction of healthy lifestyle strategies during therapy will lay the foundation for continued work in the recovery and long-term follow-up phases of survivorship. The basic principles of balanced energy intake and gradual increase in energy expenditure through strengthening and endurance exercises remain the preferred strategies for sustained effective weight loss. Increasing low energy-density foods (e.g., fiber-rich vegetables, fruits, soups, cooked whole grains); limiting portions for energy-dense foods, including fats, and limiting salt, sugar, and alcohol intake; increasing water intake; and increasing physical activity are the key elements of healthy nutrition and exercise programs for achieving a healthy weight (Doyle et al., 2006). Simple explanations for the patient and family such as the plate method (dividing the plate to show appropriate portions of different food types) will encourage portion control and the emphasis on healthy foods (Bratton & Kurtin, 2010). These same diet and exercise strategies will provide positive effects on common comorbidities in cancer survivors, such as diabetes, hypertension, arthritis, and cardiovascular disease.

Physical activity is critical to maintaining independence, avoiding injury and falls, and reducing the risk of complications of immobility, including thrombosis, osteoporosis, fractures, fatigue, insomnia, depression, infections, and skin breakdown (Doyle et al., 2006). The U.S. Preventive Services Task Force (USPSTF) and ACS recommend 30–60 minutes of moderate to vigorous exercise three to five days per week (Ehemen et al., 2012; USPSTF, 2010). Many older patients and patients with mobility limitations, such as vertebral fractures, neuropathy, stroke, pain, or fracture risk, will need assistance in developing a safe, effective, and realistic exercise plan to avoid injury and promote continued adherence. Considerations for patients undergoing active therapy will include avoidance of infections during at-risk periods (e.g., avoiding public gyms and swimming pools); adaption for underlying anemia or other factors requiring activity restrictions, such as the immediate postoperative period; pathologic fractures; and cardiac, pulmonary, or neurologic events. Patients with brain cancer present a particular challenge, as they may have limited physical control and are at increased risk for falls. Fatigue presents another challenge, as patients feel they are too tired to exercise. Unfortunately, the fatigue will likely get worse with a continued sedentary lifestyle, and patients should be encouraged to use brief strengthening exercises (e.g., using exercise bands while sitting in a chair) together with walking daily to maintain and gradually improve strength and endurance and reduce fatigue. Evaluation of a 12-month home-based diet and exercise program targeted at older adult cancer survivors found several positive outcomes, including increased quality of life, improved dietary behaviors, and increased physical activity ($p < 0.001$) (Morey et al., 2009).

Tobacco and Alcohol Use

Tobacco and alcohol use represent two of the most common risk factors for cancer as well as other chronic health problems such as chronic obstructive lung disease and cardiovascular disease. Tobacco use is responsible for more than 400,000 deaths per year in the United States and represents the single greatest cause of morbidity and mortality. The societal costs are staggering: an estimated $96 billion per year in medical expenses and $97 billion in lost productivity. Smoking cessation is a key goal for health promotion and prevention based on the risks associated with tobacco use over time and the potential for immediate and long-term health benefits of quitting. Up to 70% of smokers have expressed a desire to quit smoking (Fiore et al., 2008; U.S. Department of Health and Human Services [DHHS], 2010).

DHHS (2010) recommends a combined strategy of counseling and pharmacotherapy where appropriate. Counseling is based on consistent inquiry about tobacco use, discussion of the potential health consequences, assessment of willingness to quit, and continued reinforcement of the benefits of smoking cessation. Implementation of smoking cessation strategies includes referral to smoking cessation programs and prescriptions for smoking cessation agents such as nicotine replacement products, bupropion, or varenicline (DHHS, 2010). The use of telephone counseling programs to enhance smoking cessation has also been found to be beneficial.

Alcohol use or abuse is common in the United States with roughly one-third of adults meeting the criteria for an alcohol use-related disorder (Willenbring, Massey, & Gardner, 2009). The negative effects of alcohol misuse or abuse are well known, including physical, social, psychological, and socioeconomic consequences. Excessive alcohol use is a known risk factor for a number of cancers and other chronic illnesses and may increase the risk of treatment-related adverse events (Ganz, 2009). Together, excess tobacco and alcohol use significantly increase the risk of oral, esophageal, and lung cancers, and the continued use of either will potentially inhibit response to treatment and increase the risk of early recurrence. Similar to smoking cessation, evaluating the individual patient's use of alcohol and instituting counseling and referral strategies will promote effective discussion with the patient and family and increase the potential for successful abstinence (Willenbring et al., 2009).

Managing Comorbid Conditions and Late Effects of Treatment

Comorbid conditions are common in cancer survivors, given their average age of 71.7 years. The most common chronic diseases in this primarily older population include cardiovascular disease (coronary artery disease, hyperlipidemia, and hypertension), chronic lung disease, endocrine disorders, diabetes, and arthritis. Cancer survivors are at increased risk for exacerbation of these underlying diseases throughout the cancer survivorship continuum. Many of these illnesses will precede the cancer diagnosis, and these patients may have well-established relationships with their PCPs or other medical specialists. Age-related physiologic changes in organ function, drug metabolism, and predisposition to adverse events require consideration when initiating and monitoring therapy (see Table 13-3). Effective management of existing or treatment-related adverse events including inducing or exacerbating comorbid conditions will increase the potential for continued treatment and limit the severity of the adverse events.

Managing common chronic illnesses presents a challenge in cancer survivors. Oncologists often choose to defer to PCPs or other specialists, yet these providers may not be experienced with the late effects of many cancer treatments that have organ-specific toxicities. The best opportunity to provide optimal management of these problems is a collaborative continuum-based model of care with consistent communication among providers and a decision as to who will take the primary role in managing the individual illness. Having more than one provider make adjustments in medications or treatment regimens may increase the risk for drug interactions, patient and caregiver confusion, and ultimately adverse outcomes. Optimally, oncology professionals will become familiar with the most common consensus guidelines or at least how to access them if needed, and PCPs or other medical specialists should learn the common adverse events and late effects of cancer treatment. The threshold for symptoms may need to be adjusted depending on the prognosis, treatment plan, patient adherence to the medical regimen, and cost of therapies. Common late effects in the patient with cancer and primary care implications are included in Table 13-4.

Table 13-3. Age-Related Physiologic Changes on Pharmacokinetics and Clinical Significance

Organ/Function	Age-Related Changes	Clinical Significance
Bone marrow	Decreased red blood cell mass Hematopoietic senescence	Increased risk for myelosuppression and secondary effects Prolonged recovery
Cardiovascular	Increased incidence of cardiovascular comorbidities (congestive heart failure, hypertension)	Increased risk of acute cardiomyopathy Baseline and periodic evaluation of ejection fraction required
Gastrointestinal	Decreased gastric motility and secretion Decreased absorptive surface	Increased risk of drug-drug reactions Increased risk of reactions to oral compounds
Hepatic	Reduced drug metabolism Reduced activity of cytochrome p450 pathways Decreased splanchnic circulation	Increased risk of drug reactions Increased risk of hepatotoxicity Increased risk for drug toxicity for drugs with hepatic metabolism/clearance
Neurologic	Age-related changes in white matter Reduced sensory perception	Increased risk of central and peripheral neuropathy
Renal	Reduced glomerular filtration rate Reduced tubular reabsorption—loss of active nephrons	Increased risk for drug toxicity for drugs with renal excretion Requires careful evaluation of creatinine clearance and dose modification to reduce toxicity
Musculoskeletal	Decreased muscle mass	Shift in distribution of drugs
General	Increase in body fat, decrease in muscle mass, reduction of total body water	Shift in distribution of fat-soluble compounds
Nutrition	Protein-calorie malnutrition	Altered distribution of drugs Decreased tolerance to chemotherapy Delayed wound healing
Age-related disease attributes	Increased prevalence of multiple drug resistance phenotype Increased resistance to apoptosis Increased adhesion of neoplastic cells to the bone marrow stroma	Resistance to therapy for acute myeloid leukemia Associated with follicular lymphoma and resistance to selected treatments Associated with multiple myeloma

Note. Based on information from Balducci et al., 2009; Carreca & Balducci, 2009; National Comprehensive Cancer Network, 2010; Wedding et al., 2007.

From "Risk Analysis in the Treatment of Hematologic Malignancies in the Elderly," by S.E. Kurtin, 2010, *Journal of the Advanced Practitioner in Oncology, 1,* p. 22. Copyright 2010 by Harborside Press. Reprinted with permission.

Table 13-4. Common Late Effects of Cancer Treatment and Implications for Primary Care of the Cancer Survivor

Organ System	Common Late Effects of Cancer Treatment*	Risk Factors	Implications for Primary Care of the Cancer Survivor
Head and neck	Xerostomia	Radiation to the head and neck Surgical reconstruction Graft-versus-host disease	Dental follow-up because increased risk of dental caries. Nutrition consult to avoid weight loss
	Osteonecrosis of the jaw	Bisphosphonate administration Dental procedures	Baseline dental exam Patient and dental professional education regarding risks associated with dental procedures
	Hearing loss	Cisplatin Cranial radiation	Baseline audiology exam Referral to ear, nose, and throat with any changes Referral to neuro-otolaryngologist as indicated
	Visual changes Cataracts Retinopathy	Cranial irradiation Chronic steroids Optic neuritis	Baseline eye exam with repeat evaluation as clinically indicated Referral to retinal specialist or neuro-ophthalmologist as clinically indicated
Cardiovascular	Congestive heart failure Cardiomyopathy Coronary artery disease Atherosclerosis	Cumulative dose and combinations of cardiotoxic drugs (e.g., anthracyclines) Concurrent or prior chest irradiation Preexisting cardiovascular disease Longer duration of survival	Baseline and periodic evaluation of ejection fraction based on symptoms Coordinate care with cardiologist and primary care provider (PCP). Patient education for modifiable risk factors: tobacco use, obesity, sedentary lifestyle
	Hypertension	Vascular endothelial growth factor (VEGF) inhibitor agents Small molecule tyrosine kinase inhibitor agents Family history Obesity, sedentary lifestyle, tobacco use	Baseline evaluation, repeat blood pressure with each visit Dose modifications may be necessary for medications known to contribute to hypertension. Coordinate care with cardiologist and PCP. Patient education for modifiable risk factors: tobacco use, obesity, sedentary lifestyle
	Thromboembolism	Active cancer Tobacco use, obesity, diabetes VEGF inhibitors, immunomodulatory agents	Identification of at-risk patients Anticoagulation therapy as indicated Coordinate care with PCP, cardiologist, anticoagulation clinic. Patient education for modifiable risk factors: tobacco use, obesity, sedentary lifestyle

(Continued on next page)

Table 13-4. Common Late Effects of Cancer Treatment and Implications for Primary Care of the Cancer Survivor (Continued)

Organ System	Common Late Effects of Cancer Treatment*	Risk Factors	Implications for Primary Care of the Cancer Survivor
Endocrine	Hypothyroidism	Radiation to the thyroid gland Preexisting hypothyroidism Stem cell transplantation Radioimmunotherapy Systemic therapies: VEGF inhibitors, immunomodulatory drugs, retinoid inhibitors	Baseline testing for thyroid function, repeated as clinically indicated Thyroid replacement therapy
	Adrenal insufficiency	Chronic steroid use Adrenalectomy	Baseline testing, repeated as clinically indicated Mineralcorticoid replacement
Pulmonary	Pneumonitis Pulmonary fibrosis Restrictive lung disease	Preexisting pulmonary disease (asthma, chronic obstructive pulmonary disease, bronchitis) Radiation to the thorax/lungs Tobacco use	Baseline assessment of risk Avoidance of aggravating factors: treatment- or lifestyle-related Coordination of care with pulmonologist and PCP
Genitourinary Renal	Chronic renal insufficiency Nephrotic syndrome Incontinence	High-dose chemotherapy Radiotherapy to the renal bed Chronic graft-versus-host disease Nephrotoxic drugs	Close monitoring of renal function Avoidance of aggravating factors: medications, dehydration, IV contrast Referral to urology for urinary incontinence treatment
Gastrointestinal	Strictures Malabsorption syndrome Chronic diarrhea Incontinence Pancreatic insufficiency	Surgery Radiation to the abdomen or pelvis Bypass surgery Whipple procedure	Referral to dietitian for modified diet Review of bowel regimen for chronic constipation or diarrhea including medications and diet Endoscopy/colonoscopy for persistent symptoms
Gonadal	Infertility Testosterone deficiency	Radiation to the pelvis High-dose chemotherapy Surgical removal of the ovaries or testes	Counseling of patients of childbearing age Baseline testing, repeated as clinically indicated Replacement hormones after careful consideration of risks versus benefits

(Continued on next page)

Table 13-4. Common Late Effects of Cancer Treatment and Implications for Primary Care of the Cancer Survivor *(Continued)*

Organ System	Common Late Effects of Cancer Treatment*	Risk Factors	Implications for Primary Care of the Cancer Survivor
Nervous system	Peripheral neuropathy	Preexisting neuropathy: diabetes, drug-induced, nerve damage Cumulative doses of neurotoxic drugs: platinum compounds, thalidomide, vinca alkaloids, bortezomib, abraxane, taxanes	Careful history based on patient's daily activities for employment and enjoyment; focused neurologic exam based on reported symptoms or clinical findings Avoidance of aggravating factors: control of diabetes, smoking cessation, neurotoxic drugs Treatment of neuropathic pain Evaluation of central nervous system disease as indicated Safety evaluation
Musculo-skeletal	Osteonecrosis (joints) Avascular necrosis Osteoporosis	Preexisting bone disease: metastases, osteopenia, osteoporosis, fracture Chronic steroid use Tobacco use	Baseline evaluation of bone disease, preexisting conditions Coordination of care with PCP, orthopedics as indicated Patient education to maintain exercise, avoid tobacco and alcohol, safety guidelines

*Excluding secondary malignancies; see Table 13-2.

Note. Based on information from Bertoia et al., 2011; Bilotti et al., 2011; Dokken & Kurtin, 2010; Fadol & Lech, 2011; Felicetti et al., 2011; Ganz, 2009; Mohty & Apperly, 2010; Oeffinger & Tonorezos, 2011; Oeffinger et al., 2011; Stricker & Jacobs, 2008; Wenger, 2011.

Empowerment Strategies to Encourage Self-Management Behaviors

Cancer survivors are faced with complex decisions throughout their survivorship journey relative to their cancer diagnosis, other comorbid conditions, finances, and how they choose to participate in their care. Patients are increasingly faced with selecting among treatment options that their oncologist or other HCPs present to them. The average American reads at an eighth-grade reading level; however, most patient education materials are written well above this (Fagerlin, Zikmund-Fisher, & Ubel, 2011). Visit times to HCPs are often just 15–20 minutes, making it difficult to communicate complex ideas in a way that the patient and family will be able to understand, synthesize, and make informed decisions about their care. Patients with multiple health problems may have difficulty understanding the complexity of balancing their cancer treatment with the continued management of existing illnesses. Yet, HCPs expect patients and family members or other designated caregivers to assume a primary role in managing their illnesses, including adverse events, reporting signs and symptoms, communicating between providers, and continuing to take an active role in decision making.

Effective patient self-management requires several key elements: consistent and clear communication that allows the patient to make informed decisions, reinforcement of key messages at each visit, adjustment of visit frequency to the specific phase of survivorship and healthcare needs, integration of community programs and resources, and development of mutually determined goals (McCorkle et al., 2011). Communication of risk versus benefits is perhaps one of the most complicated processes necessary for informed decision making and consent for treatment. HCPs' descriptions are often complex and not well understood by the patient and family (Fagerlin et al., 2011). Allowing patients adequate time for review of material presented if clinically possible, providing written materials in addition to the verbal explanations, identifying community-based, national, or international resources for patient support, and incorporating members of the multidisciplinary team in the discussion with patients will provide additional support (Barry, 2011; McCorkle et al., 2011). Optimally, members of the multidisciplinary team will be well informed about the individual patient situation to avoid conflicting or confusing messages. Incorporating adult learning principles, adaptation for language barriers, and consideration of patients' spiritual and cultural needs is ideal. Rodin and colleagues' systematic review of several studies relative to patient and clinician communication conducted revealed several key elements of effective communication, including adequate description of disease stage and prognosis; open, honest, and timely communication; and increased patient participation in decision making with clinician assessment of individual preferences for information (Colosia et al., 2011; Rodin et al., 2009).

Conclusion

Given the probability of a shift in providers over time, it may be most useful to offer teaching tools and clinical guidelines for providers and patients based on the phase of cancer survivorship and at key transition points. The collaborative approach to managing the cancer survivor would therefore be adapted for the individual patient based on his or her disease, prognosis, expected survival, risk profile, lifestyle, and financial and psychosocial factors over the course of the survivorship journey. A personalized approach with message consistency across providers would likely engage the patient in self-management (McCorkle et al., 2011). This approach works well in the early course of disease when the patient is still in close follow-up and generally seen three to four times per year or more often. Patients with a poor prognosis or those under constant treatment will generally continue close follow-up with the oncology provider. The challenge is to develop an approach that is feasible in a busy clinical practice where patients who are in remission may be seen less frequently (once or twice per year).

Given the anticipated shortages in oncology specialists and PCPs, the continued support of cancer survivors will rely on nonphysician providers (NPPs) in all specialties. Advanced practice clinicians (nurse practitioners, physician assistants), patient navigators (primarily RNs), and oncology nurse specialists are critical to the continued surveillance and support for cancer survivors. ASCO's study found the use of NPPs in oncology practices to be efficient with improved provider and patient satisfaction (Towle et al., 2011). Productivity for the practices surveyed increased by 19% (Towle et al., 2011). The services most often provided by the NPPs included seeing patients during treatment visits, pain and symptom management, follow-up care after remission, patient education and counseling, emergent care, and end-of life or hospice care. Interestingly, survivorship clinics were listed as less than 20% of the services provided by the 27 practices surveyed, yet the most common services provided clearly incorporate core elements of cancer survivorship care. Perhaps the lofty goals of the survivorship movement have created some misconception about survivorship care. A simplified, collaborative, clinically practical approach to managing the cancer survivor throughout the continuum of care will not address all the patients' needs at every visit. In fact, events that occur between and after provider visits such as results of diagnostic testing; patient visits to other specialists, providers, or the emergency department; and refilling necessary medications including hormonal therapies or other chronic cancer medications may present the greatest challenge for patients and HCPs. However, over time with effective communication and participation among the providers, patients, and caregivers, a collaborative care model will limit the severity and incidence of adverse events, promote health and wellness, and reduce inefficiencies in care.

References

American Cancer Society. (2011). Cancer facts and figures 2011. Retrieved from http://www.cancer.org/acs/groups/content/@epidemiologysurveilance/documents/document/acspc-029771.pdf

Balducci, L., Colloca, G., Cesari, M., & Gambassi, G. (2009). Assessment and treatment of elderly patients with cancer. *Surgical Oncology, 19*, 117–123. doi:10.1016/j.suronc.2009.11.008

Barry, M.J. (2011). Helping patients make better personal health decisions: The promise of patient-centered outcomes research. *JAMA, 306*, 1258–1259. doi:10.1001/jama.2011.1363

Bertoia, M.L., Waring, M.E., Gupta, P.S., Roberts, M.B., & Eaton, C.B. (2011). Implications of new hypertension guidelines in the United States. *Hypertension, 58*, 361–366. doi:10.1161/HYPERTENSIONAHA.111.175463

Bilotti, E., Gleason, C., & McNeill, A. (2011). Routine health maintenance in patients living with myeloma: Survivorship care plan of the International Myeloma Foundation Nurse Leadership Board. *Clinical Journal of Oncology Nursing, 15*, 25–40. doi:10.1188/11.S1.CJON.25-40

Bober, S., Recklitis, C., Campbell, E., Park, E.R., Kutner, J.S., Najita, J.S., & Diller, L. (2009). Caring for cancer survivors: A survey of primary care physicians. *Cancer, 115*(Suppl. 18), 4409–4418. doi:10.1002/cncr.24590

Bratton, M., & Kurtin, S.E. (2010). Collaborative approach to managing a 59-year-old woman with stage IIB pancreatic cancer and diabetes. *Journal of the Advanced Practitioner in Oncology, 1*, 257–265.

Carreca, I., & Balducci, L. (2009). Cancer chemotherapy in the older patient. *Urologic Oncology, 27*, 633–642. doi:10.1016/j.urolonc.2009.08.006

Chalasani, P., Downey, L., & Stopeck, A.T. (2010). Caring for the breast cancer survivor: A guide for primary care physicians. *American Journal of Medicine, 123*, 489–495. doi:10.1016/j.amjmed.2009.09.042

Church, T.R. (2011). Screening for colorectal cancer—Which strategy is the best? *Journal of the National Cancer Institute, 103*, 1282–1283. doi:10.1093/jnci/djr300

Colosia, A.D., Peltz, G., Gerhardt, P., Liu, E., Copely-Merriman, K., Khan, S., & Kay, J.A. (2011). A review and characterization of the various perceptions of quality cancer care. *Cancer, 117*, 884–896. doi:10.1002/cncr.25644

Daniel, S., & Kurtin, S.E. (2010). Pancreatic cancer. *Journal of the Advanced Practitioner in Oncology, 2*, 141–155.

Dokken, B., & Kurtin, S.E. (2010). Collaborative approach to managing a 47-year-old male with stage IIB rectosigmoid colon cancer and new onset of diabetes. *Journal of the Advanced Practitioner in Oncology, 1*, 184–194.

Doyle, C., Kushi, L.H., Byers, T., Courneya, K.S., Demark-Wahnefried, W., Grant, B., … Andresa, K.S. (2006). Nutrition and physical activity during and after cancer treatment: An American Cancer Society guide for informed choices. *CA: A Cancer Journal for Clinicians, 56*, 323–353. doi:10.3322/canjclin.56.6.323

Eheman, C., Henley, S.J., Ballard-Barbash, R., Jacobs, E.J., Schymura, M.J., Noone, A.-M., … Edwards, B.K. (2012). Annual Report to the Nation on the status of cancer, 1975–2008, featuring cancers associated with excess weight and lack of sufficient physical activity. *Cancer, 118*, 2338–2366. doi:10.1002/cncr.27514

Fadol, A., & Lech, T. (2011). Cardiovascular adverse events associated with cancer therapy. *Journal of Advanced Practitioner in Oncology, 2*, 229–242.

Fagerlin, A., Zikmund-Fisher, B.J., & Ubel, P.A. (2011). Helping patients decide: Ten steps to better risk communication. *Journal of the National Cancer Institute, 103*, 1–8. doi:10.1093/jnci/djr318

Felicetti, F., Manicone, R., Corrias, A., Manieri, C., Biasin, E., Bini, I., … Brignardello, E. (2011). Endocrine late effects after total body irradiation in patients who receive hematopoietic cell transplantation during childhood: A retrospective study from a single institution. *Journal of Cancer Research and Clinical Oncology, 137*, 1343–1348. doi:10.1007/s00432-011-1004-2

Fiore, M.C., Jaén, C.R., Baker, T.B., Bailey, W.C., Benowitz, N.L., Curry, S.J., … Wewers, M.E. (2008). *Treating tobacco use and dependence: 2008 update*. Retrieved from http://www.surgeongeneral.gov/tobacco/treating_tobacco_use08.pdf

Ganz, P.A. (2009). Survivorship: Adult cancer survivors. *Primary Care Clinical Office Practice, 36*, 721–741. doi:10.1016/j.pop.2009.08.001

Ganz, P.A. (2011). The 'three Ps' of cancer survivorship care. *BMC Medicine, 9*, 14. doi:10.1186/1741-7015-9-14

Hahn, E.E., & Ganz, P.A. (2011). Survivorship programs and care plans in practice: Variations on a theme. *Journal of Oncology Practice, 7*, 70–75. doi:10.1200/JOP.2010.000115

Hewitt, M., Greenfield, S., & Stovall, E. (Eds.). (2006). *From cancer patient to cancer survivor: Lost in transition*. Retrieved from http://www.nap.edu/catalog.php?record_id=11468

Hollowell, K., Olmsted, C.L., Richardson, A.S., Pittman, K., Bellin, L., Tafra, L., & Verbanac, K.M. (2010). American Society of Clinical Oncology-recommended surveillance and physician specialty among long-term breast cancer survivors. *Cancer, 116*, 2090–2098. doi:10/1002/chor.25038

Kurtin, S.E. (2009). Systemic therapies for squamous cell carcinoma of the head and neck. *Seminars in Oncology Nursing, 25*, 183–192. doi:10.1016/j.soncn.2009.05.001

Kurtin, S.E. (2010). Risk analysis in the treatment of hematologic malignancies in the elderly. *Journal of the Advance Practitioner in Oncology, 1*, 19–29.

Kurtin, S.E. (2011). Leukemia and myelodysplastic syndromes. In C.H. Yarbro, D. Wujcik, & B.H. Gobel (Eds.), *Cancer nursing: Principles and practice* (7th ed., pp. 1369–1398). Burlington, MA: Jones and Bartlett.

Landier, W. (2009). Survivorship care: Essential components and models of delivery. *Oncology, 23*(Suppl. 4, Nurse Ed.), 46–53.

Mao, J.J., Bowman, M., Stricker, C.T., DeMichele, A., Jacobs, L., Chan, D., & Armstrong, K. (2009). Delivery of survivorship care by primary care physicians: The perspective of breast cancer patients. *Journal of Clinical Oncology, 27*, 933–938. doi:10.1200/JCO.2008.18.0679

McCorkle, R., Ercolano, E., Lazanby, M., Schulman-Green, D., Schilling, L.S., Lorig, K., & Wagner, E.H. (2011). Self-management: Enabling and empowering patients living with cancer as a chronic illness. *CA: A Cancer Journal for Clinicians, 61*, 50–62. doi:10.3322/caac.20093

Mohty, M., & Apperly, J.F. (2010). Long-term physiological effects after allogeneic bone marrow transplantation. *Hematology, 2010*, 229–236. doi:10.1182/asheducation-2010.1.229

Morey, M.C., Snyder, D.C., Sloane, R., Cohen, H.J., Peterson, B., Hartman, T.J., … Demark-Wahnefried, W. (2009). Effects of home-based diet and exercise on functional outcomes among older, overweight long-term cancer survivors. *JAMA, 301*, 1183–1891. doi:10.1001/jama.2009.643

Morgan, M. (2009). Cancer survivorship: History, quality of life issues, and the evolving multidisciplinary approach to implementation of cancer survivorship care plans. *Oncology Nursing Forum, 36*, 429–436. doi:10.1188/09.ONF.429-436

National Cancer Institute. (2011). SEER stat fact sheets: All sites. Retrieved from http://seer.cancer.gov/statfacts/html/all.html#risk

National Comprehensive Cancer Network. (2010). *NCCN Clinical Practice Guidelines in Oncology: Senior adult oncology*. Retrieved from http://www.nccn.org/professional/physician_gls/PDF/senior.pdf

Newhauser, W.D., & Durante, M. (2011). Assessing the risk of second malignancies after modern radiotherapy. *Nature Reviews Cancer, 11*, 438–448. doi:10.1038/nrc3069

Oeffinger, K.C., & Tonorezos, E.S. (2011). The cancer is over, now what? Understanding risk, changing outcomes. *Cancer, 117*(Suppl. 10), 2250–2257. doi:10.1002/cncr.26051

Oeffinger, K.C., van Leeuwen, F.E., & Hodgson, D.C. (2011). Methods to assess adverse health-related outcomes in cancer survivors. *Cancer Epidemiology, Biomarkers and Prevention, 20*, 2022–2034. doi:10.1158/1055-9965.EPI-11-0674

O'Toole, E., Step, M., Engelhardt, L., Lewis, S., & Rose, J.H. (2009). The role of primary care physicians in advanced cancer care: Perspectives of older patients and their oncologists. *Journal of the American Geriatrics Society, 57*(Suppl. 2), S265–S268. doi:10.1111/j.1532-5415.2009.02508.x

Pollack, L., Adamanche, W., Ryerson, B., Ehemen, C., & Richardson, L. (2009). Care of long-term cancer survivors. *Cancer, 115,* 5284–5295. doi:10.1002/cncr.24624

Potosky, A.L., Han, P.K., Rowland, J., Klabunde, C.N., Smith, T., Aziz, N., … Stefanek, M. (2011). Differences between primary care physicians' and oncologists' knowledge, attitudes and practices regarding the care of cancer survivors. *Journal of General Internal Medicine, 26,* 1403–1410. doi:10.1007/s11606-011-1808-4

Rodin, G., Mackay, J.A., Zimmerman, C., Mayer, C., Howell, D., Katz, M., … Brouwers, M. (2009). Clinician-patient communication: A systematic review. *Supportive Care in Cancer, 17,* 627–644. doi:10.1007/s00520-009-0601-y

Schulman, L.N., Jacobs, L., Greenfield, S., Jones, B., McCabe, M.S., Syrjala, K., … Ganz, P. (2009). Cancer care and cancer survivorship in the United States: Will we be able to care for these patients in the future? *Journal of Oncology Practice, 5,* 119–123. doi:10.1200/JOP.0932001

Shapiro, C.L., McCabe, M.S., Syrjala, K.L., Friedman, D., Jacobs, L.A., Ganz, P.A., … Marcus, A.C. (2009). The LIVESTRONG Survivorship Center of Excellence Network. *Journal of Cancer Survivorship, 3,* 4–11. doi:10.1007/s11764-008-0076-8

Shu, X.O., Zheng, Y., Cai, H., Gu, K., Chen, Z., Zheng, W., & Lu, W. (2009). Soy food intake and breast cancer survival. *JAMA, 320,* 2437–2443. doi:10.1001/jama.2009.1783

Siegel, R., Naishadham, D., & Jemal, A. (2012). Cancer statistics, 2012. *CA: A Cancer Journal for Clinicians, 62,* 10–29. doi:10.3322/caac.20138

Smith, R.A., Cokkinides, V., Brooks, D., Saslow, D., Shah, M., & Brawley, O.W. (2011). Cancer screening in the United States, 2011. *CA: A Cancer Journal for Clinicians, 61,* 8–30. doi:10.3322/caac.20096

Stricker, C.T., & Jacobs, L.A. (2008). Physical late effects in adult cancer survivors. *Oncology, 22*(Suppl. 8, Nurse Ed.), 33–41.

Stricker, C.T., Jacobs, L.A., Risendal, B., Jones, A., Panzer, S., Ganz, P., … Palmer, S.C. (2011). Survivorship care planning after the Institute of Medicine recommendations: How are we faring? *Journal of Cancer Survivorship, 5,* 358–370. doi:10.1007/s11764-011-0196-4

Sweed, M. (2011). Gastrointestinal and hepatobiliary toxicities of cancer treatment. *Journal of the Advanced Practitioner in Oncology, 2,* 293–304.

Towle, E.L., Barr, T.R., Hanley, A., Kosty, M., Williams, S., & Goldstein, M.A. (2011). Results of the ASCO Study of Collaborative Practice Arrangements. *Journal of Oncology Practice, 7,* 278–282. doi:10.1200/JOP.2011.000385

U.S. Department of Health and Human Services. (2010). *How tobacco smoke causes disease: The biology and behavioral basis for smoking-attributable disease: A report of the Surgeon General.* Retrieved from http://www.surgeongeneral.gov/library/tobaccosmoke/report/full_report.pdf

U.S. Preventive Services Task Force. (2010). *The guide to clinical preventive services 2010–2011: Recommendations of the U.S. Preventive Services Task Force.* Retrieved from http://www.ahrq.gov/clinic/pocketgd1011/pocketgd1011.pdf

Velicer, C.M., & Ulrich, C.M. (2008). Vitamin and mineral supplement use among US adults after cancer diagnosis: A systematic review. *Journal of Clinical Oncology, 26,* 665–673. doi:10.1200/JCO.2007.13.5905

Wedding, U., Honecker, F., Boekemeyer, C., Pientka, L., & Höffken, K. (2007). Tolerance to chemotherapy in elderly patients with cancer. *Cancer Control, 14,* 44–56. Retrieved from http://www.moffitt.org/CCJRoot/v14n1/pdf/44.pdf

Wenger, N.K. (2011). What do the 2011 American Heart Association guidelines tell us about prevention of cardiovascular disease in women? *Clinical Cardiology, 34,* 520–523. doi:10.1002/clc.20940

Willenbring, M.L., Massey, S.H., & Gardner, M.B. (2009). Helping patients who drink too much: An evidence-based guide for primary care physicians. *American Family Physician, 80,* 44–50. Retrieved from http://www.aafp.org/afp/2009/0701/p44.html

CHAPTER 14

Reducing Cancer-Related Health Disparities: What Nurses Can Do to Effect Change

Sandra Millon Underwood, RN, PhD, FAAN

Introduction

Tremendous advances have been made over the past several years relative to cancer prevention and control. Yet, despite tremendous discoveries and advances being made in within the laboratory, the clinic, and the community, decades-old disparities in cancer morbidity and mortality among population groups persist (Eheman et al., 2012). Nurse scientists and educators have artfully explored and described factors associated with the cancer-related disparities experienced by several racially, ethnically, economically, and geographically defined population groups. The critical next step is for nurses to design and evaluate strategies to address the identified needs and gaps within and beyond their immediate sphere of practice and influence.

Cancer Morbidity and Mortality in the United States

Cancer, a group of more than 100 distinct diseases, is characterized by uncontrolled growth, proliferation, and spread of abnormal cells. If the uncontrolled growth, proliferation, and spread of the more aggressive cells is not arrested, a person could die from acute complications (e.g., hemorrhage, brain compression, suffocating dyspnea), progressive deterioration in the function of normal organs secondary to metastases (e.g., respiratory insufficiency, hepatic insufficiency), or degradation of the affected individual's general health.

Cancer is the second leading cause of disease and mortality in the United States (see Table 14-1) (National Center for Health Statistics, 2011). Men have a slightly less than a 1 in 2 lifetime risk of developing cancer; among women, the lifetime risk for developing cancer is a little more than 1 in 3. According to reports disseminated

Table 14-1. Leading Causes of Death by Sex and Race/Ethnicity, United States, 2007

Ethnicity	Male	Female
All persons	Heart disease Cancer Unintentional injuries Chronic lower respiratory diseases Cerebral vascular diseases	Heart disease Cancer Cerebral vascular diseases Chronic lower respiratory diseases Alzheimer disease
White	Heart disease Cancer Unintentional injuries Chronic lower respiratory diseases Cerebral vascular diseases	Heart disease Cancer Cerebral vascular diseases Chronic lower respiratory diseases Alzheimer disease
Black	Heart disease Cancer Unintentional injuries Homicide Cerebral vascular diseases	Heart disease Cancer Cerebral vascular diseases Diabetes Nephritis, nephritic syndrome, and nephrosis
Asian/Pacific Islander	Cancer Heart disease Cerebral vascular diseases Unintentional injuries Diabetes	Cancer Heart disease Cerebral vascular diseases Diabetes Unintentional injuries
American Indian or Alaska Native	Heart disease Cancer Unintentional injuries Chronic liver disease and cirrhosis Diabetes	Cancer Heart disease Unintentional injuries Diabetes Cerebral vascular diseases
Hispanic	Heart disease Cancer Unintentional injuries Cerebral vascular diseases Diabetes	Heart disease Cancer Cerebral vascular diseases Diabetes Unintentional injuries

Note. From *Health, United States, 2010: With Special Feature on Death and Dying* (pp. 145–148), by the National Center for Health Statistics, 2011, Hyattsville, MD: U.S. Department of Health and Human Services. Retrieved from http://www.cdc.gov/nchs/data/hus/hus10.pdf.

by American Cancer Society (ACS) scientists, an estimated 1,638,910 new cases of cancer and an estimated 577,190 deaths from cancer will occur in the United States in 2012 (Siegel, Naishadham, & Jemal, 2012). The incidence estimate does not include carcinoma in situ of any site except urinary bladder, nor does it include basal cell and squamous cell cancers of the skin. Although not reporting projected incidence of basal cell and squamous cell skin cancer, Siegel et al. (2012) estimated that approximately 63,300 cases of breast carcinoma in situ and 55,560 cases of melanoma in situ would be diagnosed in 2012.

Reports disseminated by the National Cancer Institute (NCI) Surveillance, Epidemiology, and End Results (SEER) Program reveal that most common type of cancer diagnosed in men in the United States is cancer of the prostate, followed by cancers of the lung and bronchus, colon and rectum, and urinary bladder and melanoma and non-Hodgkin lymphoma (see Table 14-2) (Altekruse et al., 2010). The most common type of cancer diagnosed in women in the United States is cancer of the breast, followed by cancers of the lung and bronchus, colon and rectum, uterus, and thyroid and non-Hodgkin lymphoma. The most common cause of cancer death in men in the United States is cancer of the lung and bronchus, followed by cancers of the prostate, colon and rectum, and pancreas (see Table 14-2). Furthermore, the most common cause of cancer death in women in the United States is cancer of the lung and bronchus, followed by cancers of the breast, colon and rectum, and pancreas.

Discoveries, Breakthroughs, and Innovations in Science and Cancer Care

A host of behavioral, biologic, environmental, and genetic factors are associated with cancer risk (ACS, 2011; Doll, 1998; Doll & Peto, 1981; Harvard Center for Cancer Prevention, 1996; Landrigan, Markowitz, Nicholson, & Baker, 1995; Stein & Colditz, 2004). Although cancer was once theorized to result from viral, chemical, and hereditary causes, the discovery of two classes of genes, oncogenes and tumor suppressor genes, has broadened the understanding of cancer genesis (Cavenee & White, 1995; Cooper, 1995; Levine, 1995; Weinberg, 1996). While many cancer risk factors are modifiable and can be avoided, others are not. The unmodifiable factors most strongly associated with cancer risk are age, sex, race/ethnicity, personal history, and genetics. The modifiable factors most strongly associated with cancer risk are tobacco use, poor nutrition, physical inactivity, overweight, obesity, and unsafe sexual practices (see Table 14-3).

Over the past several decades, significant advances have been made in the areas of cancer screening, treatment, and symptom management (NCI, 2010a, 2010b). Many new screening procedures, when regularly used, have been shown to prevent the development of cancer through identification and removal or treatment of premalignant abnormalities. Breakthroughs achieved in the area of cancer treatment have led to significant declines in cancer mortality and improvements in cancer survival. For example, surgical interventions have become more precise and less drastic. Radiation therapy has grown more powerful as well as more therapeutic. Antineoplastic agents are currently being prescribed in combinations that inflict greater damage on cancer cells while sparing excessive damage to normal cells. New agents developed to minimize cancer pain and cancer fatigue and to treat expected side effects of the cytotoxic therapy have similarly affected the treatment experiences and quality of life of patients with cancer.

Disparities in Cancer Morbidity and Mortality Among U.S. Population Groups

As a direct consequence of advances and innovations made relative to cancer and control, the number of individuals in the United States reported within the ranks of cancer survivors has more than tripled from three million in 1971 to more than 11 million (ACS, 2010). Although cancer is a diagnosis that many people survive, can-

Table 14-2. Age-Adjusted SEER Cancer Incidence Rates Per 100,000 for the Top Cancer Sites by Race/Ethnicity, United States, 2003–2007

	White		Black		Asian/Pacific Islander		American Indian		Hispanic	
	Male	Female	Male	Female	Male	Female	Male	Female	Male	Female
All sites	541.5	419.6	624.0	399.1	346.5	288.9	335.8	306.3	394.8	309.2
Brain and nervous system	8.4	6.0	4.7		4.0				5.9	
Colon and rectum	55.4	40.9	68.1	52.6	45.5	34.2	43.4	40.4	44.5	31.6
Esophagus	8.0		8.9		4.1		5.2		5.1	
Female breast		126.5		118.3		90.0		76.4		86.0
Gallbladder								4.7		
Kidney and renal pelvis	17.7	10.2	21.8	10.7	10.2	5.1	21.2	14.1	17.5	10.0
Larynx			10.3						4.6	
Leukemia	16.6	10.0	12.7	7.8	8.8	6.0	7.2	5.9	11.2	8.0
Liver and intrahepatic bile duct	9.1		14.0		21.7	8.3	14.6	6.9	15.6	6.0
Lung and bronchus	76.3	54.7	101.2	54.8	52.9	38.1	52.7	39.7	41.4	25.4
Melanoma of the skin	29.7	19.1			4.1		4.1			4.7
Myeloma	6.7		14.3	10.0	4.0		4.8		6.3	
Non-Hodgkin lymphoma	24.6	17.2	17.8	12.3	15.7	10.8	12.5	10.6	18.7	14.5
Oral cavity and pharynx	15.7	6.1	16.1	5.8	10.5	5.3	9.6	5.2	8.7	
Ovary		13.5		10.2		9.8		10.9		11.0
Pancreas	13.2	10.3	16.7	14.4	10.2	8.3	10.6	10.1	10.9	10.1
Prostate	150.4		234.6		90.0		77.7		125.8	
Stomach	9.6		16.7	8.6	17.5	10.0	15.5	7.3	14.8	9.1
Testis							4.3			
Thyroid		16.0		8.9	4.4	15.2		8.5		13.3
Urinary bladder	40.4	9.8	20.7	7.6	16.0	4.0	13.3		19.2	5.1
Uterine cervix		7.9		10.1		7.5		7.7		12.0
Uterine corpus		24.4		20.6		17.3		16.8		17.6

SEER—Surveillance, Epidemiology, and End Results

Note. Based on information from Altekruse et al., 2010.

Table 14-3. Cancer Risk Factors, Recommended Lifestyle Modifications and Behaviors, and Benefit for Site-Specific Cancer

Cancer Risk Factor	Recommendations for Lifestyle Modification	Sites That Benefit From Behavior Changes
Tobacco usage	Avoid tobacco use, including cigarettes, cigars, pipes, and smokeless tobacco. Participate in a smoking cessation program. Avoid secondhand smoke.	Bladder Cervix Colorectal Esophageal Kidney Lung Oral Pancreatic Stomach
Physical inactivity	Increase activity. Engage in at least 30 minutes of moderate physical activity on most days of the week.	Breast Colorectal
Overweight and obesity	Maintain a healthy weight. Balance caloric intake from the diet with energy expenditure from physical activity.	Breast Colorectal Esophageal Kidney Uterus
Poor nutrition	Eat a healthy diet that is rich in fruits, vegetables, and whole grains. Limit consumption of red meats, cured or smoked meats, and foods and beverages that contain high fat or sugar. Limit intake of highly processed foods. Take a daily multivitamin that contains folate.	Bladder Breast Colorectal Esophageal Lung Oral Pancreatic Prostate Stomach
Excess alcohol consumption	Limit alcohol consumption to less than one drink per day for women or two per day for men. Women at high risk for breast cancer should consider avoiding alcoholic beverages entirely. Consider an alcohol treatment program for addiction.	Breast Colorectal Esophageal Oral
Multiple sexual partners	Protect oneself from sexually transmitted diseases. Engage in safe-sex habits, such as using condoms and limiting the number of sexual partners. Women, girls, men, and boys ages 9–26 years old should consider getting vaccinated against human papillomavirus.	Cervical Anorectal Esophageal Oral
Excessive sun exposure/tanning bed usage	Avoid excessive sun exposure. Stay out of the sun as much as possible. Wear hats and other protective clothing or seek shade when outdoors. Use sunscreen with SPF 15 or higher that blocks both UVA and UVB rays and carefully follow application instructions.	Oral Skin

Note. Based on information from American Cancer Society, 2011, 2012.

cer experiences have been shown to vary considerably across population groups, including race/ethnicity, socioeconomic status, and geography.

Subset analysis of data from NCI, the National Center for Health Statistics, the Centers for Disease Control and Prevention, and other entities has helped to identify population groups more likely to be diagnosed with and die from preventable cancers, to be diagnosed with late-stage disease for cancers that could be detected through screening, to receive no treatment or treatment that does not meet accepted standards of care, to die of cancers that are generally curable, and to suffer from terminal cancer without the benefit of pain control and other palliative care (Altekruse et al., 2010; Centers for Disease Control and Prevention, 2011; Cummings, Whetstone, Earp, & Mayne, 2002; Hegarty, Burchett, Gold, & Cohen, 2000; NCI, 2011; National Center for Health Statistics, 2011; Singh, Miller, Hankey, & Edwards, 2003; Smedley, Stith, & Nelson, 2003; Smith et al., 2011; Strzelczyk & Dignan, 2002; Ward, Jemal, & Cokkinides, 2004). The disparities in cancer morbidity and mortality reported among population groups distinguished by race/ethnicity, socioeconomic status, and geography are profound. For example,

- Cancer is the leading cause of death among Asian Americans and the second most common cause of death among White, Black, and Hispanic Americans (see Table 14-1).
- Among U.S. men, for all cancers combined, the cancer incidence rates are highest among Black men, followed by White, Hispanic, Asian/Pacific Islander, and American Indian/Alaska Native men (see Table 14-2). For all cancers combined, the cancer death rates are highest among Black men, followed by White, Hispanic, American Indian/Alaska Native, and Asian/Pacific Islander men.
- Among U.S. women, for all cancers combined, the cancer incidence rates are highest among White women, followed by Black, Hispanic, Asian/Pacific Islander, and American Indian/Alaska Native women (see Table 14-2). For all cancers combined, the cancer death rates are highest among Black women, followed by White, American Indian/Alaska Native, Hispanic, and Asian/Pacific Islander women.
- Blacks are more likely than other racial ethnic population groups to be diagnosed with cancer at a later stage and less likely to survive five years after a diagnosis.
- Hispanics have higher rates of infection-related cancers, such as uterine cervix, liver, gallbladder, and stomach cancer, but lower incidence rates for all cancers combined compared to Whites (see Table 14-2).
- Rates of cancer of the lung, colon, rectum, kidney, stomach, liver, cervix, and gallbladder are significantly higher in American Indian and Alaska Natives than in White populations (see Table 14-2).
- Cancer affects Asian American populations in very different ways, based on country of origin. Among Asian American subpopulations, colorectal cancer incidence rates are highest among Chinese Americans, prostate cancer incidence rates are highest among Filipino men, and cervical cancer incidence and mortality rates are highest among Vietnamese women.
- Socioeconomically disadvantaged individuals are disproportionately affected by cancer in the United States. For all cancers combined, residents of counties in the United States with a greater than 20% poverty rate have a higher death rate in men and higher death rate in women.
- Among people who develop cancer, the five-year survival rate is higher for people who live in affluent census tracts than for those who live in poorer census tracts.

- For the four cancer sites for which screening is widely recommended or practiced—colorectal cancer, female breast cancer, cervical cancer, and prostate cancer—the proportion of cases diagnosed at localized stage is lower and the proportion diagnosed at distant stage is higher in areas of higher levels of poverty compared with areas with lower levels of poverty (see Table 14-4).
- Mapping cancer trends within the United States reveals distinct areas, regions, and territories where there are significant variations in breast, prostate, lung, colon, and rectal cancer incidence and mortality.

The reasons for the staggering disparities experienced among population groups distinguished by race/ethnicity, socioeconomic status, and geography are not completely understood. Research suggests that the disparities in cancer morbidity and mortality are the result of complex interactions among individual factors (e.g., genetic endowment, lifestyle choices, health behaviors), social and economic inequalities (e.g., racism, discrimination, education, economic status), the physical environment (e.g., neighborhood conditions, exposure to toxic environments), and healthcare quality (e.g., access to care, utilization of care, provision of quality health care) (Brawley & Berger, 2008; Freeman, 2004; Freeman & Chu, 2005; Kagawa-Singer, Dadia, Yu, & Surbone, 2010; Ward et al., 2004). Yet, given what is currently known about cancer prevention, risk, screening, treatment, and symptom management, cancer disparities could be significantly reduced. Research indicates that that more than half of all cancers could be prevented if population-wide measures to reduce tobacco use, increase physical activity, control overweight and obesity, improve nutritional practices, and increase use of routine cancer screening tests were implemented (see Table 14-4) (ACS, 2011, 2012; Curry, Byers, & Hewitt, 2004; Doll, 1998; Harvard Center for Cancer Prevention, 1996; Stein & Colditz, 2004).

Health Disparities Related to Sexual Orientation and Gender Identity

Cancer-related health disparities in the lesbian, gay, bisexual, and transgender (LGBT) community are significant. The disparities are prevalent throughout the cancer continuum from screening and prevention to survivorship and end of life. Because the roughly 10% of people in the United States who identify as LGBT are essentially biologically and physiologically the same as heterosexuals, the disparities present are related to risk factors and barriers to adequate cancer screening and care (National LGBT Cancer Network, 2011).

The National LGBT Cancer Network (2011) noted that people in the LGBT community have a special cluster of risk factors that increases cancer incidence and causes delayed diagnosis. Some barriers are socioeconomic and others are behavioral. Socioeconomic barriers include discrimination in access to health insurance, housing, retirement benefits, and employment (Healthy People, 2012; National LGBT Cancer Network, 2011). Negative experiences with healthcare providers can also prevent people in the LGBT community from seeking treatment or cancer-related screening; therefore, cancer is often found at later stages (ACS, 2009; National LGBT Cancer Network, 2011).

Access to care is especially a problem among the 3% of the U.S. population who are transgender because of fear of discrimination and healthcare professionals who lack the cultural sensitivity to meet their unique needs (Stebner, 2012). People who are transgender still need health care related to their anatomical sexual character-

Table 14-4. Nationwide[1] Cancer Screening Rates by Race, Age, Income, and Education, 2008 (%)

	Breast[2]	Colorectal (fecal occult blood)[3]	Colorectal[4]	Prostate[5]	Cervical[6]
Race and ethnicity					
White	75.9	21.3	64.0	56.9	82.9
Black	79.3	23.6	58.0	59.4	86.2
Hispanic	73.5	13.1	48.2	41.3	85.2
Multiracial	72.9	15.0	47.5	37.2	81.6
Other	65.1	22.2	57.2	47.8	81.1
Age					
40–49	68.8	–	–	26.1	73.8
50–59	80.0	15.7	51.3	58.1	91.3
60–64	81.0	23.1	67.1	75.6	89.3
65+	78.5	24.6	70.7	78.4	86.2
Income					
< $15,000	63.7	17.8	52.1	40.7	71.7
$15,000–24,999	69.3	21.9	56.1	50.9	76.3
$25,000–34,999	73.8	21.5	61.3	55.4	81.3
$35,000–49,999	77.4	21.8	62.6	55.2	84.4
$50,000+	81.1	20.0	65.7	58.2	90.6
Education					
Less than H.S.	65.6	17.4	52.0	43.5	73.6
H.S. or G.E.D.	74.3	20.5	58.6	49.7	76.9
Some post-H.S.	75.8	21.2	62.0	55.1	82.9
College graduate	80.7	21.5	68.9	61.3	90.4

[1] Nationwide data reflected trends within the states, District of Columbia, Guam, and Puerto Rico.

[2] Women aged 40+ who have had a mammogram within the past two years.

[3] Adults aged 50+ who have had a blood stool test within the past two years.

[4] Adults aged 50+ who have ever had a sigmoidoscopy or colonoscopy.

[5] Men aged 40+ who have had a prostate-specific antigen test within the past two years.

[6] Women aged 18+ who have had a test within the past three years.

Note. Based on information from Centers for Disease Control and Prevention, 2008.

istics. Even if a transgender woman undergoes sexual reassignment surgery, she will retain her prostate (Advameg, 2012). Female to male surgery is less common because of cost and complexity; therefore, many transgender men will still need screening for female reproductive cancers (Advameg, 2012; Stebner, 2012).

Behavioral risk factors are often higher among people in the LGBT community than for people who identify as heterosexual (National LGBT Cancer Network, 2011). For example, obesity, tobacco use, and alcohol abuse are more prevalent in the LGBT population than in the heterosexual population. Therefore, just as in any other minority group, people who make poor health choices have increased risk of cancers associated with these choices, and people who do not have adequate access to care will likely miss opportunities to receive a cancer diagnosis at an early, treatable stage (ACS, 2009, 2010; National LGBT Cancer Network, 2011).

In regard to risk factors, an important distinction must be made between identifying as LGBT and behavioral risk factors. Sexual orientation and gender identity themselves do not predispose a person to a higher cancer risk, rather behavioral choices do. For example, multiple sexual partners and unsafe sex practices increase the risk of human papillomavirus and HIV infections, which increases the risk for certain cancers (ACS, 2009, 2010). However, LGBT does not equal promiscuity. It is important for clinicians to focus on the behavior of the individual regardless of orientation when ascertaining risk.

The first step in closing the health disparities gap between the LGBT and heterosexual communities is that more comprehensive data are needed regarding LGBT health in general and cancer specifically (Krehely, 2009; National LGBT Cancer Community, 2011). Health surveys and cancer registries usually do not include sexual identity or orientation; therefore, the actual size of the LGBT community and cancer incidence rates are based on estimation (National LGBT Cancer Community, 2011). Accurate data would go a long way to help determine the best approach to adequate cancer care in this population. Next, Krehely (2009) and Stebner (2012) suggested that sensitivity training for healthcare professionals will also help them to best treat and educate LGBT patients about cancer screening and risk factors. Liz Margolies (2012), executive director of the National LGBT Cancer Network, agrees and adds that patient information materials that are inclusive and sensitive to the LGBT community will also help to lessen the gap. Finally, economic barriers, such as access to employment and health insurance, will allow people in this community to afford the treatment and screening procedures they need (Healthy People, 2012).

Nurses Call for Action

Disparities in cancer morbidity, cancer mortality, and cancer care have long been a concern of leaders in the cancer nursing community. Well before President Nixon declared war against cancer, the excess burden of cancer experienced by racial and ethnic population groups was first reported by the Secretary's Task Force, reducing health disparities was designated a national priority, a definition for health disparities was enacted into law, and variations in healthcare access and health outcomes among diverse population groups were being denoted and discussed by nurses engaged in cancer practice (Heckler, 1985; Minority Health and Health Disparities Research and Education Act, 2000; Rettig, 1977; U.S. Department of Health and Human Services, 1991). These reports helped to increase nurses' understanding of the national cancer burden and heighten nurses' awareness of inequities in cancer care among varied population groups (Ferguson, 1948; Gillmer & Hassels, 1964; Gould, 1946; Lusk, 2005; McKee, 1946; Peterson, 1948; Strayer, 1945). For those in the profession who took notice, they also provided a prelude of challenges that were to come.

Disparities in cancer morbidity, cancer mortality, and cancer care—in this, the 21st century—continue to be reported to be a cause of great concern for clinicians, educators, and researchers throughout the nursing community. Despite advances made in science, medical technology, medicine, and nursing since the war against cancer was declared, the disparities for far too many population groups have not sufficiently narrowed. Although new knowledge has been acquired over the past 40 years in terms of understanding what cancer is and how it develops; who is at risk and why; how cancer can be prevented; how to best detect, diagnose, and treat cancer; and how to improve the quality of life for patients with cancer and survivors, many in the profession continue to question why the cancer burden is unequally borne by racially, ethnically, economically, and geographically defined population groups in the United States (see Table 14-5).

Research suggests that nurses could do much to help reduce or eliminate the cancer-related disparities experienced among U.S. population groups. Building on the foundation laid by others in the clinical, academic, and research arena, nurses have been encouraged to further their efforts to address cancer care needs of population groups at increased risk for developing and dying from cancer; to address cancer care needs of population groups at risk for being less than adequately served within the healthcare system; to identify demographic, geographic, cultural, and social phenomena that affect cancer morbidity and mortality within the states and territories; to evaluate the effectiveness, efficacy, and impact of interventions designed or tailored for use by diverse population groups; and to report promising and proven strategies to address known gaps in cancer nursing practice, nursing education, and nursing science within and beyond their immediate sphere of practice and influence.

Table 14-5. Research Exploring Cancer-Related Disparities

Cancer Type	Author	Title	Purpose/Theme
Clinical Trials			
Breast	Linden et al., 2007	Attitudes Toward Participation in Breast Cancer Randomized Clinical Trials in the African American Community: A Focus Group Study	Explore attitudes of the African American community regarding willingness to participate in breast cancer screening and randomized clinical trials.
Diagnosis			
Breast	Bibb, 2001	The Relationship Between Access and Stage at Diagnosis of Breast Cancer in African American and Caucasian Women	Identify relationships among potential access, realized access, and stage at diagnosis of breast cancer in African American and Caucasian women receiving care within an equal economic access healthcare system.

(Continued on next page)

Table 14-5. Research Exploring Cancer-Related Disparities *(Continued)*

Cancer Type	Author	Title	Purpose/Theme
Breast	Bradley, 2005	The Delay and Worry Experience of African American Women With Breast Cancer	Examine the delay in seeking treatment and worry experiences of African American women with breast cancer.
Breast	Gates et al., 2001	Caring Demands and Delay in Seeking Care in African American Women Newly Diagnosed With Breast Cancer: An Ethnographic, Photographic Study	Describe caring behaviors and demands of African American women newly diagnosed with breast cancer.
Breast	Lackey et al., 2001	African American Women's Experiences With the Initial Discovery, Diagnosis, and Treatment of Breast Cancer	Describe experiences of African American women living with breast cancer following the primary diagnosis and while undergoing initial treatment.
Breast	Reifenstein, 2007	Care-Seeking Behaviors of African American Women With Breast Cancer Symptoms	Assess delay in care-seeking for breast cancer symptoms among African American women with breast cancer symptoms.
Testicular	Gleason, 2006	Racial Disparities in Testicular Cancer: Impact on Health Promotion	Determine if there were differences in stage of testicular cancer among populations that varied by ethnicity and age.

Risk, Perceived Risk, and Risk Management

Breast	Underwood et al., 2008	Pilot Study of the Breast Cancer Experiences of African American Women With a Family History of Breast Cancer: Implications for Nursing Practice	Explore the degree to which breast cancer, breast cancer risk, and breast cancer risk management were discussed by African American women and their healthcare providers.
Not specific	Swinney, 2002	African Americans With Cancer: The Relationships Among Self-Esteem, Locus of Control, and Health Perception	Examine the relationships among self-esteem, locus of control, and perceived health status in African Americans with cancer.
Oral	Powe & Finnie, 2004	Knowledge of Oral Cancer Risk Factors Among African Americans: Do Nurses Have A Role?	Assess the knowledge of oral cancer risk factors among African Americans.

Screening

Breast	Farmer et al., 2007	Psychosocial Correlates of Mammography Screening in Older African American Women	Explore psychosocial correlates of older African American women's adherence to annual mammography screening.

(Continued on next page)

Table 14-5. Research Exploring Cancer-Related Disparities *(Continued)*

Cancer Type	Author	Title	Purpose/Theme
Breast	Fowler et al., 2005	Collaborative Breast Health Intervention for African American Women of Lower Socioeconomic Status	Describe phases of a collaborative breast health intervention designed to increase mammography screening.
Breast	Grindel et al., 2004	The Effect of Breast Cancer Screening Messages on Knowledge, Attitudes, Perceived Risk, and Mammography Screening of African American Women in the Rural South	Determine the effect of positive, neutral, and negative screening messages on knowledge, attitudes, perceived risk for breast cancer, and mammography screening among African American women.
Breast	Hall et al., 2005	Teaching Breast Cancer Screening to African American Women in the Arkansas Mississippi River Delta	Determine effectiveness of culturally sensitive breast cancer education program for African American women in the Arkansas Mississippi River Delta.
Breast	Jerome-D'Emilia et al., 2010	Feasibility of Using Technology to Disseminate Evidence to Rural Nurses and Improve Patient Outcomes	Examine feasibility of using distance education to disseminate knowledge about timely and appropriate mammography screening to rural nurses.
Breast	Kinney et al., 2002	Screening Behaviors Among African American Women at High Risk for Breast Cancer: Do Beliefs About God Matter?	Examine relationship between beliefs about God as a controlling force in health and adherence to breast cancer screening among high-risk African American women.
Breast	Russell et al., 2006	Sociocultural Context of Mammography Screening Use	Examine variations in cultural and health beliefs about mammography screening among a socioeconomically diverse sample of African American and Caucasian women.
Breast	Steele & Porche, 2005	Testing the Theory of Planned Behavior to Predict Mammography Intention	Test utility of the Theory of Planned Behavior to predict mammography intention among rural women in Southeastern Louisiana.
Breast	Swinney & Dobal, 2011	Older African American Women's Beliefs, Attitudes, and Behaviors About Breast Cancer	Identify social, cultural, and behavioral factors associated with regular participation in breast cancer screening and risk-reduction behaviors among older African American women.
Breast	Wood et al., 2002	The Effect of an Educational Intervention on Promoting Breast Self-Examination in Older African American and Caucasian Women	Test the efficacy of age- and race-sensitive breast health video in increasing knowledge about breast cancer risk and screening and breast self-examination proficiency.

(Continued on next page)

Table 14-5. Research Exploring Cancer-Related Disparities *(Continued)*

Cancer Type	Author	Title	Purpose/Theme
Breast, cervical	Welch et al., 2008	Sociodemographic and Health-Related Determinants of Breast and Cervical Cancer Screening Behavior, 2005	Identify sociodemographic and health-related determinants of breast and cervical cancer screening.
Breast, cervical, colorectal	Powe & Cooper, 2008	Self-Reported Cancer Screening Rates Versus Medical Record Documentation: Incongruence, Specificity, and Sensitivity for African American Women	Evaluate levels of incongruence, specificity, and sensitivity between self-reported screening and medical record documentation for breast, cervical, and colorectal cancer screening.
Cervical	Ackerson et al., 2008	Personal Influencing Factors Associated With Pap Smear Testing and Cervical Cancer	Explore personal influences regarding Pap smears.
Colorectal	Frank et al., 2004	Colon Cancer Screening in African American Women	Explore colorectal cancer risk factors and frequency of colorectal cancer screening among African American women.
Colorectal	Green & Kelly, 2004	Colorectal Cancer Knowledge, Perceptions, and Behaviors in African Americans	Explore colorectal cancer knowledge, perceptions, and screening behaviors of African American men and women who reside or work in urban low-income housing.
Colorectal	Griffith, 2009	Biologic, Psychological and Behavioral, and Social Variables Influencing Colorectal Cancer Screening in African Americans	Test the predictive strength of biological, psychological and behavioral, and social system factors and provider recommendations on colorectal cancer screening.
Colorectal	Gwede et al., 2010	Exploring Disparities and Variability in Perceptions and Self-Reported Colorectal Cancer Screening Among Three Ethnic Subgroups of U.S. Blacks	Explore perceptions of colorectal cancer and colorectal cancer screening behaviors among ethnic subgroups of U.S. Blacks.
Prostate	Jones et al., 2009	How African American Men Decide Whether or Not to Get Prostate Cancer Screening	Explore what prostate cancer screening means to African Americans in rural areas and how they make the decision whether to undergo prostate cancer screening.
Prostate	Parchment, 2004	Prostate Cancer Screening in African American and Caribbean Males: Detriment in Delay	Investigate health beliefs surrounding prostate health in African American and Caribbean men and reasons for delaying or avoiding prostate screenings.

(Continued on next page)

Table 14-5. Research Exploring Cancer-Related Disparities *(Continued)*

Cancer Type	Author	Title	Purpose/Theme
Prostate	Weinrich et al., 2003	Self-Reported Reasons Men Decide Not to Participate in Free Prostate Cancer Screening	Determine why men fail to take advantage of a free prostate cancer screening program.
Survivorship			
Breast	Chung et al., 2009	Breast Cancer Survivorship Program: Testing for Cross-Cultural Relevance	Assess the utility and cultural relevance of a theory-based self-management program designed to assist African American women with survivorship concerns that arise after breast cancer treatment.
Breast, prostate	Hamilton & Sandelowski, 2004	Types of Social Support in African Americans With Cancer	Determine types of social support used by African Americans to cope with the experience of cancer.
Breast	Henderson et al., 2003	African American Women Coping With Breast Cancer: A Qualitative Analysis	Determine how African American women cope with breast cancer.
Breast	Royak-Schaler et al., 2008	Exploring Patient-Physician Communication in Breast Cancer Care for African American Women Following Primary Treatment	Investigate African American breast cancer survivors' perspectives and preferred avenues for information delivery.
Not specific	Hamilton et al., 2010	Perceptions of Support Among Older African American Cancer Survivors	Explore the perceived social support needs among older adult African American cancer survivors.
Not specific	Hughes et al., 2007	Everyday Struggling to Survive: Experience of the Urban Poor Living With Advanced Cancer	Explore the meaning of dignity and the experiences of living with advanced cancer among the urban poor.
Not specific	Meghani & Houldin, 2007	The Meanings of and Attitudes About Cancer Pain Among African Americans	Describe the meaning of cancer pain and attitudes in dealing with cancer pain among African Americans with cancer.
Prostate	Maliski et al., 2010	Faith Among Low-Income, African American Black Men Treated for Prostate Cancer	Describe use of faith by low-income, uninsured African American men in coping with prostate cancer and its treatment and adverse effects.

Conclusion

Healthy People 2020, much like the reports preceding it, proclaims the elimination of disparities in cancer morbidity and mortality among U.S. population groups to be a national priority (U.S. Department of Health and Human Services Office of Disease Prevention and Health Promotion, 2009). Independently and collectively, nurses are making tremendous strides in the war against cancer. However, much more is needed if the elimination of cancer disparities is to be realized.

Nurses and other healthcare providers are strongly encouraged to make an effort to further extend their reach and venture into lesser resourced and medically underserved communities; to refine their arsenal of interventions, strategies, and approaches; and to focus their sights upstream. Doing so could allow nurses to contribute even more to efforts to reduce disparities in cancer morbidity and mortality and likewise bring the nation one step closer to the mission being declared "accomplished."

References

Ackerson, K., Pohl, J., & Low, L.K. (2008). Personal influencing factors associated with Pap smear testing and cervical cancer. *Policy, Politics and Nursing Practice, 9,* 50–60. doi:10.1177/1527154408318097

Advameg. (2012). Sex reassignment surgery. Encyclopedia of surgery. Retrieved from http://www.surgeryencyclopedia.com/Pa-St/Sex-Reassignment-Surgery.html

Altekruse, S.F., Kosary, C.L., Krapcho, M., Neyman, N., Aminou, R., Waldron, W., ... Edwards, B.K. (Eds.). (2010). SEER cancer statistics review, 1975–2007. Retrieved from http://seer.cancer.gov/csr/1975_2007/

American Cancer Society. (2009). Cancer facts for lesbian and bisexual women. Retrieved from http://www.cancer.org/Healthy/FindCancerEarly/WomensHealth/cancer-facts-for-lesbians-and-bisexual-women

American Cancer Society. (2010). Cancer facts for gay and bisexual men. Retrieved from http://www.cancer.org/Healthy/FindCancerEarly/MensHealth/cancer-facts-for-gay-and-bisexual-men

American Cancer Society. (2011). Cancer prevention and early detection facts and figures. Retrieved from http://www.cancer.org/acs/groups/content/@epidemiologysurveilance/documents/document/acspc-029459.pdf

American Cancer Society. (2012). Cancer facts and figures 2012. Retrieved from http://www.cancer.org/acs/groups/content/@epidemiologysurveilance/documents/document/acspc-031941.pdf

Bibb, S.C.G. (2001). The relationship between access and stage at diagnosis of breast cancer in African American and Caucasian women. *Oncology Nursing Forum, 28,* 711–719.

Bradley, P.K. (2005). The delay and worry experience of African American women with breast cancer. *Oncology Nursing Forum, 32,* 243–249. doi:10.1188/05.ONF.243-249

Brawley, O.W., & Berger, M.Z. (2008). Cancer and disparities in health: Perspectives on health statistics and research questions. *Cancer, 113*(Suppl. 7), 1744–1754. doi:10.1002/cncr.23800

Cavenee, W.K., & White, R.L. (1995). The genetic basis of cancer. *Scientific American, 272,* 72–79. doi:10.1038/scientificamerican0395-72

Centers for Disease Control and Prevention. (2008). Behavioral risk factor surveillance system survey data. Retrieved from http://www.cdc.gov/brfss/technical_infodata/surveydata/2008.htm

Centers for Disease Control and Prevention. (2011). *Behavioral risk factor surveillance system survey data.* Atlanta, GA: U.S. Department of Health and Human Services, Centers for Disease Control and Prevention.

Chung, L.K., Cimprich, B., Janz, N.K., & Mills-Wisneski, S.M. (2009). Breast cancer survivorship program: Testing for cross-cultural relevance. *Cancer Nursing, 32,* 236–245. doi:10.1097/NCC.0b013e318196c67b

Cooper, G.M. (1995). *Oncogenes* (2nd ed.). Burlington, MA: Jones and Bartlett.

Cummings, D.M., Whetstone, L.M., Earp, J.A., & Mayne, L. (2002). Disparities in mammography screening in rural areas: Analysis of county differences in North Carolina. *Journal of Rural Health, 18,* 77–83. doi:10.1111/j.1748-0361.2002.tb00879.x

Curry, S., Byers, T., & Hewitt, M. (2004). Fulfilling the potential of cancer prevention and early detection: An American Cancer Society and Institute of Medicine Symposium. Retrieved from http://books.nap.edu/openbook.php?record_id=10941

Doll, R. (1998). Epidemiological evidence of the effects of behavior and the environment on the risk of cancer. *Recent Results in Cancer Research, 154,* 3–21. doi:10.1007/978-3-642-46870-4_1

Doll, R., & Peto, R. (1981). *The causes of cancer.* New York, NY: Oxford University Press.

Eheman, C., Henley, S.J., Ballard-Barbash, R., Jacobs, E.J., Schymura, M.J., Noone, A.M., … Edwards, B.K. (2012). Annual Report to the Nation on the status of cancer, 1975–2008, featuring cancers associated with excess weight and lack of sufficient physical activity. *Cancer, 118*, 2338–2366. doi:10.1002/cncr.27514

Farmer, D., Reddick, B., D'Agostino, R., & Jackson, S.A. (2007). Psychosocial correlates of mammography screening in older African American women. *Oncology Nursing Forum, 34,* 117–123. doi:10.1188/07.ONF.117-123

Ferguson, M. (1948). The public health nurse and the cancer program. *Public Health Nursing, 40,* 343–346.

Fowler, B.A., Rodney, M., Roberts, S., & Broadus, L. (2005). Collaborative breast health intervention for African American women of lower socioeconomic status. *Oncology Nursing Forum, 32,* 1207–1216. doi:10.1188/05.ONF.1207-1216

Frank, D., Swedmark, J., & Grubbs, L. (2004). Colon cancer screening in African American women. *Association of Black Nursing Faculty Journal, 15,* 67–70.

Freeman, H.P. (2004). Poverty, culture, and social injustice: Determinants of cancer disparities. *CA: A Cancer Journal for Clinicians, 54,* 72–77. doi:10.3322/canjclin.54.2.72

Freeman, H.P., & Chu, K.C. (2005). Determinants of cancer disparities: Barriers to cancer screening, diagnosis, and treatment. *Surgical Oncology Clinics of North America, 14,* 655–669. doi:10.1016/j.soc.2005.06.002

Gates, M.F., Lackey, N.R., & Brown. G. (2001). Caring demands and delay in seeking care in African American women newly diagnosed with breast cancer: An ethnographic, photographic study. *Oncology Nursing Forum, 28,* 529–537.

Gillmer, R., & Hassels, A. (1964). Nurses' practices and attitudes toward cancer. *American Journal of Nursing, 64*(4), 84–85. doi:10.2307/3419058

Gleason, A.M. (2006). Racial disparities in testicular cancer: Impact on health promotion. *Journal of Transcultural Nursing, 17,* 58–64. doi:10.1177/1043659605281980

Gould, W.G. (1946). Prostitution, promiscuity, venereal disease. *Public Health Nursing, 38,* 173–177.

Green, P.M., & Kelly, B.A. (2004). Colorectal cancer knowledge, perceptions, and behaviors in African Americans. *Cancer Nursing, 27,* 206–215. doi:10.1097/00002820-200405000-00004

Griffith, K.A. (2009). Biological, psychological and behavioral, and social variables influencing colorectal cancer screening in African Americans. *Nursing Research, 58,* 312–320. doi:10.1097/NNR.0b013e3181ac143d

Grindel, C.G., Brown, L., Caplan, L., & Blumenthal, D. (2004). The effect of breast cancer screening messages on knowledge, attitudes, perceived risk, and mammography screening of African American women in the rural South. *Oncology Nursing Forum, 31,* 801–808. doi:10.1188/04.ONF.801-808

Gwede, C.K., William, C.M., Thomas, K.B., Tarver, W.L., Quinn, G.P., Vadaparampil, S.T., … Meade, C.D. (2010). Exploring disparities and variability in perceptions and self-reported colorectal cancer screening among three ethnic subgroups of U.S. Blacks. *Oncology Nursing Forum, 37,* 581–591. doi:10.1188/10.ONF.581-591

Hall, C.P., Wimberley, P.D., Hall, J.D., Pfriemer, J.T., Hubbard, E., Stacy, A.S., & Gilbert, J.D. (2005). Teaching breast cancer screening to African American women in the Arkansas Mississippi River Delta. *Oncology Nursing Forum, 32,* 857–863. doi:10.1188/05.ONF.857-863

Hamilton, J.B., Moore, C.E., Powe, B.D., Agarwal, M., & Martin, P. (2010). Perceptions of support among older African American cancer survivors. *Oncology Nursing Forum, 37,* 484–493. doi:10.1188/10.ONF.484-493

Hamilton, J.B., & Sandelowski, M. (2004). Types of social support in African Americans with cancer. *Oncology Nursing Forum, 31,* 792–800. doi:10.1188/04.ONF.792-800

Harvard Center for Cancer Prevention. (1996). Human causes of cancer: Harvard School of Public Health. Retrieved from http:// www.hsph.harvard.edu/cancer/publications/reports.html

Healthy People. (2012, February 8). Lesbian, gay, bisexual, and transgender health. Retrieved from http://www.healthypeople.gov/2020/topicsobjectives2020/overview.aspx?topicid=25#eight

Heckler, M. (1985). *Black and minority health. Report of the Secretary's Task Force.* Retrieved from http://www.eric.ed.gov/PDFS/ED263293.pdf

Hegarty, V., Burchett, B.M., Gold, D.T., & Cohen, H.J. (2000). Racial differences in use of cancer prevention services among older Americans. *Journal of the American Geriatrics Society, 48,* 735–740.

Henderson, P.D., Gore, S.V., Davis, B.L., & Condon, E.H. (2003). African American women coping with breast cancer: A qualitative analysis. *Oncology Nursing Forum, 30,* 641–647. doi:10.1188/03.ONF.641-647

Hughes, A., Gudmundsdottir, M., & Davies, B. (2007). Everyday struggling to survive: Experience of the urban poor living with advanced cancer. *Oncology Nursing Forum, 34,* 1113–1118. doi:10.1188/07.ONF.1113-1118

Jerome-D'Emilia, B., Merwin, E., & Stern, S. (2010). Feasibility of using technology to disseminate evidence to rural nurses and improve patient outcomes. *Journal of Continuing Education in Nursing, 41,* 25–32. doi:10.3928/00220124-20091222-08

Jones, R.A., Steeves, R., & Williams, I. (2009). How African American men decide whether or not to get prostate cancer screening. *Cancer Nursing, 32,* 166–172. doi:10.1097/NCC.0b013e3181982c6e

Kagawa-Singer, M., Dadia, A.V., Yu, M.C., & Surbone, A. (2010). Cancer, culture, and health disparities: Time to chart a new course? *CA: A Cancer Journal for Clinicians, 60,* 12–39. doi:10.3322/caac.20051

Kinney, A.Y., Emery, G., Dudley, W.N., & Croyle, R.T. (2002). Screening behaviors among African American women at high risk for breast cancer: Do beliefs about God matter? *Oncology Nursing Forum, 29,* 835–843. doi:10.1188/02.ONF.835-843

Krehely, J. (2009, December 21). How to close the LGBT health disparities gap. Retrieved from http://www.cancer-network.org/media/pdf/lgbt_health_disparities_gap_race.pdf

Lackey, N.R., Gates, M.F., & Brown, G. (2001). African American women's experiences with the initial discovery, diagnosis, and treatment of breast cancer. *Oncology Nursing Forum, 28,* 519–527.

Landrigan, P.J., Markowitz, S.B., Nicholson, W.J., & Baker, B.D. (1995). Cancer prevention in the workplace. In P. Greenwald, B.S. Kramer, & D.L. Weed (Eds.), *Cancer prevention and control* (pp. 393–410). New York, NY: Marcel Dekker.

Levine, A.J. (1995). Tumor suppressor genes. *Science and Medicine, 2*(1), 28–37.

Linden, H.M., Reisch, L.M., Hart, A., Harrington, M.A., Nakano, C., Jackson, J.C., & Elmore, J.G. (2007). Attitudes toward participation in breast cancer randomized clinical trials in the African American community: A focus group study. *Cancer Nursing, 30,* 261–269. doi:10.1097/01.NCC.0000281732.02738.31

Lusk, B. (2005). Prelude to specialization: US cancer nursing, 1920–50. *Nursing Inquiry, 12,* 269–277. doi:10.1111/j.1440-1800.2005.00296.x

Maliski, S.L., Connor, S.E., Williams, L., & Litwin, M.S. (2010). Faith among low-income, African American Black men treated for prostate cancer. *Cancer Nursing, 33,* 470–478. doi:10.1097/NCC.0b013e3181e1f7ff

Margolies, L. (2012, March 7). "Everyone" doesn't always mean me. Retrieved from http://www.huffingtonpost.com/liz-margolies-lcsw/lgbt-cancer_b_1322293.html

McKee, D. (1946). Visiting nurse society and cancer patient. *Public Health Nursing, 38,* 155–157.

Meghani, S.H., & Houldin, A.D. (2007). The meanings of and attitudes about cancer pain among African Americans. *Oncology Nursing Forum, 34,* 1179–1186. doi:10.1188/07.ONF.1179-1186

Minority Health and Health Disparities Research and Education Act, United States Publ. L. No. 106–525 (2000), p. 2498.

National Cancer Institute. (2010a). *Cancer trends progress report: 2009/ 2010 update.* Retrieved from http://progressreport.cancer.gov

National Cancer Institute. (2010b). The nation's investment in cancer research: Connecting the nation's cancer community. Retrieved from http://www.cancer.gov/PublishedContent/Files/aboutnci/budget_planning_leg/plan-archives/nci_2011_plan.pdf

National Cancer Institute. (2011). Atlas of cancer mortality in the United States. Retrieved from http://www3.cancer.gov/atlasplus

National Center for Health Statistics. (2011). *Health, United States, 2010: With special feature on death and dying.* Hyattsville, MD: U.S. Department of Health and Human Services, Centers for Disease Control and Prevention, National Center for Health Statistics. Retrieved from http://www.cdc.gov/nchs/hus.htm

National LGBT Cancer Network. (2011, February 5). The LGBT community's disproportionate cancer burden. Retrieved from http://www.cancer-network.org/cancer_information/cancer_and_the_lgbt_community/the_lgbt_communitys_disproportionate_cancer_burden.php

Parchment, Y.D. (2004). Prostate cancer screening in African American and Caribbean males: Detriment in delay. *Association of Black Nursing Faculty Journal, 15,* 116–120.

Peterson, R.I. (1948). Public health nursing in the cancer control program of the U.S. Public Health Service. *Public Health Nursing, 40,* 74–77.

Powe, B.D., & Cooper, D.L. (2008). Self-reported cancer screening rates versus medical record documentation: Incongruence, specificity, and sensitivity for African American women. *Oncology Nursing Forum, 35,* 199–204. doi:10.1188/08.ONF.199-204

Powe, B.D., & Finnie, R. (2004). Knowledge of oral cancer risk factors among African Americans: Do nurses have a role? *Oncology Nursing Forum, 31,* 785–791. doi:10.1188/04.ONF.785-791

Reifenstein, K. (2007). Care-seeking behaviors of African American women with breast cancer symptoms. *Research in Nursing and Health, 30,* 542–557. doi:10.1002/nur.20246

Rettig, R.A. (1977). *Cancer crusade: The story of the National Cancer Act of 1971.* Princeton, NJ: Princeton University.

Royak-Schaler, R., Passmore, S.R., Gadalla, S., Hoy, M.K., Zhan, M., Tkaczuk, K, ... Hutchison, A.P. (2008). Exploring patient-physician communication in breast cancer care for African American women following primary treatment. *Oncology Nursing Forum, 35,* 836–843. doi:10.1188/08. ONF.836-843

Russell, K.M., Perkins, S.M., Zollinger, T.W., & Champion, V.L. (2006). Sociocultural context of mammography screening use. *Oncology Nursing Forum, 33,* 105–112. doi:10.1188/06.ONF.105-112

Siegel, R., Naishadham, D., & Jemal, A. (2012). Cancer statistics, 2012. *CA: A Cancer Journal for Clinicians, 62,* 10–29. doi:10.3322/caac.20138

Singh, G.K., Miller, B.A., Hankey, B.F., & Edwards, B.K. (2003). *Area socioeconomic variations in U.S. cancer incidence, mortality, stage, treatment, and survival, 1975–1999.* Retrieved from http://seer.cancer .gov/publications/ses

Smedley, B.D., Stith, A.Y., & Nelson, A.R. (2003). *Unequal treatment: Confronting racial and ethnic disparities in healthcare.* Washington, DC: National Academies Press.

Smith, R.A., Cokkinides, V., Brooks, D., Saslow, D., Shah, M., & Brawley, O.W. (2011). Cancer screening in the United States, 2011: A review of current ACS guidelines and issues in cancer screening. *CA: A Cancer Journal for Clinicians, 61,* 8–30. doi:10.3322/caac.20096

Stebner, B. (2012, January 5). What to do when a transgender man needs his Pap smear? More OB/ GYNs become transgender friendly as awareness grows. *Daily Mail Online.* Retrieved from http:// www.dailymail.co.uk/news/article-2082909/What-transgender-man-needs-pap-smear-More-OB -GYNs-transgender-friendly-awareness-grows.html

Steele, S.K., & Porche, D.J. (2005). Testing the theory of planned behavior to predict mammography intention. *Nursing Research, 54,* 332–338. doi:10.1097/00006199-200509000-00007

Stein, C.J., & Colditz, G.A. (2004). Modifiable risk factors for cancer. *British Journal of Cancer, 90,* 299–303. doi:10.1038/sj.bjc.6601509

Strayer, M. (1945). Every nurse has a share in the war on cancer. *Trained Nurse Hospital Review, 115,* 321–323.

Strzelczyk, J.J., & Dignan, M.B. (2002). Disparities in adherence to recommended follow-up on screening mammography: Interaction of sociodemographic factors. *Ethnicity and Disease, 12,* 77–86.

Swinney, J.E. (2002). African Americans with cancer: The relationships among self-esteem, locus of control, and health perception. *Research in Nursing and Health, 25,* 371–382. doi:10.1002/nur.10050

Swinney, J.E., & Dobal, M.T. (2011). Older African American women's beliefs, attitudes, and behaviors about breast cancer. *Research in Gerontology Nursing, 4,* 9–18. doi:10.3928/19404921-20101207-01

Underwood, S.M., Richards, K., Bradley, P.K., & Robertson, E. (2008). Pilot study of the breast cancer experiences of African American women with a family history of breast cancer: Implications for nursing practice. *Association of Black Nursing Faculty Journal, 19,* 107–113.

U.S. Department of Health and Human Services. (1991). *Healthy people 2000: National health promotion and disease prevention objectives.* Washington, DC: Author.

U.S. Department of Health and Human Services Office of Disease Prevention and Health Promotion. (2009). *Developing healthy people 2020: The road ahead.* Washington, DC: Author.

Ward, E., Jemal, A., & Cokkinides, V. (2004). Cancer disparities by race/ethnicity and socioeconomic status. *CA: A Cancer Journal for Clinicians, 54,* 78–93. doi:10.3322/canjclin.54.2.78

Weinberg, R.A. (1996). How cancer arises. *Scientific American, 275,* 62–70. doi:10.1038/scientific american0996-62

Weinrich, S.P., Weinrich, M.C., Priest, J., & Fodi, C. (2003). Self-reported reasons men decide not to participate in free prostate cancer screening [Online exclusive]. *Oncology Nursing Forum, 30,* E12–E16. doi:10.1188/03.ONF.E12-E16

Welch, C., Miller, C.W., & James, N.T. (2008). Sociodemographic and health-related determinants of breast and cervical cancer screening behavior, 2005. *Journal of Obstetric, Gynecologic, and Neonatal Nursing, 37,* 51–57. doi:10.1111/j.1552-6909.2007.00190.x

Wood, R.Y., Duffy, M.E., Morris, S.J., & Carnes, J.E. (2002). The effect of an educational intervention on promoting breast self-examination in older African American and Caucasian women. *Oncology Nursing Forum, 29,* 1081–1090. doi:10.1188/02.ONF.1081-1090

CHAPTER 15

Cancer Care and Informatics

Sookyung Hyun, DNSc, RN

Introduction

In *Crossing the Quality Chasm*, the Institute of Medicine (IOM, 2001) sketched out 10 rules for redesigning healthcare delivery in the United States. The rules include responsive healthcare systems (not only for in-person visits, but also for other venues, such as the Internet and phone), customized care, patients as the source of control, knowledge and information sharing with patients, evidence-based decision making, reducing risk and ensuring safety, care transparency, anticipating patient needs, judicious use of resources and patients' time, and care cooperation among clinicians and institutions (IOM, 2001). In this context, electronic health records (EHRs) and adoption of health information technology (HIT) have been imperative to support improved health care and reduced costs.

In response to these needs, the Office of the National Coordinator for Healthcare Information Technology was established to promote the adoption of HIT and nationwide health information exchange. The American Recovery and Reinvestment Act, the Health Information Technology Act of 2009, and the Centers for Medicare and Medicaid Services Electronic Health Record Incentive Program require healthcare providers to adopt and use EHR meaningfully (Centers for Medicare and Medicaid Services, 2011). In this context, the HIT adoption in care settings offers various opportunities for oncology nurses throughout the continuum of cancer care. The following sections include an overview of health informatics, methods useful for guiding nurses in the application of informatics knowledge, HIT for the care of patients with cancer, and example informatics applications with special emphasis on the area of oncology nursing.

Overview of Health Informatics

Health informatics is the discipline that deals with health data, information, and knowledge—how they are collected, stored, retrieved, processed, and used for the advancement of health care. This section introduces several major topics in informatics, such as EHRs, electronic personal health records (e-PHRs), mobile health (mHealth), and data sharing.

Electronic Health Records

EHRs are defined as

> a longitudinal electronic record of patient health information
> generated by one or more encounters in any care delivery setting.
> Included in this information are patient demographics, progress
> notes, problems, medications, vital signs, past medical history,
> immunizations, laboratory data and radiology reports. The EHR
> automates and streamlines the clinician's workflow. The EHR
> has the ability to generate a complete record of a clinical patient
> encounter—as well as supporting other care-related activities directly
> or indirectly via interface—including evidence-based decision
> support, quality management, and outcomes reporting. (Healthcare
> Information and Management Systems Society, 2011, para. 1)

The use of EHR systems contributes to the improvement of health care by accumulating a body of evidence, increasing efficiency and quality of documentation, boosting patient safety and quality of care, and supporting clinical trials (Barretto et al., 2003; Björvell, Wredling, & Thorell-Ekstrand, 2002; Butte, Weinstein, & Kohane, 2000; Cooper, 2004; Embi et al., 2005; Moody, Slocumb, Berg, & Jackson, 2004; Robles, 2009; Tange, Hasman, de Vries Robbé, & Schouten, 1997; Vahabzadeh, Lin, Mezghanni, Contoreggi, & Leff, 2007).

Nurses are recognized as major patient data collectors and users of EHRs because they provide 24-hour patient care and coordinate the patient care that other clinicians provide (Currell & Urquhart, 2005). Nursing documentation is the record of the care planned and given to patients by professional nurses and reflects the nurses' accountability to patients (Voutilainen, Isola, & Muurinen, 2004). Nursing documentation has comprehensive roles: (a) to record patient status, (b) to communicate with other nurses or clinicians, (c) to monitor nursing practice, (d) to justify nursing interventions, and (e) to gain nursing knowledge (Southard & Frankel, 1989; Wood, 2001). Electronic nursing documentation systems in EHRs can support nurses in various ways, including providing nurses with a reminder of the specific data that need to be documented, supporting standardized assessment through the document templates, pulling information from past visits or previous shifts into current documents, and providing notification when interventions are missed (Bakken et al., 2008; Hyun, Johnson, Stetson, & Bakken, 2009; Johnson et al., 2008; Nahm & Poston, 2000). EHR use with clinical decision support systems can support patient safety and quality of care. For instance, EHR systems that have the capability of real-time clinical decision support for medication prescriptions can automatically alert clinicians to potential drug allergies, drug-drug interactions, and dosing errors. In addition, clinical decision support in EHRs can support preventive care, such as cancer screening and immunizations (Ngo-Metzger, Hayes, Chen, Cygan, & Garfield, 2010).

Electronic Personal Health Records

EHRs are created and managed by healthcare providers or institutions, whereas e-PHRs are managed by an individual. An e-PHR is

> a universally accessible, layperson comprehensible, lifelong tool
> for managing relevant health information, promoting health
> maintenance, and assisting with chronic disease management via

> an interactive, common data set of electronic health information and e-health tools. The e-PHR is owned, managed, and shared by the individual or his or her legal proxy(s) and must be secure to protect the privacy and confidentiality of the health information it contains. It is not a legal record unless so defined and is subject to various legal limitations. (Healthcare Information and Management Systems Society, 2007, p. 2)

E-PHRs include various features: online communication with care providers, appointment scheduling, and refill of medication prescriptions. E-PHRs can be a channel for sharing of EHRs, including test results when it is integrated into the EHR. In addition, e-PHRs can include the capability to import data from EHRs from multiple health institutions and can be the source of truth for an individual's record (Tang, Ash, Bates, Overhage, & Sands, 2006). Therefore, e-PHRs have the potential to benefit both patients and care providers. In terms of patients, e-PHRs can enhance communication with their care providers so that patients report problems and ask for advice to manage signs and symptoms at home. Decision support functionalities and educational functions included in an e-PHR system can empower patients so that they can engage in their care and manage their health conditions effectively. Particularly, educational tools can assist individuals with low health literacy using HIT, such as video animation and voice-over technology delivered in different languages (Hewitt, Greenfield, & Stovall, 2006; Ngo-Metzger et al., 2010; Tang et al., 2003, 2006). For care providers, e-PHRs can help to identify patient information needs, to monitor patients' health-related behaviors, and subsequently to support better clinical decisions for their patients (Tang et al., 2006).

Several research studies have been conducted on the design and development of e-PHR systems, including real-time detection and communication of adverse events during chemotherapy (Goldberg et al., 2002), symptom monitoring of chemotherapy toxicity using e-mail alerts (Basch et al., 2007), and Web-based home blood pressure monitoring with pharmacy care (Green et al., 2008).

Mobile Health

mHealth is defined as "mobile computing, medical sensor, and communications technologies for health care" (Istepanian, Jovanov, & Zhang, 2004, p. 405). Mobile technology provides individuals with ubiquitous access to multimedia resources on the Web, such as social networking sites (e.g., wikis, blogs), video sharing sites, e-mails, and text messaging. In addition, mobile devices make it easier to get health information, as mobile phones are easy to use for individuals who are less familiar with technology.

Smartphones offer more advanced computing ability and connectivity than basic phones, and the added features make them ideal for health information access. They have various capabilities, such as global positioning systems (GPSs), mobile access to the Internet, multimedia systems, and motion sensors. The percentage of Americans who own smartphones has increased from 15% in 2006 to 42% in 2009 (Carton & Crumrine, 2010). A quarter of smartphone owners use their phone rather than a computer when they go online; one-third of these people do not have a high-speed broadband connection (Smith, 2011). Clinicians' adoption of smartphones is increasing; for instance, 64% of physicians used smartphones in 2009, but an estimated 81% of physicians will use smartphones by 2012 (Manhattan Research, 2009). No information is available to show nurses' use of smartphones.

To date, thousands of healthcare applications (often referred to as "apps") and software programs have been developed and are available for healthcare consumers and professionals. In terms of health applications for nurses, applications can be categorized into several groups: references (e.g., anatomy, drugs, laboratory tests, nursing diagnosis handbook); calculators; medical dictionary, terminology, and abbreviations; and others (Handel, 2011; Phillippi & Wyatt, 2011).

Research studies on the application of mobile technology are growing in oncology care, such as the health outcome monitoring system for patients with cancer using mobile phones (Bielli et al., 2004) and mobile phone–based management of chemotherapy-related toxicity (Maguire, McCann, Miller, & Kearney, 2008; McCann, Maguire, Miller, & Kearney, 2009), as well as a number of research studies in other areas of care, such as reminders for wearing sunscreen using text messaging (Armstrong et al., 2009) and mobile behavioral coaching for patients with diabetes at primary care settings (Quinn et al., 2011). mHealth supports health promotion and health monitoring by making resources available to care providers and patients/consumers at the right time and expands communications between care providers and their patients by providing various types of voice, text, and video messages (Blake, 2008; Istepanian et al., 2004). Consequently, this ubiquitous health technology can serve underserved people with fewer resources (Akter & Ray, 2010).

Data Sharing

The National Cancer Institute Cancer Bioinformatics Grid (caBIG®) is a national network of cancer research and care in the United States. caBIG connects researchers and cancer centers to facilitate more effective and efficient research discoveries for cancer care by sharing data and resources. The network platform of caBIG is called caGrid (or the Grid). The Grid provides secure connection of caBIG resources across the network. The caBIG resources include sharable tools, database technologies, and Web-based applications for clinical trials management and life science. The tools are developed based on open-source software and are publicly available (National Cancer Institute, n.d.). In addition, caBIG is connected to international networks, such as the Oncology Information Exchange (ONIX) in the United Kingdom. The UK National Cancer Research Institute (NCRI) Informatics Initiative (n.d.) developed ONIX to support the use and sharing of data and information in cancer research by connecting resources through one Internet portal. The resources include biomedical databases, cancer research publications, data analysis tools, and research technologies. caBIG resources and tools can assist oncology nurses in providing quality care for patients with cancer by finding and sharing best practice and patient outcomes and gaining knowledge from their practice (Ozbolt & Saba, 2008).

Informatics Methods

Given the desire to deliver evidence-based care, decisions about care should be made based on evidence. Evidence can be generated and applied using informatics methods that facilitate knowledge discovery from large amounts of data, automatic data capture from EHRs, and representation of the data and information in a manner that both humans and computers can understand for further processing and sharing among different health institutions and EHR systems. In this section, such informatics methods are introduced.

Data Mining

Quality improvement, patient outcomes, and healthcare costs are more important in health care than ever. In order to understand features of care and the impact on patient outcomes, comprehensive analysis of patient data and information is desired (Hertelendy, Fenton, & Griffin, 2010; Hesse, Hanna, Massett, & Hesse, 2010). Data analysis and data mining have become more important in building nursing knowledge from large databases and promoting discovery of evidence for best practices (Berger & Berger, 2004; Goodwin, VanDyne, Lin, & Talbert, 2003; Lee & Abbott, 2003). Statistical techniques, such as logistic regression, are conventional methods that are widely used in prediction modeling to identify significant variables and construct predictive models. When compared to these classical statistical techniques, data mining techniques such as decision trees and artificial neural networks have shown to have higher prediction capabilities in classification and prediction modeling in nonlinear data relationships (Kurt, Ture, & Kurum, 2008; Liew et al., 2007; Mullins et al., 2006; Worachartcheewan, Nantasenamat, Isarankura-Na-Ayudhya, Pidetcha, & Prachayasittikul, 2010). In addition, these methods have demonstrated better performance on heterogeneous data from various sources in EHRs (Brickley, Shepherd, & Armstrong, 1998; Ellenius & Groth, 2008; Lin, Lee, Lu, & Hsu, 2006; Ridinger & Rice, 2000; Tabaton et al., 2010).

Several nurse researchers have used data mining to study various areas, including prediction of birth outcomes (Goodwin & Iannacchione, 2002), detection of older adult patients with impaired mobility (Lu, Street, & Delaney, 2006), knowledge discovery regarding urinary and bowel incontinence (Westra et al., 2011), infection prevention and patient outcomes (Park, Park, Kim, Park, & Kwon, 2006), health service use in patients with chronic conditions (Madigan & Curet, 2006), classification of smokers (Poynton & McDaniel, 2006), fall prediction (Volrathongchai, Brennan, & Ferris, 2005), and risk factor identification (Lee et al., 2011). In cancer care, research studies concerning the predictions of relapse in children with acute lymphoblastic leukemia (Podraza & Podraza, 1999), postoperative complications in patients with gastric cancer (Chien et al., 2008), classification of high-risk children with acute lymphoblastic leukemia (Pedreira, Macrini, Land, & Costa, 2009), and needs-based patient classifications for nurse staffing (Seomun, Chang, Lee, Kim, & Park, 2006) applied data mining techniques. These research studies have shown the potential for data mining as a useful method for knowledge discovery in nursing.

Natural Language Processing

Natural language processing (NLP) techniques provide a method for data capture from narratives (i.e., free text data) and create structured reports for further computer processing (Friedman, 2000). NLP techniques have shown high accuracy, sensitivity, and specificity in extracting specific clinical information from various types of clinical notes, such as discharge summaries, x-ray reports, mammograms, and visit notes in health care (Barrows, Busuioc, & Friedman, 2000; Friedman, Knirsch, Shagina, & Hripcsak, 1999; Jain & Friedman, 1997). Additionally, NLP demonstrated a real-time decision support for community-acquired pneumonia guided by specific radiology findings (Fiszman & Haug, 2000). Interestingly, when comparing nurses' narratives to physicians' narratives, nurses had a tendency to be more descriptive, whereas physicians had a tendency to be more summarizing (Hyun, Bakken, Friedman, & Johnson, 2003, 2004).

In the domain of nursing research, several researchers have applied NLP. For example, Hyun, Johnson, and Bakken (2009) captured patient safety and quality measures from oncology nursing progress notes. Hseih, Hardardttir, and Brennan (2004) extracted patterns of terms from e-mail messages. Frisch and Frisch (2011) identified nursing diagnoses from narrative nursing notes. Baldwin (2008) used NLP to support data retrieval and coding of breast cancer screening. In addition, natural language expressions of nursing-related concepts could be mapped to standard terminologies using NLP (Ravvaz et al., 2008). The International Organization for Standardization reference terminology models appear to be applicable for NLP (Bakken, Hyun, Friedman, & Johnson, 2005). NLP can also contribute to the availability of nursing data and information in EHRs for reuse in clinical decision support and patient outcomes research (Hyun, Johnson, & Bakken, 2009).

Human Factors

Design is a critical aspect for adoption and implementation of HIT systems. A human factors, or human-computer interaction (HCI), approach is to design systems in a manner that amplifies human strength in ergonomic and cognitive areas (Hesse et al., 2010; Johnson & Turley, 2006). HCI has influenced the design of user-friendly systems (Nielsen, 1993; Norman & Draper, 1986; Rinkus et al., 2005; Rubin, 1994). Examples of underlying principles in design from an HCI perspective are that the presentation order of information on the screen should be consistent with the order in which a nurse documents patient information and that information is more easily followed and remembered when the related data elements are aggregated on the computer screen (Gadd, Baskaran, & Lobach, 1998; Jaspers, Steen, van den Bos, & Geenen, 2004; Johnson & Turley, 2006).

People who design systems that support healthcare services need to have an understanding of the actual nature of care to avoid issues with user acceptance and use, user frustration, user errors, and user training, which are often related to the difference between the users' and the system designers' mental images of a system (Johnson, Johnson, & Zhang, 2005; Lundgren & Wisser, 1997; Nemeth, Nunnally, O'Connor, Klock, & Cook, 2005; Rose et al., 2005; Staggers, Kobus, & Brown, 2007; Zhang, 2005). Nurses have been engaged in developing EHR systems over past decades, initially beginning with involvement in a project team and participating in usability testing (Dix, Finlay, Abowd, & Beale, 2004; Lundgren & Wisser, 1997; Nelson, 2007). Hardiker and Bakken (2004) specified a set of requirements particularly focused on nursing data entry for EHRs. User-centered approaches can provide an opportunity to gain better understanding of an EHR system through an exploration of users' practice and tasks (Currell & Urquhart, 2003; Hyun, Johnson, Stetson, & Bakken, 2009; Moody et al., 2004). For instance, some questions cannot be answered until the characteristics of nursing documentation have been fully articulated, such as nurses' preferences for methods of electronic documentation and of clinical data and where different types of data are documented. The understanding of how nursing care is processed and documented is useful to help system designers understand the activities that should be supported by the system and identify why the systems do not work well (Martin & Sommerville, 2004; Xiao, 2005). In addition, HCI design approaches can support user efficiency and productivity, increase user satisfaction and adoption, and decrease user training costs and medical errors (Norman & Draper, 1986; Rinkus et al., 2005; Zhang, 2005).

For example, HCI design looks at whether the system is easy to navigate, easy to use, easy to learn, and easy to remember.

Informatics Applications for Oncology Care

This section introduces some informatics applications related to cancer care. Kim and colleagues (2006) demonstrated that a computerized provider order entry (CPOE) reduced errors in medication processes for pediatric chemotherapy. The research team designed and implemented their CPOE with special emphasis on a number of functions to prevent human errors in prescribing medication, such as embedded calculators, drop-down medication lists to avoid handwritten spelling errors, and pop-up alerts to enforce completion of necessary data fields. Similarly, Collins and Elsaid (2011) demonstrated an oral chemotherapy CPOE had the potential to reduce prescribing errors, including chemotherapy medication errors and adverse drug events rate. WebChoice, a Web-based support system for patients with cancer, was developed in Norway. The system included various functionalities, such as assessment and self-management intervention, information, communication, and diary sections. In a randomized clinical trial, it showed a potential to help patients better deal with their health (Andersen & Ruland, 2009; Ruland et al., 2007). Hong, Kim, Lee, and Kim (2009) developed a PDA-based home hospice information system in Korea. The system was based on the 2005 *Guidelines for Cancer Patient Management Program of the Ministry of Health and Welfare of Korea* and was able to be integrated into a home hospice service using wired or wireless technology. In a trial with visiting nurses, the system resulted in saving recording time. They anticipated the system could help nurses more effectively manage patient information and improve the quality of point-of-care.

Advanced practice nurses used an information system, called a computerized clinical information system (CCIS), to record patient care in rural areas. The CCIS supported care management and communication of patient status in a timely manner (Yancey, Given, White, DeVoss, & Coyle, 1998). Jung and Lee (2006) developed a standard nursing terminology–based nursing information system for patients with gastric cancer. Im and Chee (2011) designed a decision support system using fuzzy logic for cancer pain management. *Fuzzy logic* is a computational method that provides a manner to reach a conclusion based on imprecise input information. A collaborative project, called Workflow Information Systems for European Nursing Care (WISECARE), was initiated to improve cancer nursing practice and patient outcomes across Europe through HIT. WISECARE used clinical nursing data from collaborating institutions to quantify factors for patient care and nursing practice, including patient populations, patient outcomes, care variability, and nursing resources across Europe. The project demonstrated the impact of nursing informatics on nursing knowledge management through the integration and use of information technology (Kearney, Miller, Sermeus, Hoy, & Vanhaecht, 2000).

Informatics and Nursing Education

Advances in the Internet and information and communication technologies have created new opportunities for nursing education and practitioner training (e.g., vodcast [delivering video files] support for independent learning and mobile access to resources supporting critical thinking and problem solving) (Cimino & Bakken, 2005). This section describes examples of nursing education using applied informatics, particularly through virtual and mobile technologies.

Second Life® is a Web-based virtual world developed by Linden Lab of San Francisco, California. The virtual world imitates the real world. The user of Second Life is represented by an avatar (a three-dimensional graphic) in the virtual world. Users maneuver their avatar to visit different virtual environments, called "islands," and they have experiences that may or may not be possible in real life (Wood & McPhee, 2011). Second Life was originally developed for social networking; however, it is being explored and used for healthcare professional education, including nursing and medicine (Ahern & Wink, 2010; Hansen, 2008; Hansen, Murray, & Erdley, 2009). In nursing, a clinical scenarios–based virtual lab was created in Second Life to support students in learning clinical skills, such as analytic interpretation of clinical findings and application of interventions based on the analysis (Phillips, Shaw, Sullivan, & Johnson, 2010).

Additionally, virtual technologies have been applied to various areas of nursing education, such as use of virtual patients for development of students' clinical reasoning skills, decision-making and prescribing skills, and virtual internships for community nursing practice (Forsberg, Georg, Ziegert, & Fors, 2011; Hurst & Marks-Maran, 2011; Ward & Killian, 2011).

Mobile technologies enable user access to information resources in a timely manner, including Web-based resources and clinically relevant applications (Cimino & Bakken, 2005). Many nursing students and practitioners already use mobile devices for personal, educational, or job purposes (Phillippi & Wyatt, 2011). Nursing students record their clinical encounters in real time; view reference materials, online textbooks, or guidelines; and communicate with their instructor using e-mail and text messaging. An informatics approach using these mobile technologies has been integrated into nursing curricula and evaluated in many aspects, such as utility (Lee & Bakken, 2008), usefulness (Bakken et al., 2006), informatics competencies (Bakken, Cook, Curtis, Soupios, & Curran, 2003; Cibulka & Crane-Wider, 2011; Desjardins, Cook, Jenkins, & Bakken, 2005), student learning retention (Greenfield, 2011), and learning evidence-based practice for patient safety (Bakken et al., 2004; Currie et al., 2007).

Conclusion

This chapter has introduced a number of informatics components, such as EHR, e-PHR, mHealth, caBIG and the Grid, and informatics methods that can support data acquisition, representation, and sharing. In the rapidly changing healthcare environment, informatics is essential for supporting oncology nursing research, practice, and education. In EHRs, nursing data and information can be available to be used for multiple purposes, such as cancer care and outcomes research, generating evidence for oncology nursing practice, clinical decision support systems, and discovery of new knowledge. Patients with cancer can access their health records, and data can be shared between the patient and the care provider through EHRs and e-PHRs. Furthermore, e-PHRs have the potential to empower patients so that they can proactively participate in their care decisions and better manage their health. Mobile technologies can support cancer care and create a multitude of educational opportunities and strategies for nursing students and practitioners.

Oncology nursing should pioneer the application of informatics knowledge and methods to expand the body of knowledge for cancer care, transform the knowledge into practice, and prepare nursing students to practice in a variety of informatics-intensive healthcare settings.

References

Ahern, N., & Wink, D. (2010). Virtual learning environments: Second life. *Nurse Educator, 35,* 225–227. doi:10.1097/NNE.0b013e3181f7e943

Akter, S., & Ray, P. (2010). mHealth—An ultimate platform to serve the unserved. *Yearbook of Medical Informatics, 2010,* 94–100.

Andersen, T., & Ruland, C.M. (2009). Cancer patients' questions and concerns expressed in an online nurse-delivered mail service: Preliminary results. *Studies in Health Technology and Informatics, 146,* 149–153. doi:10.3233/978-1-60750-024-7-149

Armstrong, A.W., Watson, A.J., Makredes, M., Frangos, J.E., Kimball, A.B., & Kvedar, J.C. (2009). Text-message reminders to improve sunscreen use: A randomized, controlled trial using electronic monitoring. *Archives of Dermatology, 145,* 1230–1236. doi:10.1001/archdermatol.2009.269

Bakken, S., Cook, S.S., Curtis, L., Desjardins, K., Hyun, S., Jenkins, M., ... Soupios, M. (2004). Promoting patient safety through informatics-based nursing education. *International Journal of Medical Informatics, 73,* 581–589. doi:10.1016/j.ijmedinf.2004.04.008

Bakken, S., Cook, S.S., Curtis, L., Soupios, M., & Curran, C. (2003). Informatics competencies pre- and post-implementation of a Palm-based student clinical log and informatics for evidence-based practice curriculum. *AMIA Annual Symposium Proceedings, 2003,* 41–45. Retrieved from http://www.ncbi.nlm.nih.gov/pmc/articles/PMC1480072/?tool=pubmed

Bakken, S., Currie, L.M., Lee, N.J., Roberts, W.D., Collins, S.A., & Cimino, J.J. (2008). Integrating evidence into clinical information systems for nursing decision support. *International Journal of Medical Informatics, 77,* 413–420. doi:10.1016/j.ijmedinf.2007.08.006

Bakken, S., Hyun, S., Friedman, C., & Johnson, S.B. (2005). ISO reference terminology models for nursing: Applicability for natural language processing of nursing narratives. *International Journal of Medical Informatics, 74,* 615–622. doi:10.1016/j.ijmedinf.2005.01.002

Bakken, S., Jenkins, M., Choi, J., Hyun, S., John, R., Joyce, M., ... Soupios, M. (2006). Usefulness of a personal digital assistant-based advanced practice nursing student clinical log: Faculty stakeholder exemplars. *Studies in Health Technology and Informatics, 122,* 698–702.

Baldwin, K.B. (2008). Evaluating healthcare quality using natural language processing. *Journal for Healthcare Quality, 30*(4), 24–29.

Barretto, S., Warren, J., Goodchild, A., Bird, L., Heard, S., & Stumptner, M. (2003). Linking guidelines to electronic health record design for improved chronic disease management. *AMIA Annual Symposium Proceedings, 2003,* 66–70. Retrieved from http://www.ncbi.nlm.nih.gov/pmc/articles/PMC1480104/?tool=pubmed

Barrows, R.C., Jr., Busuioc, M., & Friedman, C. (2000). Limited parsing of notational text visit notes: Ad-hoc vs. NLP approaches. *AMIA Annual Symposium Proceedings, 2000,* 51–55. Retrieved from http://www.ncbi.nlm.nih.gov/pmc/articles/PMC2243829/?tool=pubmed

Basch, E., Artz, D., Iasonos, A., Speakman, J., Shannon, K., Lin, K., ... Schrag, D. (2007). Evaluation of an online platform for cancer patient self-reporting of chemotherapy toxicities. *Journal of the American Medical Informatics Association, 14,* 264–268. doi:10.1197/jamia.M2177

Berger, A.M., & Berger, C.R. (2004). Data mining as a tool for research and knowledge development in nursing. *CIN: Computers, Informatics, Nursing, 22,* 123–131.

Bielli, E., Carminati, F., La Capra, S., Lina, M., Brunelli, C., & Tamburini, M. (2004). A wireless health outcomes monitoring system (WHOMS): Development and field testing with cancer patients using mobile phones. *BMC Medical Informatics and Decision Making, 15*(4), 7. doi:10.1186/1472-6947-4-7

Björvell, C., Wredling, R., & Thorell-Ekstrand, I. (2002). Long-term increase in quality of nursing documentation: Effects of a comprehensive intervention. *Scandinavian Journal of Caring Sciences, 16,* 34–42. doi:10.1046/j.1471-6712.2002.00049.x

Blake, H. (2008). Innovation in practice: Mobile phone technology in patient care. *British Journal of Community Nursing, 13,* 160, 162–165.

Brickley, M.R., Shepherd, J.P., & Armstrong, R.A. (1998). Neural networks: A new technique for development of decision support systems in dentistry. *Journal of Dentistry, 26,* 305–309. doi:10.1016/S0300-5712(97)00027-4

Butte, A., Weinstein, D., & Kohane, I. (2000). Enrolling patients into clinical trials faster using RealTime Recruiting. *AMIA Annual Symposium Proceedings, 2000,* 111–115. Retrieved from http://www.ncbi.nlm.nih.gov/pmc/articles/PMC2244056/?tool=pubmed

Carton, P., & Crumrine, J. (2010, January 10). New survey shows Android OS roiling the smart phone market. Retrieved from http://www.changewaveresearch.com/articles/2010/01/smart_phone_20100104.html

Centers for Medicare and Medicaid Services. (2011, December 5). Overview. Retrieved from http://www.cms.gov/ehrincentiveprograms

Chien, C.W., Lee, Y.C., Ma, T., Lee, T.S., Lin, Y.C., Wang, W., & Lee, W.J. (2008). The application of artificial neural networks and decision tree model in predicting post-operative complication for gastric cancer patients. *Hepato-Gastroenterology, 55,* 1140–1145.

Cibulka, N., & Crane-Wider, L. (2011). Introducing personal digital assistants to enhance nursing education in undergraduate and graduate nursing programs. *Journal of Nursing Education, 50,* 115–118. doi:10.3928/01484834-20101230-07

Cimino, J.J., & Bakken, S. (2005). Personal digital educators. *New England Journal of Medicine, 352,* 860–862. doi:10.1056/NEJMp048149

Collins, C.M., & Elsaid, K.A. (2011). Using an enhanced oral chemotherapy computerized provider order entry system to reduce prescribing errors and improve safety. *International Journal for Quality in Health Care, 23,* 36–43. doi:10.1093/intqhc/mzq066

Cooper, J.D. (2004). Organization, management, implementation and value of EHR implementation in a solo pediatric practice. *Journal of Healthcare Information Management, 18,* 51–55.

Currell, R., & Urquhart, C. (2005). *Nursing record systems: Effects on nursing practice and health care outcomes* (Vol. 2005). Hoboken, NJ: Cochrane Database of Systematic Reviews.

Currie, L.M., Desjardins, K.S., Stone, P.W., Lai, T., Schwartz, E., Schnall, R., & Bakken, S. (2007). Near-miss and hazard reporting: Promoting mindfulness in patient safety education. In K.A. Kuhn, J.R. Warren, & T.Y. Leong (Eds.), *Medinfo 2007: Proceedings of the 12th World Congress on Health (Medical) Informatics* (Vol. 129, Pt. 1, pp. 285–290). Amsterdam, Netherlands: IOS Press.

Desjardins, K.S., Cook, S.S., Jenkins, M., & Bakken, S. (2005). Effect of an informatics for evidence-based practice curriculum on nursing informatics competencies. *International Journal of Medical Informatics, 74,* 1012–1020.

Dix, A., Finlay, J., Abowd, G.D., & Beale, R. (2004). *Human-computer interaction* (3rd ed.). Essex, England: Pearson Education.

Ellenius, J., & Groth, T. (2008). Dynamic decision support graph—Visualization of ANN-generated diagnostic indications of pathological conditions developing over time. *Artificial Intelligence in Medicine, 42,* 189–198.

Embi, P.J., Jain, A., Clark, J., Bizjack, S., Hornung, R., & Harris, C.M. (2005). Effect of a clinical trial alert system on physician participation in trial recruitment. *Archives of Internal Medicine, 165,* 2272–2277. doi:10.1001/archinte.165.19.2272

Fiszman, M., & Haug, P.J. (2000). Using medical language processing to support real-time evaluation of pneumonia guideline. *AMIA Annual Symposium Proceedings, 2000,* 235–239. Retrieved from http://www.ncbi.nlm.nih.gov/pmc/articles/PMC2244071/?tool=pubmed

Forsberg, E., Georg, C., Ziegert, K., & Fors, U. (2011). Virtual patients for assessment of clinical reasoning in nursing—A pilot study. *Nurse Education Today, 31,* 757–762. doi:10.1016/j.nedt.2010.11.015

Friedman, C. (2000). A broad coverage natural language processing system. *AMIA Annual Symposium Proceedings, 2000,* 270–274. Retrieved from http://www.ncbi.nlm.nih.gov/pmc/articles/PMC2243979/?tool=pubmed

Friedman, C., Knirsch, C.A., Shagina, L., & Hripcsak, G. (1999). Automating a severity score guideline for community-acquired pneumonia employing medical language processing of discharge summaries. *AMIA Annual Symposium Proceedings, 1999,* 256–260. Retrieved from http://www.ncbi.nlm.nih.gov/pmc/articles/PMC2232753/?tool=pubmed

Frisch, N., & Frisch, L. (2011). Application of language processing techniques to capture the use of nursing clinical terms from narrative statements: Report of a pilot study. *Studies in Health Technology and Informatics, 164,* 323–327.

Gadd, C.S., Baskaran, P., & Lobach, D.F. (1998). Identification of design features to enhance utilization and acceptance of systems for Internet-based decision support at the point of care. *AMIA*

Annual Symposium Proceedings, 1998, 91–95. Retrieved from http://www.ncbi.nlm.nih.gov/pmc/articles/PMC2232383/?tool=pubmed

Goldberg, R.M., Sargent, D.J., Morton, R.F., Mahoney, M.R., Krook, J.E., & O'Connell, M.J. (2002). Early detection of toxicity and adjustment of ongoing clinical trials: The history and performance of the North Central Cancer Treatment Group's real-time toxicity monitoring program. *Journal of Clinical Oncology, 20,* 4591–4596. doi:10.1200/JCO.2002.03.039

Goodwin, L.K., & Iannacchione, M.A. (2002). Data mining methods for improving birth outcomes prediction. *Outcomes Management, 6,* 80–85.

Goodwin, L., VanDyne, M., Lin, S., & Talbert, S. (2003). Data mining issues and opportunities for building nursing knowledge. *Journal of Biomedical Informatics, 36,* 379–388. doi:10.1016/j.bi.2003.09.020

Green, B.B., Cook, A.J., Ralston, J.D., Fishman, P.A., Catz, S.L., Carlson, J.D., ... Thompson, R.S. (2008). Effectiveness of home blood pressure monitoring, Web communication, and pharmacist care on hypertension control. *JAMA, 299,* 2857–2867. doi:10.1001/jama.299.24.2857

Greenfield, S. (2011). Podcasting: A new tool for student retention? *Journal of Nursing Education, 50,* 112–114. doi:10.3928/01484834-20101230-06

Handel, M.J. (2011). mHealth (mobile health)—Using apps for health and wellness. *Explore, 7,* 256–261. doi:10.1016/j.explore.2011.04.011

Hansen, M.M. (2008). Versatile, immersive, creative and dynamic virtual 3-D healthcare learning environments: A review of the literature. *Journal of Medical Internet Research, 10*(3), e26. doi:10.2196/jmir.1051

Hansen, M.M., Murray, P.J., & Erdley, W.S. (2009). The potential of 3-D virtual worlds in professional nursing education. *Studies in Health Technology and Informatics, 146,* 582–586.

Hardiker, N., & Bakken, S. (2004). Requirements of tools and techniques to support the entry of structured nursing data. In M. Fieschi, E. Coiera, & Y.C.J. Li (Eds.), *Medinfo 2004: Proceedings of the 11th World Congress on Medical Informatics* (Vol. 107, Pt. 1, pp. 621–625). Amsterdam, Netherlands: IOS Press.

Healthcare Information and Management Systems Society. (2007). HIMSS personal health records definition and position statement. Retrieved from http://www.himss.org/content/files/phrdefinition71707.pdf

Healthcare Information and Management Systems Society. (2011). EHR: Electronic health record. Retrieved from http://www.himss.org/ASP/topics_ehr.asp

Hertelendy, A., Fenton, S., & Griffin, D. (2010, Summer). The implications of health reform for health information and electronic health record implementation efforts. *Perspectives in Health Information Management, 7,* 1e. Retrieved from http://www.ncbi.nlm.nih.gov/pmc/articles/PMC2921303/?tool=pubmed

Hesse, B.W., Hanna, C., Massett, H.A., & Hesse, N.K. (2010). Outside the box: Will information technology be a viable intervention to improve the quality of cancer care? *Journal of the National Cancer Institute Monographs, 2010*(40), 81–89. doi:10.1093/jncimonographs/lgq004

Hewitt, M., Greenfield, S., & Stovall, E. (Eds.). (2006). *From cancer patient to cancer survivor: Lost in transition.* Retrieved from http://www.nap.edu/openbook.php?record_id=11468&page=1

Hong, H.S., Kim, I.K., Lee, S.H., & Kim, H.S. (2009). Adoption of a PDA-based home hospice care system for cancer patients. *CIN: Computers, Informatics, Nursing, 27,* 365–371. doi:10.1097/NCN.0b013e3181bcab43

Hsieh, Y., Hardardottir, G.A., & Brennan, P.F. (2004). Linguistic analysis: Terms and phrases used by patients in e-mail messages to nurses. In M. Fieschi, E. Coiera, & Y.C.J. Li (Eds.), *Medinfo 2004: Proceedings of the 11th World Congress on Medical Informatics* (Vol. 107, Pt. 1, pp. 511–515). Amsterdam, Netherlands: IOS Press.

Hurst, H.M., & Marks-Maran, D. (2011). Using a virtual patient activity to teach nurse prescribing. *Nurse Education in Practice, 11,* 192–198. doi:10.1016/j.nepr.2010.08.008

Hyun, S., Bakken, S., Friedman, C., & Johnson, S.B. (2003). Natural language processing challenges in HIV/AIDS clinic notes. *AMIA Annual Symposium Proceedings, 2003,* 872. Retrieved from http://www.ncbi.nlm.nih.gov/pmc/articles/PMC1480114/?tool=pubmed

Hyun, S., Bakken, S., Friedman, C., & Johnson, S. (2004). Natural language processing challenges in HIV/AIDS clinic notes. In M. Fieschi, E. Coiera, & Y.C.J. Li (Eds.), *Medinfo 2004: Proceedings of the 11th World Congress on Medical Informatics* (Vol. 107, Pt. 1, pp. 16–55). Amsterdam, Netherlands: IOS Press.

Hyun, S., Johnson, S.B., & Bakken, S. (2009). Exploring the ability of natural language processing to extract data from nursing narratives. *CIN: Computers, Informatics, Nursing, 27,* 215–223. doi:10.1097/NCN.0b013e3181a91b58

Hyun, S., Johnson, S., Stetson, P., & Bakken, S. (2009). Development and evaluation of nursing user interface screens using multiple methods. *Journal of Biomedical Informatics, 42,* 1004–1012. doi:10.1016/j.jbi.2009.05.005

Im, E.O., & Chee, W. (2011). The DSCP-CA: A decision support computer program—Cancer pain management. *CIN: Computers, Informatics, Nursing, 29,* 289–296. doi:10.1097/NCN.0b013e3181f9dd23

Institute of Medicine. (2001). *Crossing the quality chasm: A new health system for the 21st century.* Washington, DC: National Academies Press.

Istepanian, R.S.H., Jovanov, E., & Zhang, Y.T. (2004). Introduction to the special section on m-health: Beyond seamless mobility and global wireless health-care connectivity [Editorial]. *IEEE Transactions on Information Technology in Biomedicine, 8,* 405–414. doi:10.1109/TITB.2004.840019

Jain, N.L., & Friedman, C. (1997). Identification of findings suspicious for breast cancer based on natural language processing of mammogram reports. *AMIA Annual Symposium Proceedings, 1997,* 829–833. Retrieved from http://www.ncbi.nlm.nih.gov/pmc/articles/PMC2233320/?tool=pubmed

Jaspers, M.W., Steen, T., van den Bos, C., & Geenen, M. (2004). The think aloud method: A guide to user interface design. *International Journal of Medical Informatics, 73,* 781–795. doi:10.1016/j.ijmedinf.2004.08.003

Johnson, C.M., Johnson, T.R., & Zhang, J. (2005). A user-centered framework for redesigning health care interfaces. *Journal of Biomedical Informatics, 38,* 75–87. doi:10.1016/j.jbi.2004.11.005

Johnson, C.M., & Turley, J.P. (2006). The significance of cognitive modeling in building healthcare interfaces. *International Journal of Medical Informatics, 75,* 163–172. doi:10.1016/j.ijmedinf.2005.06.003

Johnson, S., Bakken, S., Dine, D., Hyun, S., Mendonça, E., Morrison, F., ... Stetson, P. (2008). An electronic health record based on structured narrative. *Journal of the American Medical Informatics Association, 15,* 54–64. doi:10.1197/jamia.M2131

Jung, K.I., & Lee, B.S. (2006). Development of the nursing information system based on the standardized nursing language system for gastric cancer patients. *Studies in Health Technology and Informatics, 122,* 109–111.

Kearney, N., Miller, M., Sermeus, W., Hoy, D., & Vanhaecht, K. (2000). Multicentre research and the WISECARE experience. Workflow Information Systems for European Nursing Care. *Journal of Advanced Nursing, 32,* 999–1007. doi:10.1046/j.1365-2648.2000.t01-1-01566.x

Kim, G.R., Chen, A.R., Arceci, R.J., Mitchell, S.H., Kokoszka, K.M., Daniel, D., & Lehmann, C.U. (2006). Error reduction in pediatric chemotherapy: Computerized order entry and failure modes and effects analysis. *Archives of Pediatric and Adolescent Medicine, 160,* 495–498. doi:10.1001/archpedi.160.5.495

Kurt, I., Ture, M., & Kurum, A. (2008). Comparing performances of logistic regression, classification and regression tree, and neural networks for predicting coronary artery disease. *Expert Systems With Applications, 34,* 366–374. doi:10.1016/j.eswa.2006.09.004

Lee, N.J., & Bakken, S. (2008). Utility of a PDA-based advanced practice nurse student clinical log to detect possible diagnostic errors related to hypertension management. *AMIA Annual Symposium Proceedings, 2008,* 1020.

Lee, S.M., & Abbott, P.A. (2003). Bayesian networks for knowledge discovery in large datasets: Basics for nurse researchers. *Journal of Biomedical Informatics, 36,* 389–399. doi:10.1016/j.jbi.2003.09.022

Lee, T.T., Liu, C.Y., Kuo, Y.H., Mills, M.E., Fong, J.G., & Hung, C. (2011). Application of data mining to the identification of critical factors in patient falls using a Web-based reporting system. *International Journal of Medical Informatics, 80,* 141–150. doi:10.1016/j.ijmedinf.2010.10.009

Liew, P.L., Lee, Y.C., Lin, Y.C., Lee, T.S., Lee, W.J., Wang, W., & Chien, C.W. (2007). Comparison of artificial neural networks with logistic regression in prediction of gallbladder disease among obese patients. *Digestive and Liver Disease, 39,* 356–362. doi:10.1016/j.dld.2007.01.003

Lin, S.P., Lee, C.H., Lu, Y.S., & Hsu, L.N. (2006). A comparison of MICU survival prediction using the logistic regression model and artificial neural network model. *Journal of Nursing Research, 14,* 306–314.

Lu, D.F., Street, W.N., & Delaney, C. (2006). Knowledge discovery: Detecting elderly patients with impaired mobility. *Studies in Health Technology and Informatics, 122,* 121–123.

Lundgren, P., & Wisser, C. (1997). Functional requirements for IT support for nursing information systems integrated in electronic healthcare record systems (EHCRS). *Studies in Health Technology and Informatics, 46,* 337–342.

Madigan, E.A., & Curet, O.L. (2006). A data mining approach in home healthcare: Outcomes and service use. *BMC Health Services Research, 24,* 18. doi:10.1186/1472-6963-6-18

Maguire, R., McCann, L., Miller, M., & Kearney, N. (2008). Nurse's perceptions and experiences of using of a mobile-phone-based advanced symptom management system (ASyMS) to monitor and manage chemotherapy-related toxicity. *European Journal of Oncology Nursing, 12,* 380–386. doi:10.1016/j.ejon.2008.04.007

Manhattan Research. (2009). Physicians in 2012: The outlook for on demand, mobile, and social digital media. Retrieved from http://manhattanresearch.com/News-and-Events/Press-Releases/physician-smartphones-2012

Martin, D., & Sommerville, I. (2004). Patterns of cooperative interaction: Linking ethnomethodology and design. *ACM Transactions on Computer-Human Interaction, 11,* 58–89.

McCann, L., Maguire, R., Miller, M., & Kearney, N. (2009). Patients' perceptions and experiences of using a mobile phone-based advanced symptom management system (ASyMS) to monitor and manage chemotherapy related toxicity. *European Journal of Cancer Care, 18,* 156–164. doi:10.1111/j.1365-2354.2008.00938.x

Moody, L.E., Slocumb, E., Berg, B., & Jackson, D. (2004). Electronic health records documentation in nursing: Nurses' perceptions, attitudes, and preferences. *CIN: Computers, Informatics, Nursing, 22,* 337–344.

Mullins, I.M., Siadaty, M.S., Lyman, J., Scully, K., Garrett, C.T., Miller, W.G., … Knaus, W.A. (2006). Data mining and clinical data repositories: Insights from a 667,000 patient data set. *Computers in Biology and Medicine, 36,* 1351–1377. doi:10.1016/j.compbiomed.2005.08.003

Nahm, R., & Poston, I. (2000). Measurement of the effects of an integrated, point-of-care computer system on quality of nursing documentation and patient satisfaction. *Computers in Nursing, 18,* 220–229.

National Cancer Institute. (n.d.). Welcome to the caBIG® Community Website. Retrieved from https://cabig.nci.nih.gov

Nelson, R. (2007). Electronic health records: Useful tools or high-tech headache? *American Journal of Nursing, 107*(3), 25–26. doi:10.1097/00000446-200703000-00015

Nemeth, C., Nunnally, M., O'Connor, M., Klock, P.A., & Cook, R. (2005). Getting to the point: Developing IT for the sharp end of healthcare. *Journal of Biomedical Informatics, 38,* 18–25. doi:10.1016/j.jbi.2004.11.002

Ngo-Metzger, Q., Hayes, G., Chen, Y., Cygan, R., & Garfield, C. (2010). Improving communication between patients and providers using health information technology and other quality improvement strategies: Focus on Asian Americans. *Medical Care Research and Review, 67*(Suppl. 5), 231S–245S. doi:10.1177/1077558710375432

Nielsen, J. (1993). *Usability engineering.* Boston, MA: Academic Press.

Norman, D., & Draper, S. (Eds.). (1986). *User centered system design: New perspectives on human-computer interaction.* Hillsdale, NJ: Lawrence Erlbaum Associates.

Ozbolt, J.G., & Saba, V.K. (2008). A brief history of nursing informatics in the United States of America. *Nursing Outlook, 56,* 199.e2–205.e2. doi:10.1016/j.outlook.2008.06.008

Park, M., Park, J.S., Kim, C.N., Park, K.M., & Kwon, Y.S. (2006). Knowledge discovery in nursing minimum data set using data mining. *Taehan Kanho Hakhoe Chi, 36,* 652–661.

Pedreira, C.E., Macrini, L., Land, M.G., & Costa, E.S. (2009). New decision support tool for treatment intensity choice in childhood acute lymphoblastic leukemia. *IEEE Transactions on Information Technology in Biomedicine, 13,* 284–290. doi:10.1109/TITB.2008.925965

Phillippi, J.C., & Wyatt, T.H. (2011). Smartphones in nursing education. *CIN: Computers, Informatics, Nursing, 29,* 449–454. doi:10.1097/NCN.0b013e3181fc411f

Phillips, B., Shaw, R.J., Sullivan, D.T., & Johnson, C. (2010). Using virtual environments to enhance nursing distance education. *Creative Nursing, 16,* 132–135.

Podraza, W., & Podraza, H. (1999). Childhood leukaemia relapse risk factors: A rough sets approach. *Medical Informatics and the Internet in Medicine, 24,* 91–108.

Poynton, M.R., & McDaniel, A.M. (2006). Classification of smoking cessation status with a backpropagation neural network. *Journal of Biomedical Informatics, 39,* 680–686. doi:10.1016/j.jbi.2006.02.016

Quinn, C.C., Shardell, M.D., Terrin, M.L., Barr, E.A., Ballew, S.H., & Gruber-Baldini, A.L. (2011). Cluster-randomized trial of a mobile phone personalized behavioral intervention for blood glucose control. *Diabetes Care, 34,* 1934–1942. doi:10.2337/dc11-0366

Ravvaz, K., Senk, P., Patrick, T.B., Coenen, A., Kim, T., Zhao, H., … Lang, N.M. (2008). Mapping nursing concepts to ontologies for evidence-based nursing. *AMIA Annual Symposium Proceedings, 2008,* 1105.

Ridinger, M.H., & Rice, J.J. (2000). Predictive modeling points way to future risk status. *Health Management Technology, 21*(2), 10–12.

Rinkus, S., Walji, M., Johnson-Throop, K.A., Malin, J.T., Turley, J.P., Smith, J.W., & Zhang, J. (2005). Human-centered design of a distributed knowledge management system. *Journal of Biomedical Informatics, 38,* 4–17. doi:10.1016/j.jbi.2004.11.014

Robles, J. (2009). The effect of the electronic medical record on nurses' work. *Creative Nursing, 15,* 31–35.

Rose, A.F., Schnipper, J.L., Park, E.R., Poon, E.G., Li, Q., & Middleton, B. (2005). Using qualitative studies to improve the usability of an EMR. *Journal of Biomedical Informatics, 38,* 51–60. doi:10.1016/j.jbi .2004.11.006

Rubin, J. (1994). *Handbook of usability testing: How to plan, design, and conduct effective tests.* New York, NY: Wiley.

Ruland, C., Jeneson, A., Andersen, T., Andersen, R., Slaughter, L., Schjødt-Osmo, B., & Moore, S.M. (2007). Designing tailored Internet support to assist cancer patients in illness management. *AMIA Annual Symposium Proceedings, 2007,* 635–639. Retrieved from http://www.ncbi.nlm.nih.gov/pmc/ articles/PMC2655776/?tool=pubmed

Seomun, G.A., Chang, S.O., Lee, S.J., Kim, I.A., & Park, S.A. (2006). A prediction model for patient classification according to nursing need: Using data mining techniques. *Studies in Health Technology and Informatics, 122,* 899.

Smith, A. (2011, July 11). Smartphone adoption and usage. Retrieved from http://pewinternet. org/Reports/2011/Smartphones/Summary.aspx

Southard, P., & Frankel, P. (1989). Trauma care documentation: A comprehensive guide. *Journal of Emergency Nursing, 15,* 393–398.

Staggers, N., Kobus, D., & Brown, C. (2007). Nurses' evaluations of a novel design for an electronic medication administration record. *CIN: Computers, Informatics, Nursing, 25,* 67–75. doi:10.1097/01 .NCN.0000263981.38801.be

Tabaton, M., Odetti, P., Cammarata, S., Borghi, R., Monacelli, F., Caltagirone, C., … Grossi, E. (2010). Artificial neural networks identify the predictive values of risk factors on the conversion of amnestic mild cognitive impairment. *Journal of Alzheimer's Disease, 19,* 1035–1040. doi:10.3233/JAD-2010-1300

Tang, P.C., Ash, J.S., Bates, D.W., Overhage, J.M., & Sands, D.Z. (2006). Personal health records: Definitions, benefits, and strategies for overcoming barriers to adoption. *Journal of the American Medical Informatics Association, 13,* 121–126. doi:10.1197/jamia.M2025

Tang, P.C., Black, W., Buchanan, J., Young, C.Y., Hooper, D., Lane, S.R., … Turnbull, J.R. (2003). PAMFOnline: Integrating EHealth with an electronic medical record system. *AMIA Annual Symposium Proceedings, 2003,* 644–648. Retrieved from http://www.ncbi.nlm.nih.gov/pmc/articles/ PMC1480088/?tool=pubmed

Tange, H.J., Hasman, A., de Vries Robbé, P., & Schouten, H. (1997). Medical narratives in electronic medical records. *International Journal of Medical Informatics, 46,* 7–29. doi:10.1016/ S1386-5056(97)00048-8

UK National Cancer Research Institute Informatics Initiative. (n.d.). Welcome to the NCRI Oncology Information Exchange. Retrieved from http://www.ncri-onix.org.uk/portal/#S1

Vahabzadeh, M., Lin, J.L., Mezghanni, M., Contoreggi, C., & Leff, M. (2007). A clinical recruiting management system for complex multi-site clinical trials using qualification decision support systems. *AMIA Annual Symposium Proceedings, 2007,* 1141.

Volrathongchai, K., Brennan, P.F., & Ferris, M.C. (2005). Predicting the likelihood of falls among the elderly using likelihood basis pursuit technique. *AMIA Annual Symposium Proceedings, 2005,* 764–768. Retrieved from http://www.ncbi.nlm.nih.gov/pmc/articles/PMC1560466/?tool =pubmed

Voutilainen, P., Isola, A., & Muurinen, S. (2004). Nursing documentation in nursing homes—State-of-the-art and implications for quality improvement. *Scandinavian Journal of Caring Sciences, 18,* 72–81. doi:10.1111/j.1471-6712.2004.00265.x

Ward, L., & Killian, P. (2011). Virtual community internships in the classroom: Testing an intervention. *Nurse Educator, 36,* 40–44. doi:10.1097/NNE.0b013e3182001e6c

Westra, B.L., Savik, K., Oancea, C., Choromanski, L., Holmes, J.H., & Bliss, D. (2011). Predicting improvement in urinary and bowel incontinence for home health patients using electronic health record data. *Journal of Wound, Ostomy, and Continence Nursing, 38,* 77–87. doi:10.1097/ WON.0b013e318202e4a6

Wood, A., & McPhee, C. (2011). Establishing a virtual learning environment: A nursing experience. *Journal of Continuing Education in Nursing, 42,* 510–511. doi:10.3928/00220124-20110715-01

Wood, D.L. (2001). Documentation guidelines: Evolution, future direction, and compliance. *American Journal of Medicine, 110,* 332–334. doi:10.1016/S0002-9343(00)00748-8

Worachartcheewan, A., Nantasenamat, C., Isarankura-Na-Ayudhya, C., Pidetcha, P., & Prachayasit-tikul, V. (2010). Identification of metabolic syndrome using decision tree analysis. *Diabetes Research and Clinical Practice, 90,* e15–e18. doi:10.1016/j.diabres.2010.06.009

Xiao, Y. (2005). Artifacts and collaborative work in healthcare: Methodological, theoretical, and technological implications of the tangible. *Journal of Biomedical Informatics, 38,* 26–33. doi:10.1016/j.jbi.2004.11.004

Yancey, R., Given, B.A., White, N.J., DeVoss, D., & Coyle, B. (1998). Computerized documentation for a rural nursing intervention project. *Computers in Nursing, 16,* 275–284.

Zhang, J. (2005). Human-centered computing in health information systems. Part 1: Analysis and design. *Journal of Biomedical Informatics, 38,* 1–3. doi:10.1016/j.jbi.2004.12.002

CHAPTER 16

Contemporary Issues in Oncology Nursing

Judith K. Payne, PhD, RN, AOCN®

The best way to predict the future is to create it.

—Peter F. Drucker

Introduction

The future of oncology nursing is in large part up to us. Oncology nurses have always been on the forefront of striving to provide quality care to our patients by setting exemplary standards of practice based on evidence when possible or best practice when evidence is lacking. Our successes are a tribute to past, current, and future oncology nurses everywhere. Through evidence-based practice (EBP), research, rigorous educational curricula in our schools of nursing, and our passion for providing quality oncology care, we have created a standard of care bar that is understandably very high. As with most expectations in health care, we need to keep raising the bar. This last chapter will provide a brief synthesis of previous content and set forth some challenges and opportunities that we are likely to encounter in the next decade.

First, a dramatic shift has occurred in how healthcare providers and members of society view cancer as a chronic rather than a terminal illness. Although a cancer diagnosis may initially present as an alarming, acute diagnosis and require rapid and aggressive treatment that can have severe life-threatening consequences, subsequent treatments and care may occur sporadically over many decades. Many patients today are "cured" following initial treatments and remain cancer free. Early detection and new and better treatments have resulted in substantial increases in the number of cancer survivors in the United States (American Cancer Society, 2011). For those individuals with cancer who have relapses, recurrences, or advanced disease at time of diagnosis, numerous effective treatment options are available for their now chronic disease. The term *chronic* can be defined as "of long duration, lasting for a long period of time or marked by frequent recurrences" ("Chronic," 2012). Although the concept of chronic illness is not new, chronicity presents a new framework for oncology healthcare providers. Various models, such as the Corbin and Strauss Model (1984), have been developed that depict dimensions of chronic illness, nursing care, and social support. The Corbin and Strauss Model proposes that nursing care differs along a trajectory of eight phases to meet patients' and families' needs. The concept of chronicity is pertinent to oncology nursing because advances in cancer care have greatly increased length of survival in many types of cancer, and therefore we provide care for patients across many phases of their illness trajectory.

Second, due to the shift of increased survivors and some cancers being treated as chronic diseases, increasingly more patients are being followed by their primary care physicians. The benefits of this are that patients can stay in their home community and see their family care providers who will monitor their ongoing health needs, such as hypertension, diabetes, and cancer, and make referrals when necessary. A challenge is that primary care providers need to seek continuing oncology education by attending conferences to stay current, consult with a specialist, or obtain a referral if needed just as they do for problems considered primary care. Perhaps the biggest challenge is for primary healthcare providers and oncology specialists to maintain good communication in order to keep patient records updated in a timely manner.

Other non-oncology healthcare environments also frequently provide care to patients with cancer. For example, the patient-centered medical home is a team-based healthcare delivery model that provides comprehensive and continuous care to patients. Emergency departments and intensive care units have always delivered care to patients with cancer during emergent and critical events. It is important that we find ways to infuse oncology-specific care into intensive care units. However, some oncology units, such as bone marrow transplant departments, have incorporated critical care equipment and skills in their repertoire of oncology care.

A third issue that is emerging is that nurse leaders and educators are reexamining the way that we educate our undergraduate, master's, and graduate students to fastidiously ensure that our students are receiving the content and experiences needed for the current healthcare environment. Indeed, the environment is very different today than when some of us were undergraduates. We need to prepare nurses for a high-tech practice environment while instilling the significance of their presence and surveillance, healing ability, caring, and human touch. Research has shown that these basic components of nursing make a formidable difference in patient care outcomes. A question that needs to be asked, or at least considered, is, Why aren't courses such as human development, nutrition, ethics and legal issues in health care, and communication required for undergraduate nursing students today? In many cases, these courses, which used to be taught frequently at the undergraduate level, are now at best "threaded" through selected courses, and quite frankly, may be leaving graduating seniors at a disadvantage by not having the knowledge or confidence to contribute equally with other healthcare providers in their practice areas. If students do not have these fundamental courses in undergraduate programs, it may be difficult to obtain and use this knowledge during their career because, as many of us know, life continues as we pursue our career goals.

For example, nutrition is a critical component of clinical practice. Recovery and healing can occur sooner when the human body is adequately nourished. Although enormous strides have been made, EBP is still lacking in the nutritional care of patients with cancer. Ethics is another example of an area that requires attention. Ethical dilemmas occur frequently in oncology practice and are at the heart of oncology. Yet many nurses and other healthcare providers have no formal education in this area of practice. The formative years as a new staff nurse, as a nurse new to oncology practice, or as an advanced practice registered nurse (APRN) are important. Early experiences begin to develop our professionalism, from novice to expert, and self-confidence continues to emerge. Except for some examples and learning that students may encounter during their undergraduate studies, most receive little content on principles of ethics in health care, including oncology.

In October 2004, members of the American Association of Colleges of Nursing (AACN) endorsed the Position Statement on the Practice Doctorate in Nursing. AACN member institutions voted to move the current level of preparation necessary for advanced nursing practice from the master's degree to the doctorate level by 2015. The doctorate in nursing practice (DNP) focuses on providing leadership for EBP (AACN, 2004). This highly anticipated change has the potential to revolutionize advanced nursing practice by providing graduate nursing students with content and knowledge to lead in the healthcare practice environment. Unfortunately, critical examination of the admission criteria, rigor of content, and type of capstone projects reinforces that not all DNP programs are equal. Philosophically, this is a nurse practice degree typically aimed at translating best evidence or science within the healthcare environment to provide quality care. Moving forward, a more standardized curriculum would help to ensure hiring practices in healthcare environments by knowing what knowledge, skills, and capacity to improve patient care outcomes that a DNP graduate can be expected to provide.

An emphasis on healthcare ethics in schools of nursing curriculum will be needed as nurses assume more responsibilities and leadership roles within healthcare institutions and the community. The highly anticipated (and recently upheld) Patient Protection and Affordable Care Act (2012) will present nurses with opportunities to have a strong voice in healthcare decisions and policy, assume positions of authority on ethics committees, and participate in strategic planning and the overall delivery of patient care. Nursing must not shy away from these opportunities. As healthcare dollars become more scarce, patient care issues will emerge that require thoughtful discussions regarding decisions such as palliative care, end-of-life care, access to care, and available resources and cost. Today more than ever, nurses need to be knowledgeable of ethical principles and legal issues related to scope of practice and understand the meaning, ramifications, and consequences when applied to their practice and to their role within an organization.

Furthermore, as nurses assume more responsibilities in health care, they need to become more knowledgeable of legal principles that affect them as individual healthcare providers as well as from an institutional perspective. The majority of nurses do not receive formal education or consistent course content on legal issues in nursing practice. This is an unfortunate lack of responsibility in nursing education. Although some schools may provide undergraduate students threads of content within a class project, student paper, or in response to student questions, few schools of nursing offer a stand-alone, separate course that provides content on legal principles and application of these principles to practice case examples. Graduate programs do a better job by offering guest lecturers who are attorneys or individuals who are knowledgeable of legal content to present APRNs with legal content and discussion of legal issues in their practice. However, undergraduate nursing students need this content as well. Omitting content on legal issues in health care is a slippery path for nursing to continue on, especially with the increased accountability and responsibility that nurses will likely have in the future.

Another opportunity where oncology nurses can excel is providing care to older patients with cancer. The number of people older than 65 is increasing rapidly. The care of older patients with cancer should be different from that of younger adult patients. For example, older patients may present with poor immune function, diminished functional status, and impaired ability of the liver to clear toxic chemotherapeutic agents. Researchers are beginning to examine age-related issues such as dose of chemotherapy for an 80-year-old woman with colorectal cancer compared to the dose for a 42-year-old woman, evaluating drug toxicity, response to treatment, morbidity and mortality, and type of nursing care provided to older adults. Unfortunately, few clinical trials have included older adults with cancer, let alone focused on older adults. Although eligibility criteria for recruitment to clinical trials for adults rarely have an upper age limit, many older patients are not approached for possible recruitment (Payne, 2010). More than 50% of adult patients with cancer are age 65 or older. Yet few oncology nurses have had education and training in geriatric care. This must be addressed in a timely manner as our society is aging.

Diversity is an important issue that oncology nurses and healthcare providers need to examine in their practice environment. Research has shown that the incidence rates of some cancer types vary by race and ethnicity. However, problems with recruiting adequate numbers of potential study participants hinder the ability to have large sample sizes for clinical trials. This has implications for cancer prevention efforts such as access, education, and additional screening. Emerging science is beginning to demonstrate that race and ethnicity are also factors in how an individual clinically responds to treatment and affect cancer mortality and morbidity rates. Researchers are also studying how race and ethnicity affect incidence of cancer, response to treatment, and overall survivor rates. However, more research is desperately needed in this area.

As underscored in previous chapters, understanding the basics of genetics and epigenetics is essential for oncology nurses as well as nurses in general. The use of targeted therapies has made understanding genetics an absolute necessity and a standard of care for oncology nurses and other oncology healthcare providers. Oncology nurses need to be knowledgeable in order to educate patients and families and to answer questions related to genetics and oncology patient care, such as heredity compared to familial risk, testing available to determine risk for cancers, and capacity of molecular-based targeted therapies to clinically improve patient outcomes. Oncology is just one of the many specialties that diagnose and treat disease based on genetics. This is an area of health care where oncology nurses can emerge as leaders and scholars in understanding and applying our unique perspective of genetics in patient care.

Cancer epigenetics, referring to gene expression patterns that are stable, carefully transmitted from parent cell to daughter cell after division, largely irreversible, and unrelated to genetic variation or mutations, began as a field of research more than three decades ago with the observation that "5-methylcytosine levels are lower in cancer cells than in normal cells" (Issa, 2008, p. 219). Waddington (1939) introduced the causal interactions between genes and their products (which bring the phenotype into being) as epigenetics, later defined as heritable changes in gene expression that are not due to any alteration in the DNA sequence (Esteller, 2008). Epigenetic alterations often are involved in the earliest stages of tumor progression, usually precede neoplastic transformation, and have been shown to affect tumor formation, suggesting that the true clinical home of cancer epigenetics and where it will likely have its greatest impact may be in prevention. Esteller offers an example of a suitable intervention for preventing early epigenetic changes as a lifelong, nontoxic dietary approach, which is an area that oncology nurses can readily intervene.

Community-based oncology practices are thriving and have access to many patients who prefer to stay close to home for their cancer care. These community-based practices have access to resources offered by the National Cancer Institute (NCI), such as NCI-sponsored research clinical trials and patient education tools, and the advantage of treating patients where they live so they can stay in their own communities. Both NCI-designated Comprehensive Cancer Centers and NCI-sponsored cancer centers are needed as research is fundamental to our understanding of disease and treatment, and convenient access to community-based practices may be the preferred choice for many patients and families.

Patients who present with mental health issues are major concerns for oncology nurses and physicians. These patients may be easily distracted and may not comprehend complicated treatment protocols and significance of subsequent symptoms. Adherence to treatment protocols can be challenging for patients with mental health problems, and it is difficult for nurses and physicians to determine patients' level of compliance. It can also be difficult to obtain informed consent, manage symptoms from treatment and disease, and provide adequate patient education. Evaluation of adequate and safe follow-up care for these patients is critical.

Another challenging area facing us is the ongoing development of healthcare reform and healthcare policy. Regrettably, many of us are not fully informed of the challenges facing oncology nurses and physicians in the very near future. It is sometimes difficult to keep abreast of changing healthcare reform and policy in addition to changing practice guidelines and protocols. However, it is our responsibility to become informed and participate at the local, regional, or national level on critical issues that will affect each and every one of us.

Future Directions

Our healthcare system works very well for some of us but not as well for others. With the institution of healthcare reform in the next few years, many changes will likely occur. Many of the changes will be favorable for nursing and will provide increased responsibilities and opportunities. The Institute of Medicine (IOM, 2010) suggested that the nursing role includes increased responsibility along with increased opportunities. IOM also recommended a substantial increase in both the number of nurses who are educated at the bachelor-degree level and the number of doctoral-prepared nurses to address the issues of a dire lack of faculty educators, researchers, and leaders in health care. This has potential to have a profound impact on practice trends and patient-related outcomes. It will also have an impact on nurses' salaries because job titles in many organizations are grouped by level of education. Thus, when the requirement becomes mandated, theoretically nurses would be ranked or grouped by level of education with physical therapists, social workers, engineers, and other occupations that require a four-year college degree. This change in group or rank could eventually raise nurses' salaries substantially.

It is feasible that we will see more nurse entrepreneurs in the future. The need for nurses who can provide for or arrange transitional care, symptom management, education, survivorship, and end-of-life care will increase. Although currently affecting only a small number of Americans, a fairly new trend is occurring within the medical profession where some physicians are entering into contracts with a selected number of patients where they negotiate a retainer fee up front for services provided. These physicians are practicing a form of medicine that involves contracting with their patients to provide medical care for them for a negotiated sum. Although oncology physicians have not practiced within this type of a healthcare delivery system, some oncology healthcare providers and oncology nurses may opt out of a routine practice arena and venture into an entrepreneur opportunity. As our society becomes older, increasing numbers of individuals will need help with their healthcare appointments, decisions, functional status, and transitional care. Oncology nurses are experts at assessment and evaluation, symptom management, patient education, and helping patients set priorities. They also tend to create and maintain collaborative relationships with their patients, colleagues, and physicians.

Health informatics has become a key component of oncology nurses' practice. Academic preparation for informatics is typically done at the graduate level. However, most healthcare institutions are moving quickly toward electronic medical records, compiling databases to better track patient care processes and outcomes and to ensure improved communication among patients, employees, and employers. One way to prepare for the future is to attend training sessions and other educational classes on topics related to informatics to remain at the forefront of an institution's list of informatics-ready staff.

EBP is the new standard of practice in many healthcare organizations. EBP is easier to successfully implement when you begin by first changing the culture of the organization; in other words, begin by changing the mindset of the staff within your organization (Payne, 2002). EBP requires staff to learn new skills such as conducting literature searches, critiquing articles, and completing an evidence table before embarking on a project. Team collaboration helps to identify a problem with clinically relevant outcomes, develop a PICO statement (P = Patient Population, I = Intervention, C = Comparison, O = Outcome), and divide the work among team members. Increasingly, reimbursement from third-party reviewers will depend in large part on whether nursing practice was supported by evidence or best practices in the case where minimal or no evidence exists. Oncology nursing research has clearly been an affirming strategy to not only improve patient care and increase the knowledge base of oncology nursing but also to increase the credibility and visibility of oncology nurses in the healthcare community. Research is one of the great pillars of oncology nursing. It is driven by practice and yet comes back to support current practice or provide evidence to promote change in practice.

The three great pillars of oncology nursing (practice, research, education) will likely form even stronger connections where *all three pillars* will work together, engaging in both formal and informal ways to better educate students, to continue to maintain an academic and clinical presence, and to conduct research relevant to oncology practice. This blend of practice, research, and nursing schools is not new; however, the strategies being employed to achieve these goals are innovative. It is common for nursing faculty and researchers to have joint appointments with a hospital or community-based service or for nurses in service positions to have adjunct appointment with academic schools of nursing. This brand of collaboration has become more customary over the past several decades, and it is becoming more the norm that nurse clinicians, educators, researchers, and administrators work together to improve the profession, institutional goals, and patient care outcomes.

The concept of community learning will become more important in the future of nursing, especially in oncology nursing. Cancer prevention strategies, such as education on nutrition, sun damage, environmental risks, and smoking cessation, are embraced by individuals and communities. Learning through community efforts is well-received by many oncology patient populations; it provides a sense of belonging to people who may be somewhat isolated and is cost effective. Much different than 40 years ago, the majority of individuals today have an increased awareness of how lifestyle choices influence the risk for cancer. Patients with cancer are typically well informed about their diagnosis, treatments, and treatment-related symptoms. Therefore, we are caring for an informed patient population who is engaged in their care.

Conclusion

We have the opportunity to chart our future. The timing of healthcare reform with the IOM (2010) report has created a perfect union of excitement and opportunity for nurses, and especially oncology nurses. Research and EBP efforts have instilled credibility and visibility for oncology patient care. Future directions include creating a stronger future by embracing our past successes, learning from past errors, and taking the lead in creating a strong, credible, and visible image of oncology nursing. Areas where oncology nurses can readily provide leadership include sustaining an evidence-based approach to patient care, conducting research to create a strong body of knowledge for translation to practice, tailoring and providing nursing care to older adults, understanding ethical and legal principles as applied to oncology patient care situations, working to improve cancer care for diverse patient populations, and keeping informed of ongoing healthcare reform and policy changes. The work that oncology nurses do is amazing. Let's raise the bar—we can do more when we all work together in a cohesive effort! The following quote says a lot about the pioneers of oncology nursing, and provides wisdom for current nurses.

> *Risk more than others think is safe.*
> *Care more than others think is wise.*
> *Dream more than others think is practical.*
> *Expect more than others think is possible.*
> —U.S. Military Academy, West Point Cadet Maxim

References

American Association of Colleges of Nursing. (2004, October). AACN position statement on the practice doctorate in nursing. Retrieved from http://www.aacn.nche.edu/publications/position/DNPpositionstatement.pdf

American Cancer Society. (2011). *Cancer facts and figures 2010.* Atlanta, GA: Author.

Chronic. (2012). In *Merriam-Webster's online dictionary.* Retrieved from http://www.merriam-webster.com/dictionary/chronic

Corbin, J., & Strauss, A. (1984). A nursing model for chronic illness management based upon the Trajectory framework. *Scholarly Inquiry for Nursing Practice, 5,* 155–174.

Esteller, M. (2008). Epigenetics in cancer. *New England Journal of Medicine, 358,* 1148–1159.

Institute of Medicine. (2010). *The future of nursing: Leading change, advancing health.* Retrieved from http://www.iom.edu/Reports/2010/The-Future-of-Nursing-Leading-Change-Advancing-Health.aspx

Issa, J. (2008). Cancer prevention: Epigenetics steps up to the plate. *Cancer Prevention Research, 14,* 219–222.

Payne, J. (2002). An integrated model of nursing using evidence-based practice. *Oncology Nursing Forum, 29,* 463–465. doi:10.1188/02.ONF.463-465

Payne, J. (2010). Clinical trial recruitment challenges with older adults with cancer. *Applied Nursing Research, 23,* 233–237.

Waddington, C.H. (1939). Preliminary notes on the development of the wings in normal and mutant strains of drosophila. *Proceedings of the National Academy of Sciences, 25,* 299–307.

Index

The letter f *after a page number indicates that relevant content appears in a figure; the letter* t, *in a table.*

A

accreditation, for APRNs, 8–10, 14, 59
adaptation, to trauma, 176
adenine, 65
adjustment disorder
  with anxious mood, 167–168
  with depression, 171
Adolescent Resilience Model (ARM), 37
adolescents
  resilience of, 37
  uncertainty in, 41
adrenal insufficiency, 204t
Advanced Oncology Certified Clinical Nurse Specialist (AOCNS®), 10
Advanced Oncology Certified Nurse (AOCN®), 10
Advanced Oncology Certified Nurse Practitioner (AOCNP®), 10
Advanced Practice Nurse in Genetics (APNG) credential, 89
advanced practice registered nurse (APRN), 5–6, 14, 160–161, 246
  Affordable Care Act and, 57–59
  competencies for, 11–12
  education programs for, 10–11, 84
  genetic testing/counseling by, 93
  gero-oncology care by, 151
  LACE model and, 8–10, 59
  measuring outcomes for, 8
  palliative care by, 158–159

reimbursement for, 7
variations in regulation of, 6–7
adverse event reporting, 116.
  See also patient safety
advisory committees, 102
advocacy, by nurses, 61–63, 102, 247
Affordable Care Act (2010), 13, 56–59, 247
ageism, 147, 149. *See also* older adults
Agency for Healthcare Research and Quality (AHRQ), 117
aging population. *See also* older adults
  cancer in, 145–149, 155
  generational shift in, 146–147, 155
alcohol use, 200–201, 215t
alleles, 69
Ambulatory Care NPSGs, 117
ambulatory treatment, 148–149
American Academy of Nurse Practitioners (AANP), 6, 9–10
American Association of Colleges of Nursing
  on doctoral training, 247
  on ethics education, 138
American Association of Critical-Care Nurses, 136
American Medical Association
  on APRN preparation, 6–7
  on ethics committees, 137
  on genetics/genomics, 88, 95
American Nurses Association (ANA), 59, 62

on ethical issues, 122, 122f, 135
on genetics nursing, 86, 88, 89f
American Organization of Nurse Executives, 135
American Recovery and Reinvestment Act, 229
American Society for Bioethics and Humanities, 135
American Society for Blood and Marrow Transplantation, 110
American Society of Clinical Oncology (ASCO)
  clinical practice guidelines of, 109
  on genetics nursing, 89f, 98
  on healthcare costs, 126
  on palliative care, 46–47
  on patient safety, 109, 113–115
  on shortage of healthcare workers, 59, 160
  Workforce Strategic Plan, 7
American Society of Human Genetics, 89f
amino acids, 67, 68f
anemia, 174
anxiety, 167–170, 172
Appraisal of Guidelines for Research and Evaluation (AGREE), 19
atherosclerosis, 203t
Atlas of Genetics and Cytogenetics in Oncology and Haematology, 89f
autonomy, 97, 123f
  futile treatment and, 130
  resilience and, 38

self-help and, 39
avascular necrosis, 205*t*
avoidance, 176
Avon Foundation, 32

B

Baby Boom generation, 146–147, 155
bachelor of science in nursing (BSN), 161
BCL6 gene, 74
Beck Depression Inventory, 171
Beck Hopelessness Scale, 180
behavior, influence on cancer, 30, 200–201, 215*t*, 219
Bellevue Hospital Training School, 2
Belmont Report (1974), 97
beneficence, 97, 123*f*
bibliographic databases, 19, 19*f*
biobehavioral/systems biology, 26*t*–27*t*, 29–30, 43*f*
biochemical genetic testing, 73. *See also* genetic testing
biologic markers. *See* biomarkers
biomarkers, 70–71
biotherapy, patient safety in, 110–111, 113–114
Boston Training School, 2
BRACAnalysis (genetic test), 74
brain tumors, 172–173
BRCA1/BRCA2 gene mutations, 67, 74, 98
breast cancer
   genetic profiling of, 74–75
   prevalence of, 213
   risk of developing, 74, 195. *See also BRCA1/BRCA2* gene mutations
   surveillance after, 195, 197–198
   survival rates for, 196*t*
Breast Cancer Navigation Kit, 32
Breast Cancer Treatment Response Inventory (BCTRI), 34
burnout, 124–125, 182–186

C

Cancer Bioinformatics Grid (caBIG®), 232
cancer diagnosis, 43*f*, 44
cancer recurrence
   resilience when facing, 38
   surveillance for, 193–198

cancer remission, 45–46
cancer screening, 43*f*, 44, 213
   community-based programs for, 32
   disparities in population groups, 218*t*
   in survivorship, 195
cancer support groups, 38, 177–178
Capps, Lois, 62
cardiomyopathy, 203*t*
caring, 3, 26*t*–27*t*, 32–33, 43*f*
Caris Target Now™ Molecular Profiling, 75
case law, 102
catheter-associated urinary tract infections (CAUTIs), 117
centromere, 66
certifications, in nursing practice, 2, 9–10, 59
certified nurse-midwife (CNM), 9
certified nurse practitioner (CNP), 9
certified registered nurse anesthetist (CRNA), 9
cervical cancer, survival rates for, 196*t*
The Checklist Manifesto, 111
checklists, for patient safety, 111–113
chemosensitivity, of tumors, 75
chemotherapy
   cognitive impairment from, 174–175
   patient safety in, 110–111, 113–114
childhood cancer
   long-term survivors of, 40. *See also* survivorship
   uncertainty in, 41
chromosomes, 65–72
chronic disease, cancer as, 146, 155, 245–246
chronic lymphocytic leukemia, 74
chronic renal insufficiency, 204*t*
CINAHL® database, 19
Clemson University, 85*t*
clinical nurse specialist (CNS), 5–6, 9, 12, 161
clinical practice guidelines (CPGs), 109, 114
clinical reasoning/decision making, 26*t*–27*t*, 31, 43*f*, 206
clinical trials, 21, 94, 127–128, 147, 151. *See also* research
coding, for genetic counseling, 95

codon, 67
cognitive-behavioral theory (CBT), 40, 169, 172, 178
cognitive impairment, 172–173
   causes of, 172–174
   interventions for, 174–175
cognitive rehabilitation, 174–175
colonoscopy screening, 32
colorectal cancer
   genetic profiling of, 75
   survival rates for, 196*t*–197*t*
Columbia University, 85*t*
communication. *See also* informatics
   barriers to, 33
   on ethical issues, 116, 135
   with older adults, 149
   patient-provider, 26*t*–27*t*, 33–34, 43*f*
   of risk vs. benefits, 206
   during transitions in care, 115–116
community settings
   healthcare delivery in, 156–157, 160–161, 248–249
   nurse advocacy in, 63
   screening programs in, 32
comorbid conditions, 156, 201, 202*t*
compassion fatigue, 182–186
competencies
   for APRNs, 11–12
   in genetics/genomics, 88
   in geriatric nursing, 150–151
computerized clinical information system (CCIS), 235
computerized physician order entry (CPOE), 114, 235
concepts, 25–28, 26*t*–27*t*
Concordia University, 161
confidentiality, 123*f*
   electronic health records and, 131–132
   in genetic testing, 99–100, 128
congestive heart failure, 203*t*
Connecticut Training School, 2
Consensus Model for Advanced Practice Registered Nurses, 9, 59. *See also* LACE model
coping, 47. *See also* resilience
Corbin and Strauss Model, of chronic illness, 245–246
core competencies. *See* competencies
coronary artery disease, 203*t*
costs, of cancer care, 126
CPT code, for genetic counseling, 95

credentialing, in genetics/genomics, 88–89
crescendo effect, 124*f*, 124–125, 133–134
critique of evidence, 19
cultural concerns, 26*t*–27*t*, 36–37, 43*f*
culture of ethics, 132–136. *See also* ethics/ethical issues
culture of learning, 109, 250–251
culture of safety, 108–109, 117. *See also* patient safety
CYP450 enzymes, 71–72
cytogenetic testing, 73. *See also* genetic testing
cytosine, 65

D

Dana-Farber Cancer Institute, 110
databases, bibliographic, 19, 19*f*
data mining, 233
data sharing, 232
DEA number, for prescriptive authority, 7
decision making. *See* clinical reasoning/decision making
deCODE, 98
delivery systems, for cancer care, 149, 155, 246
demonstration projects, in palliative care, 157–159
demoralization syndrome, 171, 179–180. *See also* depression
denial, 176
Department of Health and Human Services (DHHS), 102–103, 200–201
dependency ratios, 145
depression, 170–172, 179
desensitization therapy, 178
DHHS (Department of Health and Human Services), 102–103, 200–201
diagnosis phase, 43*f*, 44
diarrhea, 204*t*
dietary supplements, 199
Diffusion of Innovations Theoretical Model, 40
direct-to-consumer (DTC) marketing, of genetic tests, 98–99
direct traumatization, 177
discrimination

based on genetic testing, 100, 101*f*, 128
based on sexual orientation, 217–218
disparities
among population groups, 213–217, 214*t*, 218*t*
nurses' advocacy role in, 219–220
research on, 220*t*–224*t*
distress
interventions for, 181–182
moral, 123–125, 133–134, 139
psychological, 165–166, 178, 249. *See also* anxiety; depression; post-traumatic stress disorder
Dix, Dorothea, 61
DNA, 65–67, 66*f*, 68*f*
doctoral education, for nurses, 10–11, 247
doctor of nursing practice (DNP), 10–11, 247
doctor of philosophy (PhD), for APRNs, 10
donepezil, for cognitive impairment, 174
Drug Enforcement Administration (DEA) number, for prescriptive authority, 7
drug metabolism, 71–72
DTC marketing, of genetic tests, 98–99
duty to warn, in genetic testing, 99–100
dysthymic disorder, 171. *See also* depression

E

education, 246
for APRNs, 10–11, 59
on ethical issues, 138–139, 246–247
future trends in, 13, 161
in genetics/genomics, 83–88, 85*t*, 86*f*–87*f*, 89*f*–90*f*, 90–93, 248
for gero-oncology nursing, 150–151
informatics in, 235–236
on palliative care, 47–48
student loans for, 57
Education and Outreach Initiative Community Patient Navigation Program, 32

Education in Palliative and End-of-Life Care for Oncology, 47
effectiveness vs. efficacy, in research, 20–21
Electronic Health Record Incentive Program, 229
electronic health records (EHRs), 114–115, 131–132, 149, 229–230, 234, 236
electronic personal health records (e-PHRs), 230–231, 236
emotional distress, 165–166, 249. *See also* anxiety; depression
end-of-life care, 43*f*, 46–47, 156. *See also* hospice; palliative care
anxiety during, 169
demonstration projects in, 157–159
ethical issues in, 125, 125*f*, 131, 137
psychosocial intervention in, 167
epigenetics, 70, 94, 248
equipoise, 127
Essential Nursing Competencies and Curricula Guidelines for Genetics and Genomics, 84, 86, 86*f*–87*f*, 88
ethics committees, 133–134, 136–137
ethics/ethical issues, 121–122, 123*f*, 125*f*, 125–132
dilemmas in, 123–125
education on, 138–139, 246–247
with electronic health records, 131–132
in genetics/genomics, 96–99, 128–129
of healthcare costs, 126
moral courage and, 134–136
in palliative/end-of-life care, 131, 137
professional guidelines for, 122*f*, 122–123
in research, 127–128
workplace environment and, 132–136
EthnoMed, 89*f*
evidence-based practice (EBP), 17–20, 18*f*, 246, 250
clinical practice guidelines from, 109
decision making based on, 31, 72

ethical issues in, 126–127
exercise, 215*t*
    for cognitive function, 175
    during survivorship, 198, 200

F

family caregivers, 47–48
family history, 75, 76*f*, 76–79,
    77*f*–78*f*, 168–169
family pedigree, 76–77, 77*f*–78*f*
fatigue, 200
federal law, on genetics, 101
fertility, 129, 204*t*
Fibison, Wendy J., 83
fidelity, 123*f*
Foundation for Moral Courage,
    135
"4A's," for combating moral
    distress, 133
frameshift mutations, 68
Frankl, Victor E., 181
futility, 129–130
fuzzy logic, 235

G

gaps, identification of, for re-
    search, 18, 18*f*
gap table, 19
gastroesophageal cancer, 199
gastrointestinal strictures, 204*t*
Gawande, Atul, 111
G-bands, 66
gender identity, health dispari-
    ties related to, 217–219
gene alleles, 69
generalized anxiety disorder
    (GAD), 168
generalized hope, 179
generational shifts, 146–147,
    155
genes, 65–66
Gene Test Organization, 89*f*
Genetic Alliance, 89*f*
Genetics Clinical Nurse (GCN)
    credential, 88–89
genetic counseling, 75, 76*f*, 77–
    79, 90*f*, 92
    by APRNs, 93
    reimbursement for, 95–96
genetic fingerprinting, 74
Genetic Information
    Nondiscrimination Act
    (GINA) (2008), 100, 101*f*
Genetic Nursing Credentialing
    Commission (GNCC), 88
genetics/genomics, 69–70
    competencies in, 88

credentialing in, 88–89, 89*f*
ethical/legal/social issues,
    96–99, 128–129
future trends in, 92–98
nursing education in, 83–88,
    85*t*, 86*f*–87*f*, 89*f*–90*f*,
    90–93, 248
nursing research in, 94
nursing role in, 83
genetic testing, 73–75, 77, 89*f*
    direct-to-consumer, 98–99
genograms, 76–79, 77*f*–78*f*
genomes, 66
Genomic Health, Inc., 74–75
genotype, 69
germ-line mutations, 62, 74
gero-oncology. *See* aging popu-
    lation; older adults
government, nurse advocacy
    in, 62, 102
group psychotherapy, 182
guanine, 65

H

Hamilton Rating Scale, 171
handoffs, at point of transfer,
    115–116
healthcare reform, 13, 56–59,
    147–148, 249
healthcare systems, 107
health informatics, 229–232,
    250
    methods of, 232–235
    and nursing education, 235–
    236
    oncology applications, 235
health information technology
    (HIT), 229
Health Information Technology
    Act (2009), 229
health insurance, 56–59, 100,
    101*f*
Health Insurance Portability
    and Accountability Act
    (HIPAA) (1996), 96–
    97, 99
Health Resources and Services
    Administration (HRSA),
    61
Healthwell Foundation, 126
Healthy People 2020, 224
hearing loss, 203*t*
herbal supplements, 199
Herth Hope Scale, 180
historical perspectives, in nurs-
    ing, 1–3
Hodgkin disease, 74
holistic focus, in systems biol-
    ogy, 29

home care, genetics nursing
    in, 93
hope, 130, 178–181
Hopefulness Scale for
    Adolescents, 180
Hope Process Framework, 180
hospice, 43*f*, 46–47, 156. *See
    also* end-of-life care; palli-
    ative care
    genetics nursing in, 93
    Medicare benefit for, 126,
    156
Hospice and Palliative Nurses
    Association (HPNA), 62
Hospital Anxiety and
    Depression Scale, 171
HuGENeT network, 89*f*
human-computer interaction
    (HCI), 234–235
Human Genome Project, 66,
    71–73, 89*f*, 91
human rights issues, in ethics,
    125, 125*f*
human subject research, 127
HUM-MOLGEN (Listserv), 89*f*
hypertension, 203*t*
hypoactive delirium, 171
hypothyroidism, 204*t*

I

immunohistochemistry (IHC),
    95
Improving Cancer Treatment
    Education Act (2011), 62
incontinence, 204*t*
indirect traumatization, 177
infertility, 129, 204*t*
informatics, 229–232, 250
    methods of, 232–235
    and nursing education, 235–
    236
    oncology applications, 235
information gathering, coping
    enhanced by, 38–39
informative reassurance, 184
informed consent, 127–128,
    128*f*
Institute for Global Ethics, 135
Institute of Medicine (IOM) re-
    ports
    *From Cancer Patient to Cancer
    Survivor: Lost in
    Transition*, 129, 159,
    192
    Crossing the Quality Chasm,
    229
    *Ensuring Quality Cancer Care
    Through the Oncology
    Workforce*, 7, 13

To Err Is Human: Building a Safer Health System, 108
The Future of Nursing: Leading Change, Advancing Health, 3, 6, 13, 59–63, 161, 249
institutional review boards, 127
integrative health care model, 26*t*–27*t*, 39, 43*f*
integrative medicine, 39
International Council of Nurses, ethical guidelines, 122–123
International Society of Nurses in Genetics (ISONG), 88–89, 89*f*, 90–91, 96
Internet. *See also* informatics
confidentiality issues with, 131–132
genetics resources on, 89*f*–90*f*
for information gathering, 38–39
in nursing education, 235–236
intrusive thoughts, 176–177

J

job discrimination, genetic testing and, 100, 101*f*, 128
The Joint Commission (TJC)
on ethics committees, 137
on patient safety, 115–117
justice, 97, 123*f*

K

karyotype, 66–67

L

LACE model, 8–10, 14, 59
late effects, of treatment, 201, 203*t*–205*t*
learning, culture of, 109, 250–251
legal issues
in genetics/genomics, 96–99, 128–129. *See also* ethics/ethical issues
nurse training in, 247
legislation
genetics issues in, 101–102
nursing advocacy and, 62, 102

Lehman, Betsy, 110
lesbian, gay, bisexual, transgender (LGBT) community, health disparities in, 217–219
Leukemia and Lymphoma Society, 63
LGBT population, health disparities in, 217–219
licensure capacity, 6
licensure, of APRNs, 9, 58–59
literature search/review, 19, 19*f*
Living With Hope program, 180
logotherapy, 172, 181–182, 185
Long, Bethany Hall, 62
long-term survivors, 40, 45–46, 146, 191–193, 196*t*–197*t*. *See also* older adults; survivorship
lung cancer, survival rates for, 197*t*
lymphoma, 74

M

major depressive disorder, 170, 172. *See also* depression
malabsorption syndrome, 204*t*
mammography screening, 32
"mandate to care," 3
Margolies, Liz, 219
mass spectrometry, 95
mastery, over uncertainty, 41
Mature generation, 146–147
meaning-centered psychotherapy, 181
medical event reporting, 116. *See also* patient safety
Medical Genetics and Genetic Counseling Services CPT code, 95
Medicare/Medicaid
and electronic health records, 229
and genetic counseling, 95
hospice benefit, 126, 156
medication errors, 108, 110–111, 235. *See also* patient safety
meditation, for cognitive function, 175
Memory/Attention Adaptation Training, 174–175
mental health issues, 165–166, 249. *See also* anxiety; depression
messenger RNA (mRNA), 67, 68*f*
meta-analyses, 19

metastatic brain lesions, 173
Miller Hope Scale, 180
missense mutations, 68
mobile devices, 231–232, 236
mobile health (mHealth), 231–232
modafinil, for cognitive impairment, 174
Modeling and Remodeling (MRM) Theory, 33, 39
models, 26*t*–27*t*, 28
molecular testing, 73. *See also* genetic testing
mood disorder, 171. *See also* anxiety; depression
moral courage, 134–136
Moral Courage Project, 135
moral distress, 123–125, 133–134, 139
moral residue, 124*f*, 124–125
moral uncertainty, 123, 139
mortality rates, 191, 193–194, 211–213, 212*t*
disparities among population groups, 213–217, 214*t*
motivational interviewing, 40
MRM theory, 33, 39
mRNA, 67–68
Multinational Association of Supportive Care in Cancer, 109
mutations, 62, 67–69
germ-line, 62, 74
Myriad Genetics Laboratories, 74, 98

N

narrative therapy, 182, 185
National Association of Clinical Nurse Specialists (NACNS), 5, 9
National Cancer Act (1971), 2
National Cancer Institute (NCI)
Brain Tumor Progress Review Group, 173
Cancer Bioinformatics Grid, 232
and community-based practices, 248–249
on genetics nursing, 89*f*
on palliative care, 47
National Cancer Research Institute (NCRI), Informatics Initiative, 232
National Coalition for Cancer Survivorship (NCCS), 39
National Coalition for Health Professional Education

in Genetics (NCHPEG),
88, 89*f*
National Comprehensive
Cancer Network
(NCCN), on emotional
distress management, 165
National Conference of State
Legislatures Genetics
Overview, 89*f*
National Consensus Project
(NCP), 156–158
National Database of Nursing
Quality Indicators
(NDNQI), 127
National Genetics Education
and Development
Centre, 90*f*
National Human Genome
Research Institute
(NHGRI), 88, 91, 101
National Institute of Nursing
Research (NINR), 84
National Institutes of Health,
genetics nursing resourc-
es, 90*f*, 91
National LGBT Cancer
Network, 217, 219
National Nursing Centers
Consortium, 96
National Patient Safety Goals
(NPSGs), 117
National Society of Genetic
Counselors, 90*f*, 95, 98
natural language processing
(NLP), 233–234
Navigenics, 98
"near miss" reporting, 116
nephritic syndrome, 204*t*
Nightingale, Florence, 61
Nightingale model, 2
non-Hodgkin lymphoma
(NHL), 74
nonmaleficence, 97, 123*f*
nonphysician providers
(NPPs), 58, 206
noogenic neurosis, 171
novice oncology nurses, 246–247
genetic testing recommen-
dations by, 73
moral uncertainty/distress
in, 139
nucleus, 67, 68*f*
Nurse in Washington
Internship (NIWI), 62–
63, 102
nurse navigation programs,
160–161
nurse practitioner (NP), 5–7,
161
competencies for, 11–12
nurse training schools, 2

nursing competencies
for APRNs, 11–12
in genetics/genomics, 88
in geriatric nursing, 150–151
Nursing Organizations
Alliance, 102
Nursing Student Loan
Program, 57
nutrigenomics, 95
nutrition, 215*t*, 246
cognitive function and, 174
and the genome, 95
during survivorship, 198–199

O

Office of the National
Coordinator for
Healthcare Information
Technology, 229
older adults
cancer care in, 145–149,
247–248
comorbid conditions in, 201,
202*t*
future trends in care, 149–
151
healthcare reform and, 147–
148
research involving, 151
in survivorship, 155–156,
160, 191–192
oncogenes, 69, 213
Oncology Information
Exchange (ONIX), 232
oncology nurse navigator, 160–
161
Oncology Nursing Certification
Corporation (ONCC),
9–10, 59, 91
Oncology Nursing Society
(ONS), 2, 62, 150
APRN competencies pub-
lished by, 11–12, 59
APRN roles recognized by,
5–6, 9
on genetics nursing, 90*f*, 91
Legislative Action Center,
62, 102
on patient safety, 113–115
Putting Evidence Into
Practice (PEP) initia-
tive, 109
Oncotype DX®
for breast cancer, 74–75
for colon cancer, 75
operational definition, in theory, 28
order sets, for chemo/biother-
apy, 114–115, 235

osteonecrosis
of the jaw, 203*t*
of joints, 205*t*
osteoporosis, 205*t*
outcome planning phase, 43*f*,
45
outcomes, of advanced nursing
practice, 8
ovarian cancer, 74
overweight/obesity, 199–200,
215*t*

P

Pain and Supportive Care
Program, 46
palliative care, 43*f*, 46–47, 156–
160. *See also* end-of-life
care; hospice
by APRNs, 158–159
demonstration projects in,
157–159
ethical issues in, 131, 137
models for, 157
psychosocial intervention
in, 167
and survivorship, 159–160
pancreatic cancer, 199
pancreatic insufficiency, 204*t*
panic disorder, 168
p arms, 67
particularized hope, 179
patient care issues, in ethics,
125, 125*f*
patient-centered outcomes, of
advanced nursing prac-
tice, 8
Patient Health Questionnaire,
171
patient navigation model, 26*t*–
27*t*, 32, 43*f*
Patient Protection and
Affordable Care Act
(2010), 13, 56–59, 247
patient-provider relationships/
communication, 26*t*–27*t*,
33–34, 43*f*, 184
Patient Reported Outcomes
Model (PRO) model, 34
patient safety, 108–111
barriers to, 117
nursing role in, 117–118
patient/family roles in, 116
strategies to improve, 111–116
patient satisfaction, 58, 184
patient self-management, 205–
206
The Pearson Report, 7
pediatric oncology nursing, as
subspecialty, 2

pedigree, 76–77, 77*f*–78*f*
peripheral neuropathy, 205*t*
personalized medicine, 72–73, 148–149
pharmacogenetics, 71–72
pharmacokinetics, 71
phases, of cancer experience, 42–47, 43*f*, 169
phenotype, 69
phobia, 168
PICO statement, for research, 19–20, 250
pneumonitis, 204*t*
point mutations, 68
post-traumatic stress disorder (PTSD), 168, 176–178
Power as Knowing Participation in Change Tool, 42
preexisting conditions, 56–57
Preferred Reporting for Systematic Reviews and Meta-Analyses (PRISMA), 19
prescriptive authority, of APRNs, 7
President's Commission for the Study of Ethical Problems, 137
primary care providers (PCPs), managing long-term survivors, 191–193, 194*t*, 195*f*, 197–198, 246
privacy, 123*f*
    electronic health records and, 131–132
    genetic testing and, 96, 99–100, 128
problem/population, intervention, comparison, outcome (PICO) statement, for research, 19–20, 250
professional associations, nurse advocacy in, 62
Progenix, 98
ProHealth Care, 161
Project ENABLE, 157–158
Project ENABLE II, 158–159
Project Safe Conduct, 157–158
PRO outcomes model, 34
prostate cancer, 197*t*, 212–213
proteins, 67, 70, 95
proteomics, 70, 95
proto-oncogenes, 74
psychological distress, 165–166, 178, 181–182, 249. *See also* anxiety; depression; post-traumatic stress disorder
psychological trauma. *See* post-traumatic stress disorder
psychotherapeutic/psychoeducational interventions, 181–182

for anxiety, 169
for depression, 171–172
for PTSD, 178
for workplace stress, 185
PubMed, 19
pulmonary fibrosis, 204*t*

Q

q arms, 67
quality improvement (QI), 126–127
quality of life (QOL), 166–167, 175–176, 178
Quality of Life Index, 167
Quality of Life Inventory, 167
Quality Oncology Practice Initiative (QOPI), 109

R

radiation therapy, cognitive dysfunction from, 173–174
recurrence
    resilience when facing, 38
    surveillance for, 193–198
reimbursement
    for APRN services, 7
    of evidence-based practice, 250
relationships, patient-provider, 26*t*–27*t*, 33–34, 43*f*, 184
reliability, of instruments, 166
remission, 45–46
replication, of DNA, 67
reproductive issues, 129, 204*t*
research, 18*f*, 18–20, 19*f*, 250. *See also* evidence-based practice
    conduct vs. implementation of, 21–22, 22*t*
    effectiveness vs. efficacy in, 20–21
    ethical issues in, 127–128
    in genetics, 94
    on gero-oncology, 151
resilience, 26*t*–27*t*, 37–38, 43*f*
restrictive lung disease, 204*t*
ribosomal RNA (rRNA), 67, 68*f*
risk factors, 200–201, 215*t*
RNA, 67, 68*f*
Robert Wood Johnson Foundation (RWJF), 13, 59, 157
Rogers, Everett, 40
Rogers, Martha, 42, 44
Roy Adaptation Model, 40

rural settings, healthcare delivery in, 158–160, 235

S

safety. *See* patient safety
"SBAR" process, 135–136
Science of Unitary Human Beings (SUHB) model, 42, 44
Scope and Standards of Nursing Practice (ANA), 86, 86*f*–87*f*
scope of practice, 6–7, 60
screening, 43*f*, 44, 213
    for cancer survivors, 195
    community-based programs for, 32
    disparities in population groups, 218*t*
    for emotional distress, 166–167, 170–171
secondary malignancies, 156, 193–198
secondary traumatic stress disorder. *See* compassion fatigue
Second Life®, educational use of, 236
self-help/self-care, 26*t*–27*t*, 38–39, 43*f*, 185
self-management, 205–206
sexual behavior, as risk factor, 215*t*, 219
sexual orientation, health disparities related to, 217–219
shared care model, for cancer survivors, 193, 194*t*, 195*f*
shortage
    of nursing educators, 60, 249
    of oncology providers, 7, 59, 160–161
Silent generation, 146–147
silent mutations, 68
Simultaneous Care, 157–158
single nucleotide polymorphisms (SNPs), 69, 71–72, 94–95
smartphones, 231–232, 236
smoking cessation, 201. *See also* tobacco use
Snyder Hope Scale, 180
social cognitive theory, 40
social issues, in genetics/genomics, 96–99, 128–129. *See also* ethics/ethical issues
social media, 132, 231–232
Society of Gynecologic Oncology, 98

somatic mutations, 62, 74
soy supplements, 199
Speak Up initiatives, for patient safety, 116
specialization, 2, 9–10
state law
    on APRNs, 6–7
    on genetics, 101
state regulations, on APRNs, 6–7, 9
stress theory, 47. *See also* psychological distress
substruction, 32
SUHB (Science of Unitary Human Beings) model, 42, 44
suicide risk, 170, 172, 178
sun exposure, as risk factor, 215*t*
support groups, 38, 177–178
Surgical Safety Checklist, 112
surveillance, during survivorship, 193–198
Surveillance, Epidemiology, and End Results (SEER) program, 198, 212–213
survivorship, 26*t*–27*t*, 39–41, 43*f*, 45–46, 191–192, 196*t*–197*t*
    cancer surveillance in, 193–198
    comorbid conditions/late effects in, 156, 201, 202*t*–205*t*
    ethical issues in, 129
    health promotion during, 198–206
    older adults in, 155–156, 160, 191–192
    palliative care and, 159–160
    population disparities in, 213–217, 214*t*
    primary care in, 192–193, 194*t*, 195*f*, 197–198, 246
Susan G. Komen for the Cure, 63
symptom clusters, 34–35
symptom experience model, 26*t*–27*t*, 34–36, 35*f*, 43*f*
symptom management
    biobehavioral model and, 30
    biomarkers and, 71
    nursing research on, 26*t*–27*t*, 34–36, 35*f*
synthesis table, 19
systems biology, 26*t*–27*t*, 29–30, 43*f*

systems thinking, 107

T

targeted therapies, 74, 148, 248
taste alterations, 199
theories, 26*t*–27*t*, 28
Theory of Stress and Coping, 47
therapeutic empathy, 184
Thomas (U.S. Library of Congress), 90*f*
thromboembolism, 203*t*
thymine, 65, 67
tobacco use, 30, 200–201, 215*t*
transcription, of DNA, 67, 68*f*
transcultural nursing, theory of, 36
transdisciplinary model, in palliative care education, 46
transfer RNA (tRNA), 67
transgender, healthcare access and, 217–218
Transtheoretical Model, 40
trauma, psychological, 176. *See also* compassion fatigue; post-traumatic stress disorder
treatment phase, 43*f*, 44–45, 213. *See also* chemotherapy
tRNA, 67
tumor genetic profiling, 74
tumor suppressor genes, 69, 74, 213
23andMe, 98

U

Uncertainty in Illness Model, 26*t*–27*t*, 41–42, 43*f*
unclassified variant, in genetic testing, 78–79
underlying frailty, in older adults, 145
unit-based ethics conversations (UBEC), 138
University of California, San Francisco, 85*t*
University of Iowa, 84, 85*t*
University of Kansas Medical Center, 90*f*
University of Pittsburgh, 84, 85*t*
University of Washington, 85*t*
uracil, 67

U.S. Department of Energy (DOE), 90*f*
U.S. Preventive Services Task Force (USPSTF), 200
U.S. Surgeon General's Family History Initiative, 90*f*

V

validity, of instruments, 166
variant of uncertain significance (VUS), in genetic testing, 78–79
veracity, 123*f*
vicarious traumatization. *See* compassion fatigue
virtual technologies, in nursing education, 236
visual changes, 203*t*

W

Wakefield, Mary, 61–62
WebChoice, 235
Western Blot test, 95
Women's Hospital of Philadelphia, 2
Workflow Information Systems for European Nursing Care (WISECARE), 235
workforce shortage
    in nursing education, 60, 249
    in oncology care, 7, 59, 160–161
workplace
    discrimination in, 100, 101*f*, 128, 217–218
    nurse advocacy in, 61–62
    stress in, 182–186
World Health Organization (WHO)
    on palliative care, 46, 157
    on patient safety, 112

X

xerostomia, 199, 203*t*

Z

Zung Self-Rating Depression Scale, 171